Psychopathology
and Subfecundity

STUDIES IN POPULATION

Under the Editorship of: H. H. WINSBOROUGH

Department of Sociology
University of Wisconsin
Madison, Wisconsin

Samuel H. Preston, Nathan Keyfitz, and Robert Schoen. Causes of Death: *Life Tables for National Populations.*

Otis Dudley Duncan, David L. Featherman, and Beverly Duncan. Socioeconomic Background and Achievement.

James A. Sweet. Women in the Labor Force.

Tertius Chandler and Gerald Fox. 3000 Years of Urban Growth.

William H. Sewell and Robert M. Hauser. Education, Occupation, and Earnings: Achievement in the Early Career.

Otis Dudley Duncan. Introduction to Structural Equation Models.

William H. Sewell, Robert M. Hauser, and David L. Featherman (Eds.). Schooling and Achievement in American Society.

Henry Shryock, Jacob S. Siegel, and Associates. The Methods and Materials of Demography. *Condensed Edition by Edward Stockwell.*

Samuel H. Preston. Mortality Patterns in National Populations: *With Special Reference to Recorded Causes of Death.*

Robert M. Hauser and David L. Featherman. The Process of Stratification: *Trends and Analyses.*

Ronald R. Rindfuss and James A. Sweet. Postwar Fertility Trends and Differentials in the United States.

David L. Featherman and Robert M. Hauser. Opportunity and Change.

Karl E. Taeuber, Larry L. Bumpass, and James A. Sweet (Eds.). Social Demography.

Thomas J. Espenshade and William J. Serow (Eds.). The Economic Consequences of Slowing Population Growth.

Frank D. Bean and W. Parker Frisbie (Eds.). The Demography of Racial and Ethnic Groups.

Joseph A. McFalls, Jr. Psychopathology and Subfecundity.

In preparation

Maris A. Vinovskis (Ed.). Studies in American Historical Demography.

Psychopathology and Subfecundity

JOSEPH A. McFALLS, JR.
POPULATION STUDIES CENTER
UNIVERSITY OF PENNSYLVANIA
PHILADELPHIA, PENNSYLVANIA

ACADEMIC PRESS   New York   San Francisco   London
A Subsidiary of Harcourt Brace Jovanovich, Publishers

ACADEMIC PRESS, INC.
111 Fifth Avenue, New York, New York 10003

United Kingdom Edition published by
ACADEMIC PRESS, INC. (LONDON) LTD.
24/28 Oval Road, London NW1 7DX

Library of Congress Cataloging in Publication Data

McFalls, Joseph A
  Psychopathology and subfecundity.

  Bibliography: p.
  Includes index.
  1. Mental illness--Physiological aspects.
2. Sterility--Psychological aspects. I. Title.
[DNLM: 1. Psychopathology. 2. Sterility.
WP570 M143p]
RC455.4.B5M32 1979   616.8'9'07 78-67880
ISBN 0-12-484650-5

PRINTED IN THE UNITED STATES OF AMERICA

79 80 81 82   9 8 7 6 5 4 3 2 1

For my parents

Contents

Preface

My interest in the causes of population subfecundity dates back to 1971, when I was conducting research to evaluate the widely held hypothesis that changes in the prevalence of venereal disease accounted for the U.S. black fertility trend of 1880–1960. I realized then that, although subfecundity was an important population variable, it had not been widely studied. Thus, I began a research project, the earliest stages of which involved identifying and categorizing those factors that could alter human reproductive potential on the population level. Five major categories soon emerged: genetics, nutritional deficiencies, disease, psychopathology, and other environmental factors. Upon completion of this preliminary task, I concentrated on the psychopathological factors that cause subfecundity, and this monograph presents the results of that work. Works dealing with the other four categories are planned for the future.

Psychopathology was the topic completed first because it is an intriguing subject and is the one about which least is known. It became clear at the outset of the study that psychopathology is an important cause of population subfecundity because it easily fulfills the two main criteria. First, it can impair an individual's ability to reproduce by causing coital inability, conceptive failure, and/or pregnancy loss. Indeed, psychopathology is a common cause of impotence, spermatogenic failure, anovulation, and spontaneous abortion, as well as many other reproductive disorders. Second, psychopathology is highly prevalent in many parts of the world. In the United States, for instance, it is the nation's primary public health problem, affecting the majority of the population at some time during their reproductive lives. Thus, psychopathology is a fecundity depressant and is highly prevalent—the two major criteria for a cause of population subfecundity.

This book examines the relationship between psychopathology and subfecundity on both the individual and the population level. Important forms of psychopathology are studied in detail, and a determination is made as to whether, and to what extent, they cause coital inability, conceptive failure, and/or pregnancy loss. Attention is devoted to the psychosomatic and pharmacological mechanisms through which such effects occur. Prevalence data are investigated for three purposes: (a) to find out if various forms of psychopathology are prevalent enough to be of consequence on the population level; (b) to estimate the impact of each demographically important form of psychopathology on fecundity, a procedure requiring prevalence data by age and sex; and (c) to determine whether the various forms of psychopathology, collectively and individually, produce subfecundity differentials within and between populations, and over time. Although data on many populations are used, statistics on the population of the United States predominate. Finally, although the focus of this book is on subfecundity, some attention is devoted to other intermediate variables, such as birth control and coital frequency, through which psychopathology also influences fertility.

The book's principal finding is that psychopathology is an important determinant of population subfecundity and fertility, especially in developed societies and in those rapidly changing areas of developing societies where social disorganization is widespread. Moreover, because the prevalence of psychopathology in general and of its specific forms varies widely between populations, between subgroups within a population, and over time, psychopathology-induced subfecundity is seen to be a population variable and a potential contributor to fertility differentials. Some forms of psychopathology—psychic stress (neuroses, psychophysiologic disorders, and everyday stress) and alcoholism—emerged as particularly important causes of population subfecundity. Other significant causes that receive considerable attention include psychoses, sexual deviations, and drug abuse.

This book was written principally for population students, including those demographers, sociologists, economists, and anthropologists concerned with population fertility. But it is also relevant to those in medical and mental health fields such as psychiatry, psychology, reproductive biology, obstetrics and gynecology, and those dealing with infertility and psychosexual disorders. The book would also be of interest to professionals in disciplines that involve the study of both health and population, such as public health, epidemiology, and medical geography. Finally, those sociologists with particular interest in demography, marriage and the family, human sexuality, social psychiatry, and social problems may also find this book useful.

Acknowledgments

I wish to express my gratitude to those who have advised and assisted me in this research. I am especially indebted to George Masnick, John Durand, and Solomon Katz for their critical review of the first draft of this book and for the personal interest they have taken in me and my work over the years. I would also like to thank Etienne van de Walle, Vincent Whitney, Ann Miller, Richard Easterlin, Vasilios Valaoras, Edward Hutchinson, Philip Sagi, Miranda Tanfer, Lydia Christaldi, and Shobhana Thakarar, who have helped me on many occasions during my stay at the Population Studies Center. And, of course, my wife Marguerite deserves special recognition for her contributions too numerous to mention. Finally, I would like to thank my parents, who made many sacrifices to aid my education and who have always encouraged my academic pursuits.

This book was made possible in part by a training grant from the National Institutes of Child Health and Human Development and also by assistance from the Population Studies Center of the University of Pennsylvania.

Quotation Credits

The author gratefully acknowledges permission to reprint excerpts from the following works:

Bellak, L., *Manic Depressive Psychosis*. New York: Grune & Stratton, Inc., 1952. © 1952 by Grune & Stratton, Inc.

Bellak, L. and L. Loeb, *The Schizophrenic Syndrome*. New York: Grune & Stratton, Inc., 1969. © 1969 by Grune & Stratton, Inc.

Blau, M., B. Slaff, K. Easton, J. Welkowitz, J. Spingarn, and J. Cohen, The psychogenic etiology of premature births. By permission of Elsevier North Holland, Inc., from *Psychosomatic Medicine* **25**, 201, 1963.

Bogue, D., *Principles of Demography*. New York: Wiley, 1969.

Cicero, T., R. Bell, W. Wiest, J. Allison, K. Polakoski, and E. Robins, Function of the male sex organs in heroin and methadone users. By permission from the *New England Journal of Medicine* **292**, 882, 1975.

Gaulden, E. C., D. C. Littlefield, O. E. Putoff, and A. L. Seivert, Menstrual abnormalities associated with heroin addiction. By permission of the C. V. Mosby Company, from the *American Journal of Obstetrics and Gynecology* **90**, 155–160, 1964.

Green, P. and L. Rubin, Amenorrhea as a manifestation of chronic liver disease. By permission of the C. V. Mosby Company, from the *American Journal of Obstetrics and Gynecology* **78**, 141–146, 1959.

Horton, P. and G. Leslie, *The Sociology of Social Problems*. Englewood Cliffs, New Jersey: Prentice-Hall, Inc., 1978. 6th Ed., © 1978.

Israel, S., *Menstrual Disorders and Sterility*. New York: Harper & Row, 1967.

Linbeck, V., The woman alcoholic: A review of the literature. By permission of Marcel Dekker, Inc., from the *International Journal of Addiction* **7**, 567, 1972.

Mai, F., R. Munday, and E. Rump, Psychosomatic and behavioral mechanisms in psychogenic infertility. By permission from the *British Journal of Psychiatry* **120**, 199, 1972.

Masters, W. and V. Johnson, *Human Sexual Inadequacy.* Boston, Massachusetts: Little, Brown and Company, 1970.

Oliven, J., *Clinical Sexuality.* Philadelphia, Pennsylvania: J. B. Lippincott Company, 1974.

Ossofsky, H., Amenorrhea: Symptom of endogenous depression. By permission from the *Medical Annals of the District of Columbia* **41**, 744, 1972.

Palti, Z., Psychogenic male infertility. By permission of Elsevier North Holland, Inc., from *Psychosomatic Medicine* **31**, 326, 1969.

Pohlman, E., Childlessness, intentional and unintentional. By permission of The Williams & Wilkins Co., Baltimore, from the *Journal of Nervous and Mental Disease* **151**, 2, 1970.

Shader, R. and A. DiMascio (eds.), *Psychotropic Drug Side Effects.* Baltimore, Maryland: The Williams & Wilkins Co., 1970.

Tabbarah, R., Toward a theory of demographic development. By permission of the University of Chicago Press, from *Economic Development and Cultural Change* **67**, 25, 1971.

Time, The chemistry of smoking. Reprinted by permission from *Time*, The Weekly Newsmagazine; copyright Time Inc., 1977. (February 21)

WHO, The epidemiology of infertility. By permission from *WHO Technical Report Series* **582**, 1, 1975.

Note on Terminology

Subfecundity research is made difficult by the fact that several important terms are used differently within the same discipline as well as among different disciplines. So, before proceeding, it is recommended that the reader become familiar with this book's definitions of these terms.

The term *fecundity* is used here to mean reproductive ability, as opposed to actual childbearing. It refers to the ability in women to conceive and bear live children and to the ability in men to produce competent spermatozoa, that is, spermatozoa possessing the characteristics necessary to ensure fertilization of the ovum with production of a viable zygote. Coital ability is also a requisite of fecundity for both sexes unless some extraordinary procedure such as artificial insemination is an available and acceptable alternative.

It is important here to explain the difference between *genetic fecundity* and *fecundity*. Genetic fecundity is the inherited ability to reproduce and is present from the moment of conception. Within the genes is information to direct the development of organ systems such as the reproductive system—from embryonic stages, through maturation, to aging.[1] Operationally, then, the genes establish maximum reproductive potential, that is, genetic fecundity. But the ability to express this potential, that is, fecundity, may be limited by a number of nongenetic factors such as nutritional deficiencies, disease,

[1] Studies on human cells in culture reveal an innate capacity for only a set number of cell divisions, suggesting that aging is largely a gene-directed process.

environmental factors, and psychopathology.[2] Poor nutrition, for example, may delay the onset of sexual maturity and cause premature menopause. And the fecundity of even the peak reproductive years is seldom equivalent to that established by genetic fecundity, because of these factors, which are termed here *subfecundity factors.*

When an individual's ability to express maximum reproductive potential is impaired, the individual becomes *subfecund.* The degree of subfecundity is the difference between what reproductive ability would have been in the absence of any impairment (genetic fecundity) and the current ability to reproduce (fecundity). Thus, subfecundity refers to any level of reproductive ability from zero up to, but not including, full (genetic) ability for a particular age. *Infecundity* refers to the total inability to reproduce, both presently and in the future, and represents the lowest point on the subfecundity continuum.

The term *subfecundity* is also used here in a comparative sense to note a difference in the genetic fecundity of two individuals. An individual with relatively low genetic fecundity is considered subfecund in comparison to one with higher genetic fecundity. In this sense, genetic factors can also be considered as subfecundity factors, a practice followed in this book.

The reader should be aware that the terms fecundity, subfecundity, and infecundity are used differently by other demographers. Petersen (1975:196), for instance, includes as subfecundity factors a group of sexually related problems and practices, such as too infrequent coitus and excessive mastur-bation, that do not decrease reproductive ability per se, though they can reduce fertility. The Davis–Blake (1956:212) analytic framework of inter-mediate variables also uses the terms fecundity and infecundity differently than they are used in this book. In their framework, these terms relate only to the ability to conceive, whereas here they apply to coital ability and to the ability to carry a conceptus to a live birth as well.

The term *fertility* is used here in the usual demographic sense to mean reproductive performance, as opposed to ability. It denotes the actual pro-duction of live children. Although some authors (e.g., Scragg 1957) include stillbirths in the measure of fertility, this is not the usual practice and is not done here.

The reader is particularly cautioned about the meaning of the word *infertility.* Some authors use this term to include both conceptive failure and pregnancy loss. A recent WHO paper (1976) follows this procedure in its title, though in the text it sometimes uses infertility to mean only conceptive failure. Other authors (e.g., Dimic *et al.* 1972:475) use infertility to mean coital inability and conceptive failure. And demographers (e.g., Sheps and Ridley

---

[2] However, the fecundity of a small minority with inherited reproductive dysfunctions can be increased through medical procedures, such as surgery and hormone treatment.

1965:xii) sometimes use infertility to refer to women who have no live-born children, regardless of the reasons. Finally, many authors use the term infertility to mean only *conceptive failure.* This definition is the one used in this book, and it embraces any degree of conceptive capacity below normal. Thus, infertility and conceptive failure are synonymous here.

Sterility is the complete inability to conceive or to bring about conception. It is simply the lowest point on the infertility continuum. *Primary sterility* means that conception has never occurred; *secondary sterility* means that there has been one or more pregnancies but that further conception cannot be initiated (Kleegman and Kaufman 1966:5). This definition of sterility is more limited and useful than the more inclusive ones often found in the literature. For example, demographers frequently use the term sterility to mean infertility and even infecundity (as these terms are used in this book; see Kiser 1964:4929).

Pregnancy loss refers to the involuntary termination of a pregnancy that does not result in a live birth. It includes spontaneous abortions, late fetal deaths, and stillbirths, but not induced abortions or neonatal mortality. The term *pregnancy wastage* is avoided because in the literature it often includes induced abortions and neonatal mortality.

The term *population genetic fecundity* refers to the collective, genetically determined, maximum reproductive potential of a population. However, the ability of a population to express this potential—population fecundity—is usually impaired because of subfecundity factors. Thus, population subfecundity indicates that, because of such factors, a population's level of reproductive ability lies below full ability.

The genetic fecundity of two populations (or subpopulations) may differ, and it is possible to consider the population with the lower genetic fecundity to be subfecund relative to the one with higher genetic fecundity.

Introduction:
Toward an Understanding of the Fundamental Causes of Population Subfecundity

> *It is essential to involve scientists from different disciplines, such as obstetrics and gynecology, epidemiology, demography, and anthropology, in research on [population subfecundity].*
>
> —World Health Organization (1976:233)

In the middle of the nineteenth century a Russian peasant woman reputedly produced 69 children in 27 confinements (Parkes 1976:101). Although this claim is highly questionable, there is no doubt that some women have given birth to more than 20 children. Thus, maximum individual fecundity exceeds at least 20 and may be substantially higher. No population, however, has ever approached such a level of reproductivity. The most fecund population in history is probably the Hutterites, a small religious sect in North America that has an estimated fecundity of about 13 children per woman (cf. Westoff and Westoff 1971:19).[1] Population students generally recognize this level of childbearing ability as the feasible upper limit of population fertility (e.g., Coale 1969:4).

Given that the fertility of at least one population could be as high as 13 children per woman, do populations that do not ostensibly interfere with reproduction approach this level? The answer is no. Few even exceed an average of 8 children per woman. Indeed, the literature is full of reports of noncontracepting societies whose fertility rates fall well below the

---

[1]The genetic fecundity of the Hutterites ranges somewhere between 12 and 14 live births. The actual completed family size of Hutterite women is about one to three children less than this maximum theoretical number of births because most Hutterite women marry after reaching age 20, rather than at the beginning of their fecund period, and some lose husbands before they reach the end of their reproductive period (cf. Eaton and Mayer 1954:27–28).

maximum, often by more than two-thirds.[2] Clark (1969:24–27) lists about 100 such communities with unexpectedly low fertility. Such wide differences between maximum potential fertility and observed fertility can often be explained in part by underestimation of actual fertility, natural fertility factors such as intercourse taboos, and intermediate variables such as late age at marriage or undetected birth control.[3] However, a substantial portion of such "fertility deficits" is often due to another intermediate variable, subfecundity, the diminished capacity to reproduce (Hansluwka 1975:203).[4]

The Importance of Population Subfecundity

The conclusion that subfecundity can be responsible for substantial portions of these "fertility deficits" is not merely a product of deduction. Where statistics are available for populations with unexpectedly low fertility, they frequently reveal extraordinary rates of subfecundity. For instance, the World Health Organization (1976:229) notes that the proportion of women 50 years of age and older who have never borne children ranges from 20% to 40% in parts of Gabon, Cameroon, Zaire, the Central African Republic, the Sudan, and elsewhere in Africa. Moreover, the reality of the widespread subfecundity in these societies is confirmed by the fact that the inhabitants themselves are acutely aware of the problem (cf. Caldwell 1974:7).

It is proposed here that subfecundity is an important determinant of fertility, not only in societies with unexpectedly low fertility, but also in other developing, developed, and historical societies as well.

HISTORICAL IMPORTANCE

Subfecundity played an important role historically in curtailing fertility and holding down world population growth (cf. Livi-Bacci 1977:250). As Durand (1972) notes:

[2]See, for example, Bennett (1965:244), Brass and Coale (1968:135–136), Coale (1966:180, 1973:56), Harding (1970:639), Frisch (1975:20), Henin (1968:147, 1969:197), Nag (1962:8,9,71), Prothero (1972:106), Romaniuk (1968a:331–332), World Health Organization (1975:9), and Wilde (1973:26). These sources all point to subfecundity as a major reason for the unexpectedly low fertility.

[3] For a discussion of the possibility that voluntary birth control was a feature of some preindustrial populations, see Masnick and Katz (1976:39). In a more general vein, Ryder (1959:416) argues that it is dubious to assume that any society is free of fertility regulation within marriage.

[4]Subfecundity is apparently present even among the Hutterites, the population thought to be reproducing at or near the maximum rate, since the slightly increasing generational fertility is probably attributable in part to concomitant improvements in health conditions (cf. Eaton and Mayer 1954:20).

So far as one can judge from the available information about . . . loss of reproductive power through subfecundity . . . in nonindustrial populations in recent times, it would appear that few of them [historical populations] would approximate this level of eight, that a total fertility rate of six would be quite good, and that the biologically achievable total fertility rate in many [historical] populations may fall considerably lower, even as low as four [pp. 373–374].

This lower than expected fertility may be due more to subfecundity and less to other factors such as traditional birth control than is usually assumed (Frisch 1975:21). Interestingly, Razzell (1977:vi) reports that subfecundity due to smallpox may have had a sizable impact on Britain's fertility prior to 1850. And it has been suggested that genital tuberculosis may have been a signifi-cant cause of subfecundity in the highly tuberculous populations of pre-twentieth-century Europe (Gray 1977:29).

IMPORTANCE IN DEVELOPING SOCIETIES TODAY

Today subfecundity has a greater impact on the fertility of developing than on developed societies (Caldwell 1974:12). This is primarily due to two situations. First, in developing societies there are fewer social checks, such as effective contraception, operating on fertility, and thus more fertility potential for subfecundity to negate. Second, these societies are subject to greater numbers of powerful subfecundity factors than are developed ones. In par-ticular, high rates of disease and malnutrition are far more common. This situation is compounded (and perpetuated) by the relative absence of quality health care and facilities.[5] There are indications that subfecundity in these societies may have increased recently (van de Walle and Page 1969:6).

Subfecundity can have a significant effect even on the fertility of develop-ing societies thought to have excessively high fertility. For instance, the married Yoruba women in Ibadan City, Nigeria average about six children per woman. Yet by age 45, 8% are involuntarily childless and 25% have had less than four live births in a society in which four or more is the number of living

---

[5]Health conditions in many developing societies are so poor in relation to those in developed nations that the differential's true significance is difficult for some population students from the latter nations to comprehend. Perhaps the following description from Fuller (1974) of conditions at a health facility near Lagos, Nigeria, at which one of the first individuals to contract Lassa fever laid over while awaiting travel accommodations to the U.S., can provide a graphic picture of the health care situation that exists in parts of many developing nations:

The Pest House was a crumbling building set aside for contagious diseases, with rough plaster walls and the inevitable corrugated tin roof. . . . There were no fans or screens. . . . The room was dimly lit and suffocatingly hot. . . . Within minutes she became aware of the mosquitoes; hordes of them coming in through the open windows. The small sink was black with them, and with flies. There were no nets on the beds. . . . As she got into bed . . . she saw the bedbugs, wingless blood-sucking insects with a faint acrid odor. . . . A rat scurried across the floor, darted erratically back and forth, then disappeared . . . [pp. 59–61].

children considered ideal. The low fertility of these women has been attributed to subfecundity (Arowolo 1978:13). If this subfecundity were not present, the already high fertility of the whole population would rise materially. Moreover, a substantial fraction of those women with four or more children are undoubtedly also subfecund to some extent. For instance, a woman with six children may have had eight children were it not for subfecundity. Thus, the fertility of the whole population would rise even more if all subfecundity were eliminated.

IMPORTANCE IN DEVELOPED SOCIETIES TODAY

Although subfecundity factors in developed societies are not as virulent or as prevalent as those in developing societies, subfecundity is still important demographically there. Indeed, despite the fact that the major American fertility surveys of the last several decades tended to omit subfecund women, they still found extraordinarily high rates of subfecundity among their respondents. For instance, about one-third of the married white couples of reproductive age surveyed in the 1941 Indianapolis Study (Whelpton and Kiser 1946–1958) and in the 1955 and 1960 Growth of American Families Studies (Freedman et al. 1959; Whelpton et al. 1966) were considered subfecund. Harter (1970) also classified 33% of a New Orleans sample as subfecund. But since the majority of couples choose low fertility and are able to attain it through birth control, the impact of subfecundity on fertility in developed societies is not as substantial as in developing societies. However, as discussed in more detail later in this introduction, it is still important.

In sum, subfecundity is a major determinant of population fertility in developed, developing, and historical societies.

Causes of Population Subfecundity

Population students, however, know very little about the fundamental causes of subfecundity (Easterlin et al. 1976:46; Hansluwka 1975:203; WHO 1975:6). Most research to date has focused more on the measurement of subfecundity than on its causes. For instance, advances have been made in understanding how subfecundity manifests itself in terms of the elongation of birth intervals and their components (cf. Leridon 1977), but there is not much research that goes beyond these components to identify the fundamental causes of subfecundity and to quantify their impact on fertility. Thus, one authority (Hansluwka 1975) concludes, "In brief, the gaps in our knowledge are too large to permit the construction of a reasonably plausible model of the effects of health on fertility via fecundity [p. 205]."

What little knowledge does exist permits the causes of population sub-fecundity to be separated into five categories, namely: (a) genetic factors, (b) nutritional deficiencies, (c) disease, (d) environmental factors, and (e) psychopathology.[6] To be included in one of these categories, a subfecundity factor must fulfill two criteria: It must be capable of depressing individual fecundity and must be able to affect a substantial proportion of the population's potentially fecund members. Following is a brief introduction to some of the important points of information in each of the five categories and an assessment of their current status in the population literature.

GENETIC FACTORS

It has been only within the past 30 years that scientists have admitted to the possibility that human reproductive ability may be differentially influenced by heritable factors (Kleegman and Kaufman 1966:284). Yet, such a relationship could have been anticipated, for, as Kleegman and Kaufman (1966) note, "Every normal trait can have a deviation, whether it is in the number of fingers or in gametogenesis [p.284]." The most well-characterized deviations are Turner's syndrome in the female and Klinefelter's syndrome in the male. These disorders are the result of abnormalities in the sex chromosomes and are almost invariably associated with infecundity (Grieve et al. 1972:20; Kleegman and Kaufman 1966:284), since the internal sexual organs are underdeveloped (McKusick 1964:13–14). Two heritable blood traits, blood group and Rh factor, have also come under scrutiny as possible causes of subfecundity. It has been reported that spermatogenic disorders are more frequent in men with blood group A (Grieve et al. 1972:20). And some reports indicate that ABO-incompatible matings are associated with higher rates of conceptive failure (British Medical Journal 1972b:314; Grieve et al. 1972:20) and pregnancy loss (British Medical Journal 1972b:314; Takano and Miller 1972:149), although other sources (e.g., Hiraizumi et al. 1973:370) deny such a link. More certain is the observation that maternal–fetal Rh incompatibility is associated with pregnancy loss in a significant number of cases of Rh hemolytic disease (Freda 1973:72).

Differences between populations in the frequencies of these genetic traits may be responsible for differences in population fecundity. For example, since Rh factor is unevenly distributed among populations—the trait is present in 85% of Caucasians, 92% of Negroes, and nearly 100% of American Indians (Siegler 1944:430)—the frequency of Rh disease and associated subfecundity are population variables. At least one research group has

---

[6]There are intercategory differences, however, in the quantity and quality of research. Nutritional deficiencies, for example, have been the subject of the most and the highest quality research, and genetic factors have been the most neglected.

suggested that such differences in the genetic fecundity of populations are responsible for differences in population growth. After reporting that blood group A males are more often oligospermic and azoospermic, Grieve and his associates (1972:22) relate that the A gene has a higher frequency in slowly expanding European populations (40%) than in rapidly expanding ones such as India (25%).[7]

Research in genetic fecundity has not been plentiful, but preliminary findings suggest that it is a potentially significant factor in population fecundity. Nevertheless, there is little to indicate that population students are aware of this field of research,[8] as the assumption is often made in the population literature that the genetic fecundity of populations does not differ (see page 11).

NUTRITIONAL DEFICIENCIES

Nutritional deficiencies can also cause population subfecundity. Severe undernutrition is a potent subfecundity factor, reducing male and female conceptive ability. Malnutrition is a far less powerful direct cause of subfecundity. Although it can delay the onset of sexual maturation and can probably cause premature menopause, strong evidence that it can significantly depress fecundity in the interim is lacking. But malnutrition's indirect effect on fecundity is extremely important. Since malnutrition weakens the body's immunological defenses, it increases the frequency, severity, and duration of disease, including some that are potent causes of subfecundity. For instance, malnutrition is one of the most frequent precipitators of active tuberculous disease in infected persons, and one type of tuberculosis, genital TB, is an important cause of subfecundity. Malnutrition in early life is also responsible for contracted pelvis, a skeletal deformity frequently seen in the tropics. Contracted pelvis is commonly associated with obstructed labor and resulting high rates of fetal loss. The instrumental interference required in such cases is often nonsterile and predisposes to severe postpartum infections and subsequent sterility. It is also likely that malnutrition affects population fertility behaviorally, by, for example, decreasing coital frequency.

Nutritional deficiencies have been the subject of comparatively more

[7]Maintenance of a stable A gene frequency, if such persons are relatively infertile, necessitates a postconception selective advantage for the A genotype. Such an advantage has been reported by Hiraizumi and his associates (1973:370).

[8]Discussion in the population literature of the relationship between genetic factors and population fecundity is confined almost entirely to a few speculations that genetic factors may produce fecundity differentials (e.g., Freedman 1963:49; Nag 1962:148). A few students, for instance, suggest that super-high fertility groups such as the Hutterites may have largely "bred-out" their subfecund strains (cf. Clark 1969:17–18; Eaton and Mayer 1954:31). Another speculation is that the genetic fecundity of low fertility modern populations may be declining due to an increase in the proportion of genotypes with reduced reproductive powers (cf. Davis, 1966:182–183).

research than the other categories of subfecundity factors. Interest in recent years has been especially keen.[9] Nevertheless, much remains to be learned.

DISEASE

The role of disease in subfecundity has barely moved beyond the speculative, and there is little in the way of vigorous research. In addition, the fixation many population students have with venereal disease as the almost exclusive disease-related cause of subfecundity has all but obscured the role of other potentially significant diseases, such as genital tuberculosis, filariasis, and postpartum and postabortal sepsis.

ENVIRONMENTAL FACTORS

A host of environmental conditions may affect population fecundity. These include natural factors such as altitude, latitude, and temperature, and also the by-products of industrialization, most notably chemical pollutants. Every year more and more chemicals are being designated as causes of subfecundity. Just recently, for instance, high rates of sterility have been noted in men working in the manufacture of certain pesticides (DBCP) and fire retardants (TRIS). And wives of men working in one plastics industry (PVC) have rates of spontaneous abortion and stillbirth twice the normal, a situation attributed to sperm abnormalities in their husbands. One threatening aspect of environmental factors is their increasing proliferation and prevalence, which can only continue due to ongoing technological development, population growth, industrialization, and urbanization. Whatever the current impact of environmental factors on population fecundity and fertility, it will be far more substantial in the future.

However, with the exception of altitude,[10] study of environmental factors as causes of subfecundity has been almost totally neglected in the population literature.

PSYCHOPATHOLOGY

Psychopathology is a potentially important cause of population subfecundity, since it can impair individual fecundity and is prevalent in many populations. However, aside from a few remarks suggesting that increases in psychopathology due to the stress of modern living may reduce the fecundity

[9]For an excellent review, see Moseley (1977).

[10] The effect of altitude on fecundity has received more attention than any other environmental factor. See, for example, Stycos (1963), Heer (1964, 1967), James (1966), Whitehead (1968), Bradshaw (1969), and Abelson et al. (1974).

of developed societies, the relationship between psychopathology and sub-fecundity is all but ignored in the population literature.

Subfecundity Factors: Their Treatment in the Population Literature

Thus, population students have devoted little attention to the fundamen-tal causes of subfecundity. Many of the discussions that do exist are deficient and can be characterized in one of three ways.

First, the possibility is raised that a specific factor is a cause of a popula-tion's low fertility, but then it is quickly *dismissed without evidence being brought to bear*. Petersen (1975:200), for instance, suggests that sexual deviations may have a negative effect on population fecundity and fertility but concludes otherwise without reference to any empirical research relevant to the relationship. Similarly, Blake (1961), in trying to answer the question of why the Jamaican birth rate was so modest for such a poor agrarian country, notes that "the answer is sometimes sought in sterility and spontaneous abortion on the grounds that Jamaican women are especially subject to fibroid tumors and that venereal disease is prevalent on the island [p. 13]." However, she quickly discounts venereal disease (VD) by stating that "proof is hard to find" and cites Roberts (1957:207–215) as the source for this appraisal. However, consulting Roberts, it is found that he is primarily dis-cussing the relationship between the control of syphilis and mortality. Robert's research was not designed to address the issue of whether VD was an important determinant of the fertility level. It is also noteworthy that Roberts was discussing syphilis, not all venereal diseases. Gonorrhea may have been important even if syphilis was not. It is also characteristic of the usual treatment of subfecundity factors by population students that Blake focused primarily on VD to the exclusion of other diseases and health factors. Even if VD did not turn out to be an important cause of the unexpectedly low fertility, perhaps other factors, such as schistosomiasis or filariasis, were important.

The second way the relationship between subfecundity and its funda-mental causes is treated in the population literature is *speculative* in nature. Hypotheses are advanced that are incidental and conjectural, and these are frequently followed by little, if any, discussion. It is clear in such instances that the authors are interested only in covering all possibilities and have no intention of ever rigorously exploring the hypothesis. As will be seen in Chapter 1, discussion of the relationship between subfecundity and psychopathology in the population literature is confined to such speculative hypotheses.

The final form taken by discussion of the causes of subfecundity in the population literature is that of the *residual* hypothesis. These hypotheses are interjected into the discussion when other research hypotheses are tested and found wanting. An example of such treatment is the "VD hypothesis" used by many authors to explain the trend in U.S. black fertility from 1880 to 1960. The "VD hypothesis" is discussed in more detail later.

What these three treatments—the suggestion but quick rejection without evidence approach, the speculative hypothesis, and the residual hypothesis—all have in common is that they are used in place of rigorous research. As such, these devices have retarded the growth of knowledge concerning the identity and importance of the fundamental causes of population subfecundity.

Reasons for Deficient Research

There are at least three reasons why research into the fundamental causes of population subfecundity is scarce and often deficient. First, there is a strong social science bias among many fertility specialists involved in population research, which directs attention away from the fundamental causes of subfecundity. Second, the thinking of many population students is still hampered by erroneous fecundity assumptions. Finally, collaboration between population students and health scientists is rare, leading to a paucity of research on subfecundity that is readily usable by population students. These three reasons are discussed in turn.

THE SOCIAL SCIENCE BIAS

The conspicuous lack of systematic study accorded the fundamental causes of population subfecundity suggests the existence of a social science bias. Since the vast majority of population students are trained in the social sciences, it was probably inevitable that social variables would be overemphasized in explanations of fertility. Interestingly, though subfecundity factors are currently the stepchildren of fertility research, they dominated fertility theories as recently as the early twentieth century but then began to be gradually deemphasized. In fact, Carr-Saunders was one of the first prominent scientists to recognize the influence of social as well as biological (subfecundity) factors, and his book, *The Population Problem: A Study in Evolution* (1922), signaled the change from the predominantly biological to the social science approach toward fertility research. (Bogue 1969:19). Unfortunately, the pendulum swung from one extreme to the other. The ensuing infusion of the social science outlook became so pervasive that fertility research is now largely divorced from its original biological perspective (WHO 1969:5), and, consequently, valuable inputs into the general theory of fertility are being forfeited. As noted above, interest in some subfecundity factors, especially in nutritional deficiencies, has recently been rekindled, though most subfecundity factors continue to receive no attention whatsoever. Indeed, as Henry (1965) observes, "It is only in recent years that obvious [biological] facts were successively introduced into demography and employed to construct a coherent theory of natural fertility and the processes of family building [p. 340]."

Biases are difficult to nail down. However, perhaps the following passage by Hawthorn (1970) provides a glimpse of the social science bias: "A theoretical fecundity rate would be of interest to biologists who can match it against observed socially-unregulated fertility rates. Demographers . . . are interested in comparing the latter with socially-regulated ones [p. 11]." If Hawthorn's statement is considered normatively, a social science bias is evident, particularly as he separates and defines the disciplinary interests of demographers and biologists. Actually, such discrete boundaries do not exist, and any comprehensive explanation of the entire natality process would require the integration and synthesis of pertinent knowledge from many disciplines, including the biological sciences. Demographers must be concerned with more than simply the social checks, as Hawthorn's statement suggests. They must also investigate the biological checks (subfecundity factors), collaborating whenever possible with health scientists.

The social science bias may also be evident in the common practice of pitting subfecundity factors against sociocultural ones as explanations for fertility levels and trends.[11] What generally happens is that the author concludes that the sociocultural factors are far more powerful than the subfecundity ones and in the process explicitly or implicitly lays the foundation for a rationalization to ignore the latter. However, such either/or treatments misrepresent reality. Subfecundity factors must be treated simply as one of many possible causes of fertility phenomena, not as juxtaposed to all sociocultural factors collectively. As Katz (1972:364–365) argues, what is needed to explain fertility trends and behavior is a holistic approach that ties together both subfecundity and sociocultural factors and that recognizes their independent and interactive effects on fertility.[12]

In sum, the social science bias deflects attention away from subfecundity factors toward the more familiar and tractable social science ones and thus

[11]See, for example, Grabill *et al.* (1958:348), Parkes (1976:102), Ryder (1959:401), Farley (1970b:189), Coale (1973:61), Freedman (1963:55), Petersen (1975:196), and Llewellyn-Jones (1974:129).

[12]See also Omram (1971:509) for another discussion of the need for a multidisciplinary approach to population theory.

retards the development of a more balanced, interdisciplinary approach to the study of population fertility.

FAULTY FECUNDITY ASSUMPTIONS

The second reason for deficient research concerning the fundamental causes of population subfecundity is that the thinking of many population students is still hampered by two erroneous fecundity assumptions. The first assumption is that genetic fecundity is approximately equal in all populations. This is a common operating assumption within demography, as Ryder (1959) recognizes: "It has become relatively routine research practice to assume that the fertilities of populations being compared do not differ in genetic fecundity [p. 418]."

Coale (1969:4–5) and his associates, for example, utilized this assumption in the construction of measures used to document fertility levels and trends in Europe. In that project, the highest rates of age-specific fertility on reliable record—those of married Hutterite women—were used to measure the extent to which various European populations approached maximum potential fertility (genetic fecundity). This convention assumes that the genetic fecundity of these populations is approximately the same and is equal to that of the Hutterites. Although these researchers, and others who employ this assumption, may agree that it is invalid,[13] it is frequently used because the lack of knowledge of genetic influences on population (and individual) fecundity makes the practice strategically sensible. But in the meantime, there is little evidence that population students are keeping abreast of progress in this area or, in fact, are even cognizant of the importance of genetic fecundity to population research. Thus, the continual use of this assumption retards the progress of fertility research.

The second assumption is that the amount of subfecundity due to nongenetic factors is approximately the same in all populations, and, thus, subfecundity is not a cause of fertility differentials. As Ryder (1959), a critic of this assumption, observes: "The larger assumption is also commonly made that differences in fertility between populations are solely the consequence

---

[13] Hollingsworth (1977) also has doubts about using the Hutterites' fecundity and fertility as a standard for other populations. In his words:

> Again, the use of the Hutterites, the population with the highest natural fertility recorded, as providing a standard fertility schedule is somewhat questionable. Was there genetic selection for high fertility amongst them, which might partially invalidate comparisons with less fertile populations? An average fertility level, rather than an extreme one, might perhaps give more appropriate comparisons. This, of course, would need devising and some general agreement to use it, but the Hutterites are really a highly unusual group. It is rather like standardizing mortality by the experience of the group with the heaviest mortality ever recorded [p. 553].

of differences in fertility regulation [p. 418]." An example of this assumption in the literature is the following statement by Bogue (1969): "It is important to emphasize that differences in fecundity . . . seem to be almost equal among the world's population and are not a major factor in accounting for the international differences in the world's birth rates [p. 676]." But this second assumption is unreasonable because populations experience different sets of subfecundity factors, sets that can vary both in the number and in the strength of component factors, and the set of subfecundity factors experienced by one population may be such that fecundity is virtually unaffected, whereas the set experienced by another population may be capable of depressing fecundity to the point where fertility levels are affected. Thus, the second fecundity assumption is more deleterious to the study of fertility than the first because, although population differences in genetic fecundity are probably not so great that any fertility differentials would arise, differences in the amount of subfecundity can be appreciable and can be an important variable in explaining differential fertility rates.

However, if these two assumptions are accepted, that is, that genetic fecundity is equal and that the amount of subfecundity is the same, then population fecundity would be a constant. And, since some populations have very high fertility, which necessitates high fecundity, it would follow that the fecundity of all populations is high. Thus, taken together, the two faulty fecundity assumptions support the idea that the fecundity of all populations is high and constant. Indeed, these assumptions are generally operationalized through this idea.

The idea that fecundity is high and constant dates back at least to Malthus, who declared in his famous essay that human fecundity was so great that, if a population grew unchecked, it would increase faster than the means of subsistence. Although Malthus recognized that faulty diet, disease, and other health factors checked population growth, he was of course referring to the mortality rather than to the fertility side of the vital equation. However, the idea of high and constant fecundity can more likely be traced to the demographic transition theory.[14] In the theory's heyday, it was widely thought that fertility was high in all pretransitional societies. As Bourgeois-Pichat (1967) critically writes, "It has long been assumed that before birth control began in the sense we use this expression today, there was no control at all of fertility. It followed that fertility was high or more or less at the same level everywhere [p. 160]." This high and constant level of fertility implied and necessitated high and rather constant fecundity. As economic development occurred, fertility fell. But high fecundity was still assumed and consequently was not considered an important differential fertility determinant.

[14]For a general discussion and critique of demographic transition theory, see Coale (1973:53–72), Dumond (1975:713–721), Teitelbaum (1975:420–425), and Durand (1967:1–12).

However, in the last two decades, evidence has been assembled that contradicts this view of fertility patterns. Demographers now generally accept the theory that the fertility levels of pretransitional populations were quite variable. Unfortunately, the implications of the transition theory have not receded as quickly. The idea that fecundity is high and constant still lingers long after its supporting theoretical premises collapsed under the scrutiny of empirical research. Such lingering ideas constitute a deterrent to systematic research on the determinants of fecundity.

Among even those population students who recognize the variability of fecundity, there remains the inclination to presume that this variability is not relevant to the natality of contracepting, low fertility, developed societies. The rationale is that modern birth control methods are sufficient to maintain the same fertility rate regardless of subfecundity factors. Even Tabbarah (1971), who helped topple erroneous aspects of transition theory and believes strongly that subfecundity factors influenced pretransitional fertility, writes: "Since C (the desired number of children) is admittedly determined by social, economic, and psychological factors, fertility in the industrial countries may be said to be a socioeconomic phenomenon [p.269]." In similar fashion, Bourgeois-Pichat (1967) states: "One of the main features of the so-called demographic revolution has been precisely to change not only the level of fertility but also its nature. Having a child has become more and more the result of the couple. . . . *Fertility has left the biological* and social field to become part of behavioral science [p. 163, emphasis added]." Tabbarah and Bourgeois-Pichat are in large part correct. There is no doubt that subfecundity factors lose much of their importance in the face of widespread and effective birth control, but, as will be discussed, they do not become inconsequential.

However, in discussions of the determinants of fertility in developed societies, subfecundity is ignored. Again the same erroneous fecundity assumptions crop up. Tabbarah (1971:264), for example, operationalizes these assumptions by assigning to women in developed societies the minimum possible birth interval, roughly equal to that of the Hutterites. It is not at all clear, however, that the Hutterites, or any other super-high fertility group for that matter, are representative of the populations of developed societies. The latter probably have lower genetic fecundity and undoubtedly have far more subfecundity judging from the survey evidence noted above that indicates widespread subfecundity among American women. Thus, it is not likely that the populations of developed societies could duplicate the Hutterite performance even if they had the desire to do so.

Furthermore, despite efficient birth control, it is improbable that the level of fertility would be maintained in developed societies if subfecundity factors were eliminated. Even if the rate did remain the same, there would be shifts in the parity distribution. Involuntarily childless couples or those at other parities who had fewer children than desired due to subfecundity would increase their fertility. Moreover, within developed societies, there are frequently significant subgroups not practicing effective birth control whose fertility would rise if subfecundity were not present. Indeed, a case could be made that many subfecundity factors are disproportionately prevalent among such groups. As Freedman (1963) notes, "Health conditions and poor nutrition may affect the fecundity of the whole society or may affect the lowest stratum with *special force* as a result of the operation of the economic distribution system [p. 51; emphasis added]."

Some might argue that most subfecund women in developed societies still have the number of children they desire; it just takes them longer. Thus, it would be reasoned that subfecundity would not affect completed fertility. This position denies the reality that substantial fractions (10% is not unusual) of ever-married women in developed societies are involuntarily and permanently childless and that, in addition, large numbers of parous women are infecund. It also ignores the effect of the timing of fertility on completed family size. For example, many women in the United States are now postponing childbearing until their late twenties and early thirties. This not only gives them fewer years to achieve their desired fertility but also requires that they do so in the face of the lower fecundity characteristic of these years due to normal aging and the accumulated subfecundity from causes such as disease. Thus, in reference to the much-speculated-upon possibility that many U.S. women are about to try to have their first two children late in their reproductive careers, Conrad Taeuber (cited in Blackman 1975) made the following comment: "It's a pretty cloudy crystal ball. If women have these two children, we're bound to see the number of births go up. . . . But there is some reason to believe that some women will be disappointed and find they can't have these children [p. 2]."

It is also important to recognize that subfecundity factors can have indirect effects on population fertility. First, they may influence fertility behaviorally through any of the other Davis–Blake (1956) intermediate variables. They can, for instance, influence the chances of marrying or maintaining a stable sexual union, or they may be responsible for contraceptive use, changes in coital frequency, sterilization, or voluntary abortion.[15] Syphilis provides a good example of such a factor. Infected persons, as well as those

---

[15] Identification of diseases harmful to the fetus and better detection of these diseases in pregnant women, together with readily available abortions, have undoubtedly raised the rates of voluntary fetal wastage for many disorders. For example, maternal rubella infection is associated with an increased risk of spontaneous abortion (Barrett–Connor 1969:277), but the induced abortions requested by infected women who fear their offspring might be malformed by this virus account for far greater amounts of pregnancy wastage. Even inadvertent vaccination of pregnant women with the attenuated virus, though not conclusively known to cause malformations, is a frequent cause of induced abortion. In one series 50% of vaccinated women sought abortions, yet not one of the continued pregnancies ended in congenital rubella (Kuhr 1973:1357).

trying to avoid the disease, often use prophylactic procedures during coitus that are secondarily contraceptive. The discovery of syphilis during the frequently mandatory premarital blood test may force postponement or even cancellation of marriage. And before antibiotics the prospect of giving birth to a child with congenital syphilis was likely a reason for voluntary abortion. Finally, syphilis is almost certain proof of one partner's infidelity and undoubtedly increases the frequency of separation and divorce.

Second, subfecundity factors can indirectly affect population fertility by influencing the timing of early fertility. Delays in early childbearing due to subfecundity can provide women with the opportunity to develop a life style other than that of becoming the mother of a large family (Presser 1971:336). And the presence of subfecundity during the early reproductive years may allow progress to be made toward learning effective birth control ability, which would reduce the amount of unwanted fertility or permit the aforementioned woman who is changing her reproductive goals to achieve her revised ones (Masnick and McFalls 1976:224). Syphilis is also illustrative of this type of subfecundity factor. The disease, which is usually contracted early in reproductive life, causes high rates of pregnancy loss during the 2 years following initial infection. However, even untreated syphilis has little effect on pregnancy outcome after this period, and no direct effect on completed fertility would be anticipated among couples with low or moderate family size desires. But the 2-year respite during the peak reproductive years provided by the disease gives a woman the opportunity to revise her reproductive goals.

Thus it is clear that subfecundity not only affects fertility directly but can also, as described earlier, have indirect effects through other intermediate variables, such as birth control. These latter considerations cannot be overlooked when considering the impact of subfecundity on the fertility of both developed and developing societies. Subfecundity, birth control, and mate exposure all affect the fertility level. These factors should be viewed both in terms of their independent effects and in terms of how they interact with each other. Because these relationships have rarely been untangled, generalizations about the importance of subfecundity with respect to the fertility of developed and developing societies are largely conjectural.

Finally, population students must not be deluded by the notion that populations considered "healthy" are necessarily healthy or have low incidences of reproductive dysfunction. The islanders of Tristan Da Cunha, for instance, were thought to be extraordinarily healthy. However, closer examination revealed that this was not an accurate assessment. As Lewis *et al.* (1972) note:

> It was because of their reputation for good health that the Medical Research Council survey was orginally conceived. Its initial object was to measure the

> levels of health of this unique population. But it became apparent that the islanders were not paragons of good health. There was a peculiar chronic asthmatic state that affected almost half the people, a low resistance to respiratory infection, a high incidence of roundworm infestation, and other conditions that might be found typically in an underdeveloped country; there was, moreover, serious dental deterioration, and the suggestion of widespread congenital anomalies [pp. 386–387].

In sum, the two faulty fecundity assumptions and their product, the idea that fecundity is high and constant, continue to exert an influence on the work of many population students. Unfortunately, they seriously discourage systematic research concerning the causes of subfecundity and their impact on fertility.

INSUFFICIENT COLLABORATION BETWEEN POPULATION AND HEALTH SCIENCES

The final reason why research into the causes of population subfecundity is scarce and often deficient is that collaboration between population students and health scientists has been rare. As Tabbarah (1971) observes: "Unfortunately, systematic research in this field which would throw light on the quantitative or statistical relationships between different diseases and fecundity is still inadequate, apparently because it requires the collaboration of demographers and medical personnel, which has not yet been forthcoming [p. 268]." Similarly, Weisbrod et al. (1973) note: "There have been no studies in which economists have combined their talents with sociologists and anthropologists, let alone with physicians, engineers, and administrators in the public health field. Yet, as Gunnar Myrdal points out, there is a pressing need for much more specific and carefully supported knowledge about facts and causal relationships with respect to health conditions in the less advanced, poorly developed countries of the world where these conditions dominate the quality of life [p. 17]."

Because of the social science bias and misunderstanding stemming from adherence to the faulty fecundity assumptions outlined above, few population students consider it necessary to seek out collaboration with health scientists. Moreover, many population students seem to take the attitude that the fact that health scientists are not encouraging them to enter joint research is evidence that these scientists believe that subfecundity factors are insignificant determinants of population fertility or that once health-related information of potential interest to population students is developed it will be made available to the latter in a readily usable form via the population literature. The truth is, however, that few health scientists are concerned with the population fecundity ramifications of their research. In reporting their research in the medical literature, they routinely frustrate hopeful population students by their reluctance to explore the demographic implications of their findings. Thus, though population students behave as if the study of the fundamental causes of population subfecundity were outside their province, there seems little willingness on the part of health scientists to assume the burden. In order to determine the importance of the effect of subfecundity factors on fertility, population students will either have to seek help from health scientists or, as Clark (1969) concludes, "assemble information from diverse fields such as biology and medicine [p. i]" themselves.

This section and the two preceding ones outlined the reasons why population students seldom study subfecundity factors. It should be understood, however, that these three reasons, namely, the social science bias, the faulty fecundity assumptions, and the lack of collaboration, were discussed separately for presentation purposes only. Actually, all three are somewhat different expressions of the same phenomenon, which could be described simply as a general and routinized lack of concern about the fundamental causes of population subfecundity. Although these reasons exert remarkable influence, they are sometimes subtle and are often overlooked. They are detectable, however, in discussions that attempt to discount the importance of subfecundity's impact on population fertility. Appendix A provides an example and a detailed critique of one such discussion by Donald Bogue (1969:724–726).

The Legacy of Deficient Research

The past lack of rigorous research into the fundamental causes of subfecundity has led to two important research problems. First, population students do not know what factors are actually capable of materially affecting population fecundity. They are often unable to specify causality even when they are sure subfecundity is an important fertility determinant. For example, in trying to establish the causes for the unusually low fertility of the Afro–Arab population of Zanzibar Town, Blacker (1962:265) was almost certain that sterility played a major role, but he was unable to specify the cause of the sterility. Venereal disease and malaria, two of only a handful of specific factors capable of impairing fecundity that are commonly known by population students, were not sufficiently prevalent to be major determinants. Blacker was apparently at a loss to suggest and investigate any other cause of subfecundity; his analysis was truncated, and the causes of the subfecundity in Zanzibar Town remain obscure. There is a clear need, therefore, to *identify* the important causes of population subfecundity in order to aid hypothesis formation. And, as Hawthorn (1970) aptly states, "Until we know the biological factors contributing to fecundity we shall not be able to interpret properly the checked performance that we in fact observe almost everywhere, and in particular, we shall not be able to disentangle these biological factors from social ones [p. 11].''

The second research problem stemming from the past lack of research is that little or nothing is known concerning even the approximate *quantitative* relationship between subfecundity and its suspected causal factors. Thus, even in studies in which a subfecundity factor has been identified and is known to be important, it is usually impossible for population students to estimate its absolute importance or its significance relative to other factors. Lessa and Myers (1962:250), for example, in a study of the 1904–1949 fertility decline in Ulithi, reached the conclusion that it was due to widespread gonorrhea. However, their conclusion would have been more convincing if they had estimated the impact of the disease on individual fertility and, together with prevalence data and other information, related these findings to the fertility trend. Without such quantitative estimates, it is easy to misinterpret the causal strength of such factors. Perhaps gonorrhea was only half as powerful as Lessa and Myers believed, and other factors escaped unnoticed because the effect of gonorrhea was overstated. Without quantification, there is no certain way to check the validity of conclusions.

A good illustration of why it is necessary to estimate the quantitative impact of subfecundity factors on fertility centers on the ''VD hypothesis'' that has been used to explain the U.S. black fertility trend from 1880 to 1960. Essentially, this hypothesis stipulates that the prevalence of VD increased among blacks from 1880 to 1936, thereby severely reducing their fecundity and subsequent fertility. In addition, the hypothesis attributes the subsequent black natality rise to a fall in VD prevalence that resulted from the discovery of superior treatment methods and to their simultaneous application to large numbers of people through the creation of government VD control programs. This hypothesis was first introduced in a speculative fashion, with no accompanying attempts at validation (cf. Grabill *et al.* 1958:217; Thompson and Whelpton 1933:284). Then Farley (1970a), having investigated other explanations and found them wanting, advanced it as a residual hypothesis.

Both in its speculative and in its residual forms, the VD hypothesis suggests that venereal disease was the principal architect of the black fertility trend. However, no adequate attempt was made to measure the quantitative impact of these diseases on fecundity and to relate such information to the fertility trend. Once this effort was made (McFalls 1973), it became clear that VD was actually a minor though probably still significant determinant of the fertility trend. This finding not only placed the role of VD in its proper perspective but also drew attention to the fact that a new explanation for the black fertility trend was required.

If population students are to be able to identify subfecundity factors and to quantify their impact on population fecundity and fertility, more than the casual approach forwarded by Stone (1954) will be required: "For the demographer and social scientist concerned with the problems of human populations, an acquaintance with some basic biological factors which influence human fertility may be of interest [p. 731]." Rather, population students must study potential factors in depth, determining whether and to what extent they can cause coital inability, which is frequently overlooked as a form of subfecundity (e.g., Hansluwka 1975:203; WHO 1975:6), conceptive failure, and/or pregnancy loss. Such determinations, which should be made for men[16] as well as for women, require an understanding of the factor[17] that can only be gained from intensive research into the medical literature or consultation with appropriate health specialists. Failure to proceed in this manner often leads to disappointing results.

One study that did not proceed in this manner was that of Weisbrod and his associates (1973), which investigated the health impact of parasitic diseases, particularly schistosomiasis (*S. mansoni*), on the island of St. Lucia. This study was based on the widely accepted view that schistosomiasis causes mass chronic invalidism. The research hypothesis was that the purported physical and mental defects associated with the disease would have a quantifiable negative effect on natality, as well as on mortality, academic performance, and numerous economic variables. Before conducting the study, the authors checked the literature to verify the a priori sensibility of their research hypothesis—that schistosomiasis affects demographic and social variables through chronic ill health. But they found little supporting evidence and argued that there had been "extremely little careful research on these matters."

---

[16]It should be noted that less is known about the effect of subfecundity factors on the fecundity of men than on that of women. Data for men are not as plentiful, as the male factor in subfecundity was ignored prior to 1930 (Nag 1962:120) and even today, especially in developing societies (Ojo 1968:210), where men do not often present for study as they are reluctant to admit responsibility for a couple's subfecundity. Thus, it is difficult to know the relative importance of male and female subfecundity, which would of course vary by time and place. However, experts have estimated that male subfecundity is responsible for from 20 to 60% of the subfecundity in various populations (cf. Llewellyn-Jones 1974:111; Milojkovic *et al.* 1966:828; and Nag 1962:120).

[17]Though neonatal mortality is not a component of subfecundity, it should also be investigated in studies of subfecundity factors for several reasons. First, since some research focuses on perinatal mortality, it may be impossible to separate neonatal from late fetal mortality. Second, information about neonatal mortality is often better than that on late fetal mortality. Since death that occurs before and after delivery can often be ascribed to the same etiology (Babson and Benson 1971:10), knowledge that a factor causes neonatal mortality is sometimes also useful in inferring a probable impact on pregnancy loss. Finally, population students investigating the causes of unexpectedly low fertility observed in some societies may jump to the conclusion that the fertility deficit is entirely due to subfecundity if there is an obvious and prevalent subfecundity factor present. Any neonatal mortality caused by such disease might be ignored. This could be a problem, since observed "fertility deficits" can be the result of the underreporting of children who die very young. Thus, some information on neonatal mortality would help population students avoid this error (cf. Shapiro *et al.* 1968:42).

Thus, they had to underpin their research hypothesis with remarks made almost 25 years earlier about schistosomiasis causing mental retardation and being the possible cause of the physical defects observed in Egyptian army recruits (Weisbrod *et al.* 1973:11).

In their initial discussion of the effects of schistosomiasis on natality, the authors gave three reasons for expecting a negative impact. They felt that a deteriorating general health in severe cases would increase conceptive failure and pregnancy loss,[18] that parasites would "irritate the system" and "divert essential nutrients away from childbearing," and that in persons of ill health the probability of marrying and the frequency of intercourse would be reduced. But their data did not show the anticipated negative relationship between schistosomiasis and fertility and, in fact, showed a slightly positive one (Weisbrod *et al.* 1973:65). In order to square this unexpected finding with the study hypothesis, they then contended that chronic invalidism could indeed lead to higher natality rates. They reasoned that schistosomiasis, rather than lowering coital frequency, as they previously thought, might actually increase it, since coitus might become one of the few sources of gratification in the otherwise limited existence of persons weakened by these parasites. But all this is just speculation and is not grounded in a scientific understanding of the disease and its consequences.

Further research failed to show any negative effect of schistosomiasis on mortality, academic performance, or economic variables (Weisbrod *et al.* 1973:81). The question was then raised as to whether schistosomiasis was severe enough in St. Lucia, but the researchers were advised that the island was a representative area of moderate severity (Weisbrod *et al.* 1973:84). They finally concluded that schistosomiasis, even when moderately severe, has only a modest effect on physical and mental health (Weisbrod *et al.* 1973:89). In sum, the data did not support their original hypothesis—that schistosomiasis would, because of assumed deleterious effects on health, adversely affect demographic and social variables. Thus, the researchers in the St. Lucia study were incorrect when they initially identified schistosomiasis as a cause of physical and mental illness grave enough to be reflected in demographic and social variables.

On the other hand, Farley did not accurately quantify the impact of a correctly identified subfecundity factor, venereal disease, which he advanced

---

[18]The most widely held view on the relationship between schistosomiasis infection (specifically *S. haematobium* infection) and pregnancy loss centers on the notion that the disease is a cause of ectopic pregnancy (cf. Aal *et al.* 1975:403; Spingarn and Edelman 1966:715; WHO 1975:15; Zinsou *et al.* 1966:281). This view has lately been challenged by a group of researchers who report that the deposition of schistosome ova in the female genital tract does not usually produce inflammatory or structural changes capable of producing extrauterine implantation (Gelfand *et al.* 1970:784, 1971:849).

as the major factor in the 1880–1936 U.S. black fertility decline (1970a:222–226). Unlike other proponents of the VD hypothesis, Farley, at least with respect to syphilis, did attempt to go beyond the fact that syphilis causes subfecundity via pregnancy loss to an understanding of just how much subfecundity it could produce. Unfortunately, his conclusions were based on data from early sources that estimated that "a syphilitic woman, untreated, has only one chance in six of bearing a live healthy infant (Moore 1941:474, as cited in Farley 1970a:222)." However, recent sources, whose data are based on a more scientific understanding of the pathological changes associated with each stage of syphilitic disease, limit fetal infection, even in untreated women, to the 2 years following initial infection (early syphilis) (Kissane and Smith 1967:58).[19] Such findings substantially reduce the impact of syphilis on population fecundity and seriously challenge the VD hypothesis.

Thus, the most recent and most reliable sources must be used whenever possible. And a scientific understanding of the biological effects of the factor must be attempted. Questions to be asked in the case of a subfecundity factor from, for instance, the disease category include: Does the disease have different stages? How does the effect on fecundity differ between stages? Does the effect on fecundity invariably occur, or is it a feature of a particular complication? Do reinfections occur? Can immunity develop? Is there the possibility of spontaneous cure? What is the nature and effectiveness of treatment? By answering these and other pertinent questions with regard to venereal disease, McFalls (1973) was able to clarify the effect of VD on the individual and to offer a more accurate and conservative interpretation of the importance of VD in the natality history of the black population.[20]

In sum, there is a clear need for research that would identify those factors capable of causing population subfecundity and that would help determine the quantitative impact of such factors on population fecundity. This research requires in-depth study of subfecundity factors.

---

[19]Some recent material may also be misleading. For instance, Brown et al. (1970:26, 27), in their monograph *Syphilis and Other Venereal Diseases,* note that syphilis causes abortions and stillbirths but fail to mention that such outcomes are limited to early syphilis.

[20]When relating a subfecundity factor to the fertility of a particular population, many aspects of the social setting must also be taken into consideration. For example, in evaluating the VD-hypothesis argument that the rise in black fertility that began in 1936 was due to a fall in VD prevalence that resulted from the discovery of superior treatment methods in the 1930s and their simultaneous application to many blacks through the creation of government VD programs, McFalls (1973:9–12) showed how important it was to determine whether these VD programs and new treatment methods were actually available to blacks and how blacks responded to these developments in those places where they were available. The answers to these questions indicated that most blacks did not benefit from these programs and treatment methods until after the fertility rise was well under way, a finding that seriously undermined the plausibility of this part of the VD hypothesis.

A Current Research Project

Not enough basic information is available in the health sciences litera-ture to fully meet the requirements of such research. But much information, albeit scattered and often conflicting, is there that could increase the under-standing of population students concerning these matters; it has not, how-ever, been made available to them in a readily usable form. Thus, a recent WHO group (1975:230) concerned with population subfecundity recom-mended that, before any resources are committed to new research on popu-lation subfecundity, all currently available sources of information should be carefully reviewed.[21]

At the time this recommendation was made, this author had already spent several years on such a research project. The project's first major objective is to identify factors that can cause population subfecundity. Such factors must not only be capable of depressing individual fecundity but must also be sufficiently prevalent to merit consideration on the population level. This identification process is not as elementary as it may appear. Indeed, there is disagreement whether even major public health threats, such as malaria, have this potential.[22]

The project's second major objective is to provide information with which population students can judge the quantitative impact of subfecundity factors on individual and ultimately on population fecundity. Thus, popula-tion students with a particular population and a specific subfecundity factor in mind would have a ready resource with which to test quickly and accu-rately their hypotheses concerning the importance of the subfecundity factor as a determinant of the population's fertility. If, for example, proponents of the VD hypothesis had had access to the kind of population-related discus-sions on syphilis and gonorrhea that this project will provide, their research time might have been shortened and faulty conclusions based on misinfor-mation might have been avoided.

This project also makes note of subfecundity factors that individually are not potent enough to substantially depress a population's fecundity but that have a substantial collective effect when acting in concert with other similar factors.[23]

[21]These sources include demographic data, vital statistics, clinical records, disease reports, and so forth.

[22] Ironically, the very diseases that may prove to have the most significant impact on popula-tion fecundity are the ones about which least is known. It must be recognized that most research on disease is carried out in developed nations and in centers on diseases that affect them. Diseases such as schistosomiasis that are rare in developed nations receive very little attention, and research on diseases such as tuberculosis, which have been almost eradicated in developed nations but which are still widespread in developing nations, has come to a virtual halt.

[23]Generally, the effect of such factors on population fecundity is not strong enough to be discernable in statistical series on fertility that are subject to contrary influences (Romaniuk 1968b:219).

This project also advances the idea that subfecundity factors and result-ing fecundity levels are important population variables. It is proposed that populations experience diverse sets of subfecundity factors whose number, mix, and prevalence within a set are variable. Therefore, there is no compel-ling reason to assume that any two populations, each experiencing a unique set of subfecundity factors, have the same level of fecundity, even if these populations share a similar characteristic, such as being a "developed na-tion."[24]

In sum, this project will provide a set of criteria designed to help popula-tion students identify the causes of subfecundity and, when possible, to estimate their potential quantitative impact on population fecundity. To ac-complish these objectives, potential subfecundity factors are studied in depth. A determination is made as to whether, and to what extent, they can cause coital inability, conceptive failure, and/or pregnancy loss. Attention is devoted to the mechanisms through which such effects occur. Prevalence data are also investigated for three purposes: (a) to find out if the factor is prevalent enough to be of interest on the demographic level; (b) to estimate the impact of a demographically important factor on population fecundity, a procedure requiring prevalence data by age and sex; and (c) to determine whether the factor produces subfecundity differentials within and between populations, as well as over time.

Although this project focuses principally on factors that can directly depress fertility by causing subfecundity, it also recognizes, as noted, that these same factors can affect population fertility through other intermediate variables. They can, for instance, influence the chances of marrying or of maintaining a stable union or may affect contraceptive use, voluntary abor-tion, sterilization, or coital frequency.[25] Some attention will be devoted to

---

[24]If population fecundity is thought of as a continuum, the Hutterites would establish the upper extreme and the population of the Bas-Uele district of Zaire would perhaps represent the lower extreme. Among the latter, subfecundity is rampant, as is evidenced by the nearly 50% childless-ness rate for women 30–34 years of age during the 1960s (Romaniuk 1968a:328). In contrast, only 2% of one cohort of ever-married Hutterite women are childless (Eaton and Mayer 1954:20). The Hutterites are probably genetically super-fecund, virtually all individuals being the offspring of parents with eight or more children; they are prosperous enough to provide each individual with a nutritionally adequate diet and have a social system that ensures that each person receives it; they avail themselves of one of the world's most advanced health care systems, which minimizes disease and its consequences; they have extraordinarily low rates of psychopathology; and, as members of simple rural and farm communities, they avoid most of the environmental factors that depress fecundity (cf. Eaton and Mayer 1954; Eaton and Weil 1955). In contrast, many of the inhabitants of Bas-Uele endure poverty levels that deprive them of proper nutrition and health care; subfecundity-producing diseases such as malaria are endemic and epidemic; and the devastating social forces at work in this rapidly changing society likely ensure substantial rates of psychic stress and other forms of psychopathology. Virtually all other populations experience a degree of sub-fecundity somewhere along the continuum bounded by the high fecundity Hutterites and the low fecundity inhabitants of Bas-Uele.

[25]It is worth stressing that coital *frequency* is not a determinant of subfecundity, though it is a factor in natural fertility. A person may be highly fecund, for example, but have low fertility due to

these other ways in which subfecundity factors depress fertility for two reasons. First, it is important that population students be aware that some subfecundity factors also depress fertility as much or even more so via non-subfecundity intermediate variables, so that they can differentiate between the two causal paths. Second, little is written in the population literature about these nonsubfecundity relationships, and thus there is a genuine need for this information.

The research project described above is ongoing and is expected to continue for several more years. Its findings with respect to the five principal categories of subfecundity causes—genetic factors, nutritional deficiencies, disease, environmental factors, and psychopathology—will be presented separately. This book deals with the psychopathology category. Chapter 1 provides the background; Chapters 2–10 discuss the relationship between various forms of psychopathology and population subfecundity; and Chapter 11 provides further conclusions and discussion regarding this relationship.

---

infrequent coital exposure. But, although low and even too high coital frequency may depress fertility (cf. Amelar *et al.* 1977:206), it is a behavioral phenomenon independent of an individual's innate capacity to reproduce and is not of central interest to this project.

1

Psychopathology and Subfecundity: An Introduction

I would like to say that if there is any basis for the present day emphasis on the importance of psychosomatic medicine, it would be strange indeed if psychological factors were altogether absent in all cases of involuntary infertility. If psychological factors are important in physical health they probably are also important in the emotionally-laden fields of sex and reproduction.

—Clyde V. Kiser (1964:4928)

All people have mental illness of different degrees at different times.

—Karl Menninger (1963:32)

Psychopathology can impair individual fecundity. It can cause coital inability, conceptive failure, pregnancy loss, in fact, virtually every kind of reproductive disorder.

Psychopathology is also highly prevalent in many parts of the world. In the United States, for instance, one review (Dohrenwend and Dohrenwend 1969:10–11) of the epidemiological literature reports estimates of psychological morbidity in study populations as high as 64%. A preliminary report of the President's Commission on Mental Health states that between 20 and 32 million Americans require mental health care. The Commission also found that at any given time one-fourth of the nation's population are experiencing psychic stress that produces varying degrees of depression and anxiety (Shearer 1977:12). According to Knowles (1976), "There exists a steadily expanding number of the 'worried well.' . . . One out of every four people is 'emotionally tense' and worried about . . . ability to cope with modern life. At least 10 percent of the population suffer from some form of mental illness, and one-seventh of these receive some form of psychiatric care [p. 62]." Psychiatric patients currently occupy 37% of all hospital beds in the United

States (Mauss 1975:324).[1] In short, mental illness is the nation's primary public health problem.

Since psychopathology is both ubiquitous and a fecundity depressant, it is only natural for population students to ask: Can psychopathology depress population fecundity (and fertility) and, if so, to what extent?

Review of the Literature

In the first half of the twentieth century, some observers were convinced that psychopathology could lower population fecundity even to the extent of depopulation. Most of their studies were on primitive societies. For instance, Pitt-Rivers (1927:142–148) believed that depopulation in Melanesia was due in large part to a declining birth rate caused mainly by a psychopathological factor, namely, "the loss of zeal in life." This factor was thought to reduce the fecundity of both men and women and also to lead to decreased sexual activity. Similar theories relating subfecundity in central Africa to psychopathology were legion. One commonly accepted idea was that contact with Europeans created in certain tribes emotional conditions or psychological trauma potent enough to inhibit reproduction (Romaniuk 1968b:219). Indeed, Roberts (1927), according to Scragg (1957:5), summarized anthropological thought of the day by stating that the root of depopulation "lay with the curious despair which dominated the native mind and colored his every action and thought [p. 5]."

The etiology of depopulation among primitives, though much debated, is still a subject on which there is little agreement (Petersen 1975:380). Currently, however, there is scarcely any support for the theory that psychopathology played a major role. After making a comprehensive survey of studies arguing for a link between psychopathology and depopulation, Hunt and associates (1949:10) concluded that such a link was nonexistent. Similarly, Romaniuk (1968b:219) believes that the contribution that depopulation–psychopathology theories make to the knowledge of the effects of biological factors on population fecundity is "nugatory." Finally, Scragg (1957), having found no indication of the presence of fecundity-affecting psychological factors in two societies whose depopulation was previously attributed to them, suggests that psychological "factors must be

---

[1] A decade ago, mental patients occupied approximately one-half of all hospital beds (Horton and Leslie 1978:526). The decline from 50 to 37% does not signify a decrease in the prevalence of mental illness, since outpatient treatment for mental illness has increased more that inpatient treatment has declined. These trends are due largely to the development of psychoactive drugs, tranquilizers and antidepressants, which enable the mentally ill to remain more in the community.

completely discarded and considered to be myth presented by anthropologists in the absence of any adequate physical explanation at the time [p. 116]."

Nag, however, takes a more moderate position. He recognizes that psychopathology has been overemphasized by some writers in explaining the fertility reduction in certain nonindustrial societies but does not believe that psychopathology was of no importance whatsoever (Nag 1962:146,129). His conclusion is simply that "there is indirect evidence to suggest that psychological factors are not of major importance in affecting the fecundity of peoples in nonindustrial societies [p. 148]" or that "at least they are of much less importance than was previously suspected by some authorities [p. 129]."

Nag's refusal to entirely dismiss psychopathology as a fecundity depressant in nonindustrial societies may stem from his apparent familiarity with modern psychogenic research. He reports that "the intensive medical research on sterility carried out in the last one or two decades has resulted in the recognition of emotional factors, such as anxiety, repressed hostility, and neurotic or psychotic tendencies, as possible causes of sterility [p. 127]." Nag, like Davis and Blake (1956:234), believes that these forms of psychopathology are to be expected more in industrial than in nonindustrial societies and concludes that their effect on fecundity in industrial societies cannot be denied (Nag 1962:129, 146). However, probably because he recognizes that psychopathology is not altogether absent in nonindustrial societies, Nag cautiously allows that it may affect fecundity there also.

Anthropologists, such as Nag, are not the only scientists not working directly in this type of research who believe that psychopathology can affect population fecundity. The geographer Prothero (1972: 106) notes, for example, that medical–psychological factors may help explain the unexpectedly low fertility found among certain nomadic populations. Mosley (1977:7), an epidemiologist, believes that the 40% decline in the crude birth rate of Bangladesh during the 1974–1975 famine was attributable largely to a reduction in the conception rate, which was due in part to the anxiety associated with the crisis conditions. Clark (1969:5), an economist, speculates that the high fecundability of newly marrieds and those resuming fertile intercourse with a desire to conceive may be due partially to positive psychogenic factors or, alternatively, to the absence of negative ones. Similarly, Eaton and Mayer (1954:31), a sociologist and a psychiatrist, respectively, suggest that the extraordinarily high fertility of the Hutterites may result partially from the relative absence of psychosomatic subfecundity. Sociologist Cutright (1971, Chap. 3:11) notes that psychic factors may help determine a population's average age at menarche. Another sociologist, Hawthorn (1970), states that "especially in the area of fertility, it is almost certain that maternal psychological stress can have some effect on fecundity and the ability to bring a conception to term: have, that is, physiological effects [p. 119]."

A few demographers also allow that psychopathology may affect population fecundity. For example, Davis and Blake (1956) raise the possibility that "the nervous tension and artificial modes of life characteristic of urban—industrial populations may lower fecundity [p. 234]." Similarly, Freedman (1963:55) suggests that the stresses associated with urban life may decrease population fecundity in special situations. And, finally, Thomlinson (1976:170) remarks that psychological tension is a significant fecundity-depressing factor.

It is especially noteworthy, however, that the psychopathology—fecundity hypotheses in the 10 references above are all incidental or speculative. They are advanced alone, without discussion, and seemingly with little enthusiasm. The reader gets the impression that these hypotheses are mentioned simply to ensure that all possible fecundity-depressing factors are at least noted, even if their importance is largely unknown and is not likely to be tested in population research. Hawthorn's statement is a particularly germane example of this treatment, being the final sentence in his monograph *The Sociology of Fertility.*

Those population students who acknowledge the potential effect of psychopathology on population fecundity probably do so because of their awareness that psychopathology is a proven fecundity-depressant on the individual level and is widespread in many populations. This awareness is fostered by health scientists, who occasionally discuss the subject briefly in the population literature (cf. Stone 1954:740; WHO 1969:22). However, though a few population students are willing to acknowledge the potentiality of this relationship, virtually no research has been carried out concerning it. Indeed, in the early 1960s Freedman (1963:82) reviewed the population fertility literature and found that there were only a small number of psychological studies of any kind relating to fertility and that their orientation was scattered. Moreover, the psychological variables considered usually dealt with the process by which reproductive norms are learned or with the attitudes, motivations, or personality traits that affect such norms or actual fertility (Freedman 1963:66). A typical example of these studies is one by Centers and Blumberg (1954) that found that the major differences between voluntarily childless couples and those desiring children were psychological rather than sociological. In short, Freedman found studies that dealt with normal psychological factors and not psychopathology and studies that focused on fertility, not fecundity.[2]

---

[2]The Indianapolis Study (Whelpton and Kiser 1946–58:Vols. I–V) and the Princeton Study (Westoff *et al.* 1961) attempted to relate to fertility mild forms of personality problems verging on

Unfortunately, in the decade and a half since the Freedman review, the situation has remained essentially the same. Though more than a few psychologists have become interested and involved in population research since the 1960s (Sills 1973:V) and especially in the last 5 years (Campbell 1976:iii), they too have been attracted mostly to topics relating normal psychology to family planning or fertility (Fawcett 1973:vii). With only a few exceptions these psychologists as well as other population students still ignore the relationship between psychopathology and fecundity. Even recent, specialized, population-related works dealing mainly with psychology and reproduction, such as Newman and Thompson's *Population Psychology: Research and Educational Issues* (1976) or Fawcett's systematic review of the literature, *Psychology and Population* (1970) or his edited volume, *Psychological Perspectives on Population* (1973), do not include discussion of this topic.[3] In the preface of the latter work, the editor states that his intention is to provide readers with a "state of the art" report for a field still in its infancy. If the study of psychology and fertility is still in its infancy, by way of comparison, the demographic study of psychopathology and fecundity has barely been conceived.

Research Problems

Why do population students fail to study the relationship between psychopathology and fecundity? Probably for the same reasons that they do not adequately investigate the fundamental causes of subfecundity in general. These three reasons, namely, the social science bias, faulty assumptions about fecundity, and insufficient population–health sciences collaboration, are discussed in the Introduction. In addition, population students are discouraged from studying this relationship by a variety of research problems. First, it is difficult to specify psychopathology variables. Experts on

---

neurosis. Only slight relationships were found, and the results were basically disappointing. It should be noted that the dependent variable in these studies was fertility, not fecundity. Indeed, subfecund women were excluded from these studies by design. Thus, the results of these surveys shed no light on the relationship between psychopathology and fecundity.

These studies tend to exclude subfecund women not only by design (by not interviewing childless and one-child women, by placing limits on the amount of past pregnancy loss allowed, and so forth) but also indirectly, as a by-product of other features of the research, such as interviewing efficiency. For instance, such studies rarely interview psychopathological individuals—the alcoholics, psychotics, drug addicts, unmarried homosexuals, etc.—individuals who make poor respondents. However, it is in such individuals that the relationship between psychopathology and fecundity (and fertility) would be most vivid.

[3]One exception is Flapan (1976:45), who argues for studies to be designed that can answer such questions as "Do childbearing conflicts contribute to subsequent problems of conception or the occurrence of miscarriages and spontaneous abortions?"

psychopathology still have not agreed on what to include as psychopathology[4] or on how to classify its various forms (cf. Clinard 1968:451; Perry and Perry 1976:404; Suinn 1970:42). Second, little is known about the effects of various forms of psychopathology on individual fecundity, though research on these relationships has expanded in the last decade. Finally, psychological morbidity statistics are grossly inaccurate. To this point, Kramer and associates (1972) remark:

> The development of annual morbidity rates for mental disorders is a problem that has defied satisfactory solution. Standardized basic instruments required to develop such data are not available: case finding techniques for detecting persons in the general population with mental disorders, differential diagnostic techniques for assigning each case to a specific diagnostic group with a high degree of reliability, and methods for establishing dates of onset and termination of specific disorders. Until such instruments become available and procedures and programs are developed for their application to population groups, it is difficult to see how systematic morbidity statistics on the mental disorders can be collected [p. 1].

It is because of these shortcomings, both past and present, that psychological morbidity statistics are particularly ill-suited to dealing with trends (Wrong 1977:92). Thus, it is clear that, before it is practical to investigate thoroughly the population dimensions of the psychopathology–fecundity relationship, needed primary research, both substantive and methodological, must be performed by scientists in the appropriate health fields. Kiser (1964:4929) recognized this need more than a decade ago, leading to a plea on behalf of social scientists for better data on the question. The same plea could be made strongly today.

Despite these difficulties, however, it is only prudent to keep abreast of the relevant psychopathology literature, to identify findings of potential or actual demographic significance, and to incorporate these findings into population theory as they occur rather than en masse at some later date. Even if intensive study is presently impractical, it behooves population students to develop and maintain a current population perspective on the psychopathology–fecundity relationship rather than to continue the current practice of the periodic repetition of one line speculations of the sort "The nervous tension of urban life might depress fecundity," and so forth.

---

[4]See Horton and Leslie (1978:527), Kendler (1963:495), Mechanic (1969:2), and Mauss (1975:324). Clinard (1968:451) provides an interesting example of how experts differ on what to include as psychopathology. He points to an experiment conducted by Leighton in which six psychiatrists were asked to assess whether each of the same 50 men were mentally "ill" or "well." There was much variation in their judgment. In fact, one psychiatrist placed five men in the "sickest" category, whereas another considered the same five men to be "well."

Objectives and Methodology

Ryder (1959:427) once observed that the ability of psychopathology to decrease fecundity is "mysterious." The purpose of this investigation is to dissolve as much of that mystery as possible by providing an overview of available knowledge concerning the relationship between psychopathology and subfecundity.

This investigation has two principal objectives. The first is to identify those forms of psychopathology that can cause population subfecundity, that is, forms capable of depressing individual fecundity that are prevalent enough to merit consideration on the population level. The second objective is to determine how much subfecundity each form of psychopathology can produce. This determination, however, can only be a first approximation, due to the problems discussed above.

To achieve these objectives, the forms of psychopathology are studied in depth. The capacity of these conditions to produce coital inability, conceptive failure, and/or pregnancy loss is determined, and attention is devoted to the mechanisms through which such effects are thought to occur. (The absence of this approach is considered a major failing of the aforementioned published arguments concerning the impact of psychopathology on the fecundity of depopulating societies.) In addition, prevalence data are investigated for three reasons: (a) to find out if the form of psychopathology is prevalent enough to be of interest on the population level; (b) to estimate the approximate impact of the condition on population fecundity, a procedure requiring prevalence data by age and sex; and (c) to determine whether the psychopathological factor produces subfecundity differentials within and between populations, as well as over time. Although data on many populations are used, statistics on the population of the United States predominate.

Finally, though the focus of this investigation is on subfecundity, some attention is also devoted to other intermediate variables, such as birth control, through which the various forms of psychopathology can influence fertility.

A more detailed discussion of the objectives and methodology of this study can be found in the Introduction.

Types of Subfecundity-Producing Psychopathology

The major groups of psychopathology are disorders of psychogenic origin, disorders of organic origin, and mental retardation (Suinn 1970:43).

This investigation is confined to consideration of the first group, the psychogenic disorders, because of time and resource limitations. However, this is the key group to study because these disorders are the most prevalent and are the ones referred to in the psychopathology–population fecundity hypotheses.[5] Disorders of psychogenic origin include the psychoneuroses, psychophysiologic disorders, psychoses, and personality disorders.

PSYCHONEUROSES, PSYCHOPHYSIOLOGIC DISORDERS, AND EVERYDAY STRESS: PSYCHIC STRESS

Psychoneuroses or neuroses are emotional disturbances in which certain fixed symptoms are used to cope with anxiety and conflict. They essentially represent defense mechanisms that are being overly relied upon in efforts to avoid rather than to deal directly with life's difficulties. Not all neuroses can affect fecundity. One that can is conversion reaction, sometimes called hysteria, in which bodily symptoms are manifested without the presence of any identifiable organic pathology (Suinn 1970:222). In one such symptom, anorexia nervosa,[6] amenorrhea is a frequent feature. As amenorrhea is usually associated with anovulation, fecundity is affected.

Psychophysiologic disorders are certain conditions in which organic changes in the body are attributed principally to emotional disturbance. These conditions are the end effects of the intimate interrelationship between mind and body, that is, the inseparable interaction between emotional conflict and the endocrine and autonomic nervous systems.[7] The individual suffering from a psychophysiologic disorder is thought to have failed to develop a successful defense against anxiety. Unlike most psychoneurotics, the psychophysiologic person has failed to find a way to discharge tensions, channeling them instead through bodily organs (Suinn 1970:251–252). Reproductive organs are common targets especially among women (cf. Bardwick 1971:72), although the choice of organ involvement remains a mystery.

There is considerable controversy as to whether or not psycho-

---

[5]The study of mental retardation may also be profitable, since the disorder is highly prevalent (6 million Americans were retarded in 1967; Suinn 1970:443) and undoubtedly has an impact on population fertility for a variety of reasons. For instance, retarded individuals have a lower chance of marrying. If retarded persons are subfecund, they might have a substantial impact on population fecundity because of their sheer numbers. This would be an interesting research topic. For a discussion of some issues concerning the fertility and sexuality of the mentally retarded, see Bass (1978).

[6]Anorexia nervosa is observed primarily in young women and is characterized by a refusal to eat (Suinn 1970:234).

[7]The autonomic nervous system is that part of the nervous system that innervates the glandular component and smooth muscles of the internal organs. These reflexes are purely involuntary, and their stimuli may be in the external environment or may arise within the body (Copenhaver 1964:184–185).

physiologic disorders can be clearly differentiated from neuroses that have physiologic repercussions. Differences in the neurological pathways effecting the physical response have been cited (cf. Kendler 1963:504). Others (e.g., Suinn 1970:252) believe that the difference lies only in the fact that the physical symptoms in the neurotic help to relieve anxiety, whereas in the psychophysiologic person they are simply responses to stress and do not serve as a psychological defense. The distinction between the two is still unsettled (Cameron 1971:751), and as a result there is often no clear-cut distinction made between these neuroses and psychophysiologic disorders in the literature dealing with psychopathology and subfecundity.

Everyday stress is included in this study as a form of psychopathology,[8] since it is powerful enough to produce adverse psychosomatic symptoms (cf. Handlon 1962), including those capable of negatively affecting the male (cf. Milojkovic *et al.* 1966) and female (cf. Bardwick and Behrman 1967) reproductive systems. Everyday stress is also caught up in the gray area of nonspecificity already discussed. Too often authors focus on symptoms such as tension, worry, anxiety, and so forth, which are common to neuroses, psychophysiologic disorders, and everyday stress, or on the psychosomatic mechanism (discussed later) through which they all principally affect fecundity. Therefore, by necessity, neuroses, psychophysiologic disorders, and everyday stress are treated as one in Chapters 2–5 of this book, and for convenience this amalgamation is referred to as "psychic stress."

PSYCHOSES

Psychoses are conditions characterized by profound disturbance and disability, often entail loss of contact with reality and sensory distortions, and may exist without the patient's being aware of the nature and severity of the disturbance. Only two groups of psychoses may have the potential to affect population fecundity: schizophrenia and manic-depressive psychoses. Chapter 6 of this book focuses on these two disorders.

PERSONALITY DISORDERS

Personality disorders are the final major group of psychogenic disorders.[9] These are conditions characterized by the tendency to act out conflict

[8]Because of differing theoretical perspectives, authorities cannot agree on whether or not to include everyday stress as psychopathology (Mechanic 1969:5–6). However, some kinds of everyday stress can be formally classified as transient situational disturbances (cf. APA 1968:48).

[9]Historically, there have been a number of other names assigned to the conditions labeled here as personality disorders; these include constitutional psychopathic inferiority, character disorders, moral feeblemindedness, sociopathy, and conduct disorders.

through behavior that violates society's code of conduct. Little if any anxiety is experienced, and impaired personality development rather than severe emotional stress is the apparent cause (Suinn 1970:43). Personality disorders share a common criterion of abnormality, that is, bizarreness, and those who exhibit such behavior are thought to be unable to easily inhibit forbidden responses (Buss 1966:31,430).

Personality disorders include antisocial reactions, dyssocial reactions, sexual deviations, and drug abuse (Suinn 1970:273). However, only the latter two are capable of significantly affecting fecundity, and this investigation is confined to them.

Sexual deviation is behavior in which gratification of sexual impulses is obtained by practices other than intercourse with a legally consenting, genitally mature person of the opposite sex. On the basis of prevalence and subfecuntity-producing ability, only one form of sexual deviation, homosexuality, has the potential to affect population fecundity. Therefore Chapter 7, on sexual deviations, focuses mainly on homosexuality.

Drug abuse is the other personality disorder capable of impairing population fecundity. Psychopathologists[10] and the public[11] normally regard only the use of such drugs as narcotics and hallucinogens or the nonmedicinal use of tranquilizers, barbiturates, and amphetamines as drug abuse. Alcohol and tobacco are generally not regarded as drugs at all (NCMDA 1973:10), and their excessive use is not considered drug abuse (Mauss 1975:238). Alcohol and tobacco are viewed as fundamentally different from the other psychoactive drugs on the basis of the cultural meanings ascribed to their use, even though they are clearly similar to these drugs in both circumstances of use and general effect. Following the well-reasoned practice of the National Commission on Marihuana and Drug Abuse, this study categorizes alcohol and tobacco as drugs and considers their excessive use as abusive to the individual and to society.[12]

The discussion of drug abuse in this book is divided into three chapters. Chapter 8 is devoted to alcohol or, more particularly, to alcoholism; Chapter 9 deals with tobacco smoking, especially in the form of cigarettes; and Chapter 10 focuses on illicit drug abuse, with special emphasis on the following drugs or drug groups: barbiturates and tranquilizers, stimulants, marihuana, other hallucinogens, and narcotics.[13]

[10]The *Diagnostic and Statistical Manual of Mental Disorders* (1968) of the American Psychiatric Association, for instance, specifically excludes from its "drug dependence" category alcohol and tobacco. The former is considered separately as a nondrug. The latter is ignored entirely. However, a new classification system is currently being devised by the APA that, according to early drafts, will place alcohol and tobacco abuse in the "drug-use disorders" category.

[11]For a discussion of the public's attitude toward alcohol and tobacco as drugs and as drugs of abuse, see NCMDA (1973:9–11) and Mauss (1975:237–238).

[12]For an excellent discussion of what is a drug, consult Goode (1973:5–8).

[13]The reader should be aware that there are other drugs, used medicinally and rarely taken otherwise, that can also negatively affect fecundity.

The Psychopathology–Subfecundity Relationship

Psychopathology and subfecundity are related in many ways, the principal ones being shown in Figure 1.1. In this illustration, an arrow suggests a causal connection between two variables, with the dependent variable being at the head of the arrow. Alcoholism is used as the specific form of psychopathology in this instance.

Example A portrays a direct causal relationship from alcoholism to subfecundity. Example B shows an intervening causal relationship. In this case, alcoholism leads to disease, which, in turn, leads to subfecundity. Example C

(A) DIRECT CAUSAL

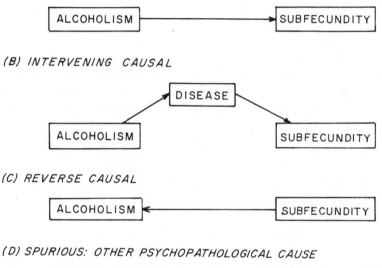

(B) INTERVENING CAUSAL

(C) REVERSE CAUSAL

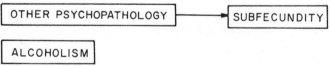

(D) SPURIOUS: OTHER PSYCHOPATHOLOGICAL CAUSE

(E) SPURIOUS: OTHER NONPSYCHOPATHOLOGICAL CAUSE

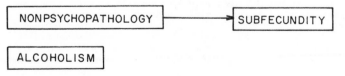

Figure 1.1 *Examples of the ways psychopathology can be related to subfecundity.*

is a reverse causal model in which it is the subfecundity that causes the alcoholism.[14] Example D illustrates the possibility that some other form of psychopathology, for instance, psychic stress, may cause the subfecundity. In this example, alcoholism is only a coincidental finding and does not depress fecundity. Example E is the same as D except that the causal factor is now a nonpsychopathological factor, such as a genetic disorder, rather than a psychopathological one. These five examples are not the only relationships possible, and, of course, even these can be combined to make more complex systems. But they do illustrate the principal ones.

The relevance of these different relationships depends on the nature of the research question. If the question were "What percent of alcoholics are subfecund?" there would be no need to know the nature of the relationships involved. If the question were "What is the effect of psychopathology, including alcoholism, on fecundity?" it would be necessary to identify and delete relationships such as C and E. If the question were "What is the effect of alcoholism on fecundity?" relationships C, D, and E would have to be eliminated. Finally, if the question were "What is the direct effect of excessive alcohol on reproductive failure?" that is, without considering intervening mechanisms such as cirrhosis of the liver, only relationship A would be relevant; that is, relationships B, C, D, and E all must be identified and eliminated.

Though all of these questions are pertinent to the study of population fecundity, the bulk of this investigation concerns itself with questions of the third type, that is, with what the effects of psychic stress, alcoholism, psychoses, and so forth on fecundity are. Thus, relationships of the sort C, D, and E are irrelevant and should be ignored. However, many of the sources that this investigation had to rely on did not or could not identify the exact nature of the relationship between subfecundity and the psychopathology under discussion. Much of the evidence, therefore, is merely associative, and it is difficult to determine just how much subfecundity is actually due to the psychopathology. The conclusions of this investigation are tempered in accordance with this lack of specificity.

---

[14]Subfecundity can, and not uncommonly does, cause psychopathology. As is discussed later in this investigation, subfecund individuals tend to become alcoholics, drug addicts, and heavy smokers more than does the general population.

Pohlman (1970) draws attention to another interesting example of this phenomenon. He notes that unintentionally childless (subfecund) couples may become subject to psychopathology (psychic stress) as a result of their subfecundity. In his words:

> All of the social pressures toward parenthood just noted spill over onto the heads of the sterile and help to make them feel miserable, although they are partly excused because (poor souls) they are unable to have children. They may, nevertheless, often feel sexually undemonstrated and imperfect, lacking in adult adequacy and unnatural. Marital conflict and attempts to blame each other may result [p. 10].

The preceding has shown that psychopathology can cause subfecundity directly or through an intervening variable. The following discussion will characterize the exact mechanisms by which these causal relationships are established.

INTERVENING CAUSAL RELATIONSHIP

In this relationship, psychopathology is an indirect cause of subfecundity. Here psychopathology causes a disease, nutritional deficiency, or some other condition that is then the direct cause of subfecundity. Much of the subfecundity observed in individuals with personality disorders is caused in this way. For example, because homosexual men have many sexual contacts, they have markedly higher rates of venereal disease, a well-known fecundity depressor. And drug abusers and alcoholics often have life styles that predispose them to malnutrition and to diseases such as tuberculosis, both of which are associated with fecundity impairment.

DIRECT CAUSAL RELATIONSHIP

Psychopathology can also be a direct cause of subfecundity. Two mechanisms have been identified: a pharmacological mechanism and a psychosomatic mechanism.

Pharmacological Mechanism The existence of a pharmacological effect on subfecundity is easy to conceptualize, and such an effect may often be directly observed through experimental methods. Naturally, a pharmacological mechanism is chiefly at work in psychopathology involving drug abuse. Some examples are: the impotence caused by decreased testosterone levels that are the result of the action of alcohol on the glandular tissue of the testes; reduced fertilizing capacity caused by the toxic effect of alcohol on the germinal epithelium of the testes; and the higher rates of pregnancy loss in smoking mothers due to nicotine-induced constriction of blood vessels, with a subsequent drop in oxygen levels in fetal tissues.

Psychosomatic Mechanism The second, more elusive, mechanism by which psychopathology may directly cause subfecundity is the psychosomatic mechanism. This mechanism is operating when psychological phenomena alter the body's physiological processes. A knowledge and understanding of the operation of the psychosomatic mechanism is essential to an appreciation of the potential for psychopathology to alter fecundity.

In the past, such a mechanism was considered unlikely, since psychological and physiological processes were believed to be separate and distinct. But now this bifurcation is believed to be too simplistic (Israel 1967:196), since there is a growing recognition that almost every psychological process has physiological expressions. As Kleegman and Kaufman (1966) note, "Psychological and physiological processes are like interwoven threads in a tapestry. There is no division between the two, only a constant interaction and each emotional state has a physiological correlation [p. 289]."

That normal psychological states can have pronounced effects on physiology is readily perceptible. Individuals can easily recognize that their thoughts, feelings, or emotions sometimes produce noticeable physiological reactions, such as blushing and perspiration. Physiological responses to various psychic states can be detected and measured by instruments like the polygraph, and it is even possible to psychically alter the functioning of body systems via a technique known as biofeedback. Probably another example of the psychosomatic mechanism is the apparent ability of humans to postpone natural death. Actuarial statistics show that deaths are less frequent before and during holidays and higher afterwards, a phenomenon known as the "death dip."

The psychosomatic mechanism involves not only normal physiological effects but also pathological ones. Indeed, the field of psychosomatic medicine grew out of the realization that a very large percentage of human physical ailments are of mental origin (Guilford 1952:189). As Horton and Leslie (1978) observe: "Various medical estimates define from one-half to three-fourths of all physical disorders as being wholly or partly caused by emotional disturbances. Today there is scarcely any disorder—not even cancer—from which emotional factors are definitely excluded as being of no importance [p. 604]."[15] Headaches, neck pains, nausea, stomach ulcers, intestinal tract ulcers, mucous colitis, asthma, and allergies are just a few of the problems that are often caused by mental disorder rather than by injury or disease. A sudden drop in the stock market or the termination of a love affair can exacerbate a latent peptic ulcer or reawaken a tuberculous lesion (Dubos 1978:76). And myriad health studies have shown that single, widowed, and divorced individuals are far more likely to fall prey to disease than are married ones, a demonstration of the power of social isolation and loneliness to bring about physical deterioration psychosomatically (cf. Lynch 1977).

[15]A recent book by Lawrence LeShan, *You Can Fight for Your Life: Emotional Factors in the Causation of Cancer,* has sparked widespread interest in the relationship between psychic stress and cancer. Earlier work by other researchers is now being reexamined to determine if chronic emotional stress really is a carcinogen. Much of this work has shown that a rather specific personality profile—nonaggressive, socially-isolated persons who keep their emotions to themselves—is connected with cancer. One of the most convincing findings is that loss of a central relationship often predates the appearance of cancer symptoms. Two biochemical mechanisms have been proposed to explain the psychic stress–cancer relationship. One proposal is that hormones, the production of which rises in response to stress, may be the chemical link between anxiety and malignancy. Another is that the suppressed immunity associated with depression allows malignant cells that otherwise would have been destroyed to flourish (McQuerter 1978:19).

In the psychosomatic mechanism the changes that accompany stress are initiated and controlled by the brain and are mediated by either the autonomic nervous system or the endocrine system. The familiar changes in heart rate and the perspiration and blushing that often accompany acute stress are examples of responses mediated by the autonomic nervous system, a functional division of the nervous system that sends electrical messages from the brain to certain organs, telling them to react in a prescribed manner. Nerve fibers of the autonomic nervous system terminate on the heart muscles (directing changes in heart rate), on the secretory cells of certain glands (causing perspiration, for example), and on the smooth muscles of the internal organs and the blood vessels (causing blushing, for example) (Copenhaver 1964:223). Physiological responses to stress may also be the result of changes in endocrine function. Such changes may occur by two routes. The less important route is the outpouring of hormones as the result of autonomic nervous stimulation. This occurs only in one endocrine gland, the adrenal, and, in fact, in only a portion of that, the adrenal medulla, which produces the hormone epinephrine (Copenhaver 1964:584–585). The other portion of the adrenal gland, the adrenal cortex, and the other endocrine glands are not under autonomic nervous system control but are controlled by hormones produced by the master gland, the pituitary. The release of the pituitary hormones is, in turn, directed by the brain and is modulated, via a feedback mechanism, by existing hormone levels in the blood.

The elucidation of the exact mechanism by which the brain influences hormone secretion began in the 1950s. Two discoveries—that blood flowed to the pituitary from an adjacent portion of the brain, the hypothalamus, and that chemicals produced by the hypothalamus, hypothalamic-releasing factors, stimulate the pituitary—allowed a new understanding of the functioning of the endocrine system. It was determined that cells in the hypothalamus, upon receiving electrical signals from the rest of the brain, release chemicals that are carried by the blood to the pituitary, where they affect the secretion of pituitary hormones (Rossi 1977:10). The acknowledged scope of the psychosomatic mechanism was greatly enlarged and the mechanism itself was largely legitimatized by this discovery that psychological states can influence hormone secretion.

The role of the psychosomatic mechanism in subfecundity is multifarious. Autonomic nervous system-mediated responses include (a) responses of the involuntary muscles that are found in most of the reproductive organs (fallopian tubes, uterus, vagina, sperm ducts, penis, etc.), with the exception of the ovary and testis; and (b) responses of the organs of secretion (seminal vesicles, prostate, cervix, etc.). An example of each response is: (a) the muscular spasms that can occur in the sperm ducts of men under stress and can interfere with semen transmission and fertilizing capacity; and (b) the secretion in some stressed women of abnormal cervical mucus that is hostile to spermatozoa and thereby reduces conceptive ability.

Endocrine-mediated responses are intimately involved with the workings of the hypothalamic–pituitary–gonadal axis. The hypothalamus produces gonatropin-releasing factors that stimulate the pituitary to produce the gonadotropic hormones that influence the ovary and testis. One of these gonadotropic hormones, follicle-stimulating hormone, directs the growth of the ovarian follicle and spermatogenesis. Another, luteinizing hormone, stimulates the production of estrogen by the ovary and testosterone by the testis. Estrogen is responsible for maturation of the ovarian follicle and ovulation, and both estrogen and testosterone are responsible for maintenance of the accessory reproductive organs and the secondary sex characteristics (Copenhaver 1964:568). Since the hypothalamus is the primary control site for gonadal growth and function (Steinberger *et al.* 1977:278), any interference with the workings of the hypothalamic–pituitary–gonadal axis can have vast repercussions on reproductive potential. Stress is capable of such interference. Under conditions of emotional stress, hypothalamic function is altered such that gonadotropic-releasing factors are not available to act on the pituitary, and hypogonadotropism results (Amelar *et al.* 1977:74). Stress-related alterations in hypothalamic function may be responsible for the abnormal hormone levels observed in some homosexual men. And this mechanism may play a role in the psychoses also, since abnormalities in hormone levels and spermatogenesis have been noted in schizophrenic men. But certainly the mechanism is most frequently encountered in the neuroses, psychophysiological disorders, and everyday stress. Common examples are the spermatogenic failure and anovulatory cycles observed in stressed individuals and the amenorrhea associated with severe trauma, such as internment in concentration camps.

Psychosomatic Subfecundity: An Overview and Critique

Since the psychosomatic mechanism is so important to psychopathology-induced subfecundity, a brief overview and critique of the status of this mechanism is in order. As early as 1797, Buchan understood, albeit in a rudimentary fashion, the potential of psychic disturbances to impair fecunidty (Noyes and Chapnick 1964). He noted: "Barrenness is often the consequence of grief, sudden fear, anxiety, or any of the passions which tend to obstruct the mental flux. When barrenness is suspected to proceed from affectations of the mind, the person ought to be kept as easy and cheerful as possible, all disagreeable objects are to be avoided, and every effort taken to amuse and entertain the fancy [p. 555]." If Buchan's insight had gained acceptance into the medical theory of his day, perhaps medical knowledge about psychosomatic subfecundity would be more advanced than it is today.

Unfortunately, however, what notions existed about psychosomatic subfecundity prior to the twentieth century were more the province of the supernatural than of science.[16] The Judeo—Christian tradition, for example, viewed much of male and female subfecundity as a divine curse or punishment (cf. Johnson 1968:2; Thomlinson 1976:169). This viewpoint led even Malthus (1798) to ask, in his *Essay on the Principal of Population,* "Is it some mysterious interference of Heaven which . . . strikes the men with impotence and the women with barrenness?"

Some primitive tribes still believe that the supernatural can affect fecundity. The Bantu have a common belief that sterility is caused by spirits (Bennett 1965:250), as do the Trobriand Islanders (O'Loughlin 1974:5). Similarly, according to Ashanti views, religious shortcomings and sorcery are the principal causes of subfecundity (Meuwissen 1967:224). It is also the assumption among some preliterate tribes that certain taboo violations will cause spontaneous abortion. Abortions resulting from nondeliberate taboo breaking are reportedly widespread. And in one tribal group, the Maoris, women deliberately break the taboo in order to terminate their pregnancies (cf. Dunbar 1962:137). Belief systems such as these are not confined to primitive societies, however. There is evidence that they exist even among certain populations in advanced countries (Ferreira 1965:108; Petersen 1975:239).

Even though the notion that the supernatural can produce subfecundity is dismissed by scientists, this does not mean that such beliefs do not have their imputed effect. Modern medicine is well acquainted with both the patient's ability to generate the symptoms of disorders they believe they should have and the therapeutic effect of placebos. It is also recognized that the effectiveness of any treatment is partially dependent on the authority with which it is prescribed and, thus, the faith that patients have in it (Petersen 1975:238). These phenomena help to explain how the primitive belief systems can actually affect fecundity, even though they are based on false notions. The mechanism involved is not supernatural but psychosomatic. In susceptible individuals, the psychological impact of the curse (anticipated punishment) leads to a form of emotional stress that causes subfecundity psychosomatically.

Today, there is an upsurge of interest in psychosomatic subfecundity.

[16]For discussions of the imputed relationship between the supernatural and subfecundity, see Ferriera (1965:108–109), Tupper and Weil (1968:758), Penrose (1971:112), and Kroger and Freed (1951:282).

Many researchers are now convinced that psychic disorders can exert a powerful influence on virtually every function of the reproductive system (Bardwick 1971:70; Kleegman and Kaufman 1966:288). Women especially are thought to experience a variety of psychosomatic dysfunctions astonishing in their variability and frequency. A partial list of dysfunctions cited in the literature include vaginismus, dyspareunia, amenorrhea, pseudocyesis, anorexia nervosa, obstetrical complications, conceptive failure, and habitual spontaneous abortions. In men psychosomatic dysfunctions of the reproductive system include impotence, dyspareunia, premature ejaculation, ejaculatory incompetence, and spermatogenic failure.

However, though there are many sources in the literature that contribute to the belief in psychosomatic subfecundity in humans, few contain rigorous proof of a cause and effect relationship (Noyes and Chapnick 1964:543). In fact, less is known about psychosomatic subfecundity than about perhaps any other potentially major cause of reproductive dysfunction. There are several reasons for this lack of knowledge. First, the systematic study of the field of psychosomatics is a relatively recent development (Ferreira 1965:108), and this is particularly true with respect to the subfecundity aspects. Second, current methods of inquiry are inadequate (Rutherford (1965:114). In fact, methods designed to measure psychological states utilize only indirect indicators of these conditions, and researchers do not have accurate measures of even common psychological disorders, such as depression or anxiety (Aitken 1972:287). Finally, rigorous research often requires multidisciplinary collaboration. One authority (Aitken 1972:285) suggests that such research would best be carried out by a team including a psychologist, a physician, a biochemist, and a physiologist. This requisite is usually impractical.

The result of these and other problems is that the literature on human psychosomatic subfecundity abounds with theories, overstated etiological hypotheses, general clinical impressions, and the like but is seriously deficient in systematic research and hypothesis testing (Aitken 1972:285; Buss 1966:424; Grimm 1967:5; Johnson 1968:74; Mai 1969:31; Noyes and Chapnick 1964:555). Perhaps the single most important failing of this body of literature is that few studies contribute data about cause and effect, since they are designed to demonstrate, at most, an association or correlation between psychological and physiological factors (Aitken 1972:28; Grimm 1967:18; Mai et al. 1972:203; Noyes and Chapnick 1964:487; Seward et al. 1965:534). Most studies have demonstrated only that differences in psychological states may have either caused, accompanied, or resulted from physiological events (Grimm 1967:37). Indeed, given the strong desire of most persons for children, there is no reason to ignore the possibility that reproductive failure causes the psychic disorder rather than vice versa (Kleegman and Kaufman

1966:293; Richardson 1967:viii). Mai (1969) puts the problem this way: "If personality or psychiatric variables are found in infertile couples, it must then be decided whether these did in fact contribute to the infertility or whether they may have resulted from it. This problem of cause and effect is, of course, a constant one in research in the psychosomatic diseases [p. 35]." A mutually reinforcing system between subfecundity and psychopathology is also distinctly plausible.

Despite these research problems and the primitive state of the knowledge, there is an overwhelming consensus among mental health professionals and experts on reproductive dysfunction that psychopathology can psychosomatically cause or contribute to subfecundity in both men and women (Ferreira 1965:112; Kleegman and Kaufman 1966:296; Noyes and Chapnick 1964:547; Rutherford 1965:114). This causal relationship is considered by most experts to be axiomatic. The studies in the literature do show remarkable consistency in demonstrating an association, albeit of undetermined nature, between psychopathology and subfecundity. This association was found in childless persons, as well as in those with children, and whether functional or organic features dominated (Seward et al. 1965:535). Other reasons for belief in a causal relationship are based on evidence from many scientific experiments on animals and countless clinical observations on humans (Kleegman and Kaufman 1966:296; Rutherford, 1965:114).

In sum, most experts agree that psychopathology can cause subfecundity psychosomatically, but there is less agreement concerning both the frequency with which this phenomenon occurs and the magnitude of the effects.

2

Psychic Stress and Coital Inability

The role of psychic stress in coital inability is well established (Seward *et al.* 1965:533). Psychic stress can produce or facilitate several psychosexual disorders that impede coitus, including impotence, vaginismus, and dyspareunia. These disorders lower fecundity and are of primary interest to this study. Incidentally, other psychosexual disorders, such as premature ejaculation, ejaculatory incompetence, frigidity, and inorgasmy, may also reduce fecundity, but they operate primarily through conceptive failure. They are discussed in Chapter 3.

Impotence

It is through impotence, the inability to achieve and/or maintain an erection sufficient to accomplish successful coital connection (Kaufman 1967:133; Masters and Johnson 1970:137), that psychic stress has its greatest impact on subfecundity due to coital inability. Although impotence can be due to a wide variety of nonpsychic causes, psychic stress is an important etiological factor (Abse 1966:133; Palti 1969:326). In fact, according to most authorities, psychic stress is responsible for about 90% of impotence (cf. Braiman 1970:738; Cooper 1972:548; Gonick 1976:191; Hastings 1960:430; Kaufman 1967:135; Kinsey *et al.* 1948:323; London 1972:611;

Melchiode 1976:98; Money 1967:276). There is even evidence that much of the impotence seen in old age is psychogenic (Kinsey *et al.* 1948:323). Several clinical series also indicate that the great majority of cases are caused by emotional disturbances. Of 22 couples who were subfecund due to male impotence, Kleegman and Kaufman (1966:294) report that only 2 cases were not psychogenic. Similarly, Dubin and Amelar (1972:580) found only 6 cases of organic impotence among 27 impotent men.

However, not all authorities are convinced that nearly 90% of impotence is psychogenic (Knight 1978:8). For instance, Johnson (1968:37) cautions that there is a tendency to automatically ascribe a psychological origin to impotence cases that have no obvious physical explanation, thus somewhat inflating the proportion of impotence considered psychogenic. Oliven (1974) has even stronger reservations concerning the conventional wisdom that 90% of impotence is psychogenic. Labeling this view as the "myth of the 90 percent," he states:

> It is no longer possible uncritically to accept the dictum that most cases of impotence are psychogenic. Diagnosis by exclusion, even after painstaking organic search, remains an inadequate rationale for assignment to psychogenicity. In the face of mounting new insights into sexual functioning . . . such assignment no longer seems an acceptable "out" in case of apparent zero findings. The oft-cited figure of 90 percent (psychogenic causes of impotence) which found its way into the medical literature in the 1950s needs finally to be buried: it simply does not correspond to what cases are seen in clinics and offices which take a little trouble and have no axes to grind [p. 371].

Oliven and Johnson are correct in pointing out that, in a substantial proportion of impotence cases, the cause remains obscure. Nevertheless, the consensus remains that, if not 90%, at least the overwhelming majority of impotence cases are psychogenic (cf. Amelar *et al.* 1977:204).

Psychogenic impotence may be due to stress of either long-standing or situational origin (Money 1967:276). A review of the literature indicates that impotence can be caused by many psychic stress factors (cf. Cooper 1972:548; Gregory 1968:348; Johnson 1968:73; Oliven 1974:384–388; and Talkington 1971:28). Fear and guilt are the most common causes of impotence (Abse 1966:133; Kaufman 1967:142–144), but depression over aging, an unsatisfactory marriage, business and financial worries, and other anxieties can also be etiological factors (Pearlman and Kobashi 1972:300).

PRIMARY IMPOTENCE AND ITS ETIOLOGY

Impotence can be classified as either primary or secondary. A man with primary impotence is one who has never been able to achieve and/or maintain an erection sufficient to accomplish successful coital connection.

Masters and Johnson (1970:137–138) report that multiple etiological factors are usually at the root of primary impotence, the most frequent of which are untoward maternal influences, psychosocial restrictions originating with religious orthodoxy, involvement in homosexual functioning, and personal devaluation from prostitute experience. They also note (1970:144) that there frequently is a psychosexually traumatic incident associated with the virginal coital experience. But such environmental factors or a traumatic episode during the first coital experience do not invariably lead to primary impotence. At present, however, scientists really have no concept of the specific psychodynamic factors that render some but not all young men, failing in the first coital connection, susceptible to continuing coital failure (Masters and Johnson 1970:145).

SECONDARY IMPOTENCE AND ITS ETIOLOGY

The male with primary impotence does not just fail in his initial coital encounter; the dysfunction is present with every subsequent opportunity. In contrast, the male with secondary impotence has experienced successful intromission at least once, either during the initial coital episode or during a later opportunity. The typical pattern is success with the initial coital connection and continued effective performance with the first fifty, hundred, or even thousand or more coital opportunities. At some time, however, an episode of failure occurs that in certain men is the harbinger of secondary impotence (Masters and Johnson 1970:157).

The cultural belief that the male must accept full responsibility for establishing successful coital connection has placed the psychological burden for the coital process upon him. The level of cultural demand for effective male sexual performance is important in the etiology of secondary impotence. Thoreau's observation that "nothing is so much to be feared as fear" is particularly apt with respect to the etiology of secondary impotence. Masters and Johnson (1970) put it this way:

> Any biophysical or psychosocial influence that can interfere with a male partner's ability to achieve and to maintain an erection can cast a shadow of conscious doubt upon the effectiveness of his coital performance, and, in due course, upon his concept of the state of his masculinity. Once a shadow of doubt has been cast, even though based only on a single unsatisfactory sexual performance after years of effective functioning, a man may become anxious about his theoretical potential for future coital connection. With the first doubt raised by any failed attempt at sexual connection in the past comes the first tinge of fear for the effectiveness of any sexual performance in the future [p. 160].

The fear of impotence can be raised in the always susceptible minds of men in most cultures by a variety of psychological, circumstantial, environmental, physiological, or even iatrogenic factors. Masters and Johnson (1970:160) cite the existence of a prior state of premature ejaculation as by far the most frequent potentiator of secondary impotence and indicate that the second most common factor is the occurrence of an incident of acute inges-tion of alcohol or alcoholism itself. Environmental factors of importance include the existence of a serious imbalance in parental relationships, either maternal dominance, paternal dominance, or a one-parent family, as well as homosexuality and religious orthodoxy (Masters and Johnson 1970:169, 175). Iatrogenic factors refer to the negative effect of consulted therapeutic opin-ion. Careless or incompetent professionals, including physicians, psy-chologists, marriage counselors, lay analysts, and clergymen, can inadver-tently either initiate the symptoms of secondary impotence or amplify and perpetuate the condition (Masters and Johnson 1970:188–192). There are many physiological factors leading to impotence, including diabetes and arteriosclerotic vascular disease (Amelar *et al.* 1977:207).

When considering the etiology of secondary impotence, Masters and Johnson continually stress not only the multiplicity of etiological influences but also the phenomenon that most men exposed to parallel psychosexual pressures and similar environmental damage shrug off these impediments and live as sexually functional males. It is the susceptibility to these influ-ences that ultimately leads to sexual inadequacy. But, unfortunately, little is known about this.

ABSOLUTE AND RELATIVE IMPOTENCE

Psychogenic secondary impotence may be absolute or relative (Kaufman 1967:144). Absolute impotence refers to the inability to perform coitus in any situation. Relative or periodic impotence refers to impaired potency under a particular set of circumstances and is due to the ineffectiveness of a particu-lar type of psychic stimulus to provoke sexual arousal. This selective sexual inadequacy largely excludes an organic basis for the condition and points to some form of psychic aberration (Johnson 1968:55).

Some factors accounting for relative impotence are monotony, hostility toward the partner or toward women in general, and unattractiveness of the mate (Kaufman 1967:144). Many men are impotent with women of their own social or economic background but are potent with women they regard as "degraded," such as prostitutes or casual acquaintances (Braiman 1970:739). Relative impotence due to fear, ambivalence, or negative attitudes toward pregnancy and subsequent paternity is a classic example of psychogenic subfecundity. Infertility specialists are familiar with cases of impotence oc-curring after contraception is terminated (Kleegman and Kaufman 1966:294) or only at the expected time of ovulation (Mai 1969:33). A typical manifestation of this phenomenon relates to the drugs capable of inducing ovulation that were introduced into clinical use in recent years. Couples are instructed to perform coitus according to a specific time schedule, and this "sex by the clock" procedure has given rise to a new condition of "periodic impotence" that exists only on those days on which intercourse is prescribed. On other days impotence does not occur (Palti 1969:326).

TREATMENT

Both primary and secondary impotence can be treated, but success to date has been limited. Masters and Johnson (1970:367) report more success than most, with a success rate for primary cases of 59% and, for secondary cases, 69%. Lief and his associates have also achieved a high rate of success, curing 65–70% of their patients (Knight 1978:18). However, few currently have access to such successful treatment programs, and conventional treatment is often ineffective (Smith et al. 1972:524).

PREVALENCE

Impotence is probably the most frequent male psychosexual disorder in any age group, including young adulthood (Braiman 1970:738). Sloan and Africano (1976:13) report that impotence is "epidemic and as prevalent as the common cold." Kaufman (1967:142) states that psychic factors cause impotence at some time in most men and that the man who has never had a sexual failure is a statistical rarity. But much of the impotence these authorities are alluding to is of a transient nature and of little significance in terms of influencing population fecundity. Similarly, although the incidence of impotence in elderly men is estimated to be over 50% (Kaufman 1967:135), too few of these men are mating with fecund women to have much of an impact on population fecundity either. To assess the importance of psychogenic impotence as a cause of population subfecundity, the prevalence of nontransient impotence in men during the normal reproductive ages must be determined.

How many men in their reproductive ages suffer from nontransient impotence? No one knows exactly, for there are no prevalence figures by age for any population. All that is possible is to estimate prevalence by piecing together data from surveys and clinical studies. In one survey of 4108 men, Kinsey et al. (1948:236) found that .1% were permanently impotent at age 20, about 1% at age 30, and about 2% at age 40. These figures probably underestimate the prevalence of impotence because of the restrictive definition of impotence used (relative impotence was not included) and because at that time impotent men were probably less likely to voluntarily discuss their sexual history than were their nonimpotent counterparts. In another more recent survey of 2801 men seen in their urological practice, Pearlman and Kobashi (1972:299) found impotence among 2.5% of men in their twenties, 1.5% in their thirties, and 4.7% in their forties. They compare their figures directly to Kinsey's and to those of other authors and do not suggest that men visiting a physician due to a possible urological problem are likely to have a higher incidence of impotence than do men in general. Unfortunately, they give no indication of their criteria for impotence.

These two surveys, though far from adequate for judging the prevalence of impotence in the United States, do indicate that it may be as high as 1–2% for men in their twenties and thirties and 3–5% for those in their forties. The prevalence of relative impotence must be added to these estimates.

Vaginismus

Vaginismus is a syndrome that affects a woman's sexual response by severely, if not totally, impeding coital function (Hirsch 1972:448). It is almost always psychogenic (Oliven 1974:420). Masters and Johnson (1970) describe vaginismus as follows:

> Anatomically this clinical entity involves all components of the pelvic muscula-
> ture investing the perineum and outer third of the vagina. Physiologically, these
> muscle groups contract spastically as opposed to their rhythmic contractural
> response to orgasmic experience. This spastic contraction of the vaginal outlet is
> a completely involuntary reflex stimulated by imagined, anticipated, or real
> attempts at vaginal penetration [p. 250].

Vaginismus can cause subfecundity by impeding coital function (Hirsch 1972:448; Kleegman and Kaufman 1966:289). In vaginismus, constriction of the vaginal outlet may be so severe that penile penetration is impossible. Vaginismus can make it impossible to consummate a marriage (Masters and Johnson 1970:251). It has been encountered frequently in nonconsummated marriages as well as in unions with rarely occurring coitus (Oliven 1974:420). In addition to causing subfecundity in the woman herself, vaginismus may depress the fecundity of her partner. The syndrome is highly associated with primary impotence, each disorder probably antedating the other with equal frequency (Masters and Johnson 1970:251–252; Oliven 1974:420). More-over, secondary impotence resulting from long-denied intromission due to vaginismus is not at all uncommon (Masters and Johnson 1970:256).

Subfecundity produced by vaginismus is frequently prolonged. Onset is most often early in the sexual life of a woman and frequently persists for indefinite periods (Oliven 1974:420). Moreover, as with many other psychosexual disorders, women tend either never to seek treatment for vaginismus or to wait for many years before doing so. As Hirsch (1972) informs us, "The patient who suffers from vaginismus seeks medical help often only after years of serious ailment, overcoming eventually her feelings of shame of a nonconsummated marriage, when things have reached a critical point in her matrimonial life [p. 448]."

It is also worth noting that vaginismus, in addition to causing subfecundity, can lower fertility in other ways. For example, Kroger and Freed (1951:314) report that vaginismus has been responsible for the dissolution of innumerable marriages.

ETIOLOGY

According to Kroger and Freed (1951:315), most psychiatrists agree that vaginismus is a defense mechanism against sexual intercourse. Thus, the observation by Masters and Johnson (1970:250) and others (Hirsch 1972:448; Kroger and Freed 1951:316; Oliven 1974:420–421) that vaginismus is a classic example of a psychosomatic illness. Its causes have variously been ascribed to fear and anxiety that date back to childhood or to teenage experiences (Hirsch 1972:448) and to such Freudian concepts as penis dread and oedipal conflicts (Kroger and Freed 1951:316). Oliven (1974:420–421) stresses the importance of male impotence in the etiology of vaginismus, and Masters and Johnson (1970:250) also cite male sexual dysfunction as the most important cause. They further list, in descending order of frequency, the excessively severe control of social conduct inherent in religious orthodoxy, specific episodes of prior sexual trauma, and prior homosexual identification.

TREATMENT

Vaginismus is eminently treatable from both the psychological and physiological points of view. With full cooperation from both members of the sexually dysfunctional marital unit, Masters and Johnson (1970:264–265) have achieved 100% success.

PREVALENCE

The prevalence of vaginismus is unknown. There are no census or survey data available and, as mentioned earlier, many women do not seek treatment, and thus go undetected. Physicians often uncover these problems in the course of normal examinations when the woman's obviously disordered behavior regarding aspects of her reproductive system is displayed. On the whole, vaginismus is probably a relatively rare problem. At least this is the opinion of Kole (1975:13). However, one British authority, Prudence Tunnadine, believes that thousands of married British women do not engage in sexual relations with their husbands because of vaginismus, but this is only a guess (Shearer 1975:4). The prevalence of vaginismus probably varies from society to society. The French gynecologists Faure and Sireday emphasized the fact that vaginismus is more prevalent wherever the old custom of forced marriages still prevails (Kroger and Freed 1951:315).

Dyspareunia

Dyspareunia is difficult or painful coitus. It is a psychosexual dysfunction affecting both men and women. Dyspareunia in the male is discussed first.

MALE DYSPAREUNIA

Dyspareunia is considered to be a subfecundity factor for, if severe enough, coitus may cease entirely and for practical purposes be impossible. Many men with this condition are distracted from and even denied effective sexual functioning by pain during or after coitus (Masters and Johnson 1970:288). Dyspareunia may range from minor irritation to crippling pain (Masters and Johnson 1970:289). One symptom may be a sharp, stabbing pain in the groin during coitus severe enough to compel the individual to abandon attempts at coitus (Johnson 1968:54). Dyspareunia can eventually lead to inhibition in sexual drive and may also result in impotence (Johnson 1968:54).

Etiology Male dyspareunia can be either a physiologic or a psychophysiologic disorder (Masters and Johnson 1970:266). Sexual repression may be an important etiological factor, Smith and Auerback having drawn attention to the frequent occurrence of penile and testicular pain in sexually repressed males (Johnson 1968:53). But the proportion of dyspareunia that is psychogenic is unknown. In one small clinical series discussed by Johnson (1968:54), evidence of local disease or abnormality to account for dyspareunia was found in only one of six men. This was interpreted to mean that the condition in the vast majority of these men was largely a psychophysical manifestation of emotional conflicts and apprehensions. Masters and Johnson (1970:294), however, emphasize the physiological as well as the psychological causes and stress that the former are often ignored and should be ruled out before assignment of a case to the latter.

Prevalence Dyspareunia is a less common complaint in men than in women (Masters and Johnson 1970:294), although there are no prevalence figures available. In a study of 76 men referred to a London hospital for assorted sexual disorders, 55 were found to be impotent, whereas only 6 complained of dyspareunia (Johnson 1968:43,54). Thus, among this referred population at least, dyspareunia was about one-tenth as prevalent as impotence. Whether this proportion holds for the population of Great Britain as a whole is impossible to tell. In any event, after a review of the literature on psychosexual disorders, the impression one gets is that dyspareunia is not a common problem in the male.

FEMALE DYSPAREUNIA

Dyspareunia in women can take many different forms, varying from postcoital vaginal irritation to severe immobilizing pain with penile thrusting (Masters and Johnson 1970:268). Dyspareunia can lead to subfecundity in women in the same ways it does in men. In severe cases, coital activity may cease altogether. Vaginismus occasionally develops also (Masters and Johnson 1970:258). Aside from its subfecundity effects, dyspareunia, together with the stresses that caused it, can exert negative influences on a couple's fertility via many other Davis—Blake intermediate variables, such as marital disruption or surgery.

Etiology Dyspareunia can be due to a variety of purely physiologic factors (Siegler 1944:42). Coital pain, for example, may be caused by scars from obstetrical incisions during childbirth, criminal abortion techniques, or rape episodes (Masters and Johnson 1970:268). Etiological factors also include vaginal infections, sensitivity reactions to various chemicals (including those contained in contraceptive creams, jellies, suppositories, foams, douching preparations, and the rubber used in the manufacture of diaphragms and condoms), radiation, menopause, insufficient vaginal lubrication, traumatic laceration of uterine support, pelvic infection, endometriosis, tumors, and surgery (Masters and Johnson 1970:268–288).

Dyspareunia may also result from psychic stress (Kleegman and Kaufman 1966:289; Taylor 1969:42), and a substantial though unknown fraction does. Although Taylor (1969:4) notes that most cases of dyspareunia have a recognizable organic cause and Oliven (1974:269) observes that psychogenic factors are too often and too indiscriminately named as causes of dyspareunia in females, most workers concede that the distribution of causation between psychopathological and other causes remains uncertain.

A sexually dysfunctional woman may use the symptomatology of pain as a means of completely avoiding or at least reducing markedly the number of unwelcome sexual encounters in her marriage. Masters and Johnson (1970) expand on this point as follows:

> Once convinced that there is no recourse for reversal of her dysfunctional status, the sexually inadequate partner in any marriage manufactures excuse after

excuse to avoid sexual confrontation. As women have long since learned, a persistent, aggressive male partner can overwhelm, neutralize, or even negate the most original of excuses to avoid sexual exposure. However, presuming any degree of residual concern for or interest in his partner as an individual, the husband is rendered powerless to support his insistence upon continuity of sexual contact when the wife complains of severe distress during or after sexual connection [p. 267].

Psychic stress in conjunction with a minor form of local pathology may together be sufficient to cause dyspareunia. Oliven (1974) offers the following two examples:

Some women to whom intercourse is chronically unwelcome are distressed more easily, more severely and more persistently by minor degrees of local pathology which would not deter a loving, unruffled or lusty mate; here dyspareunia becomes part of a subconscious avoidance reaction. Women with this type of psychogenically augmented pain are particularly apt to feel sexually incapacitated and to prescribe abstinence from coitus for themselves. . . . Pain which is indirectly psychogenic can be experienced by the woman who does not develop genital moisture at the critical time because the proceedings mean little to her; the resulting chafing reinforces her aversion and vice versa [p. 270].

Prevalence There are no data available on the prevalence of female dyspareunia, for the same reasons there were none concerning vaginismus. Masters and Johnson (1970:266) do estimate that psychogenic dyspareunia develops "countless thousands of times," presumably among U.S. women, but this information is not sufficient to yield a prevalence estimate.

Clinical studies may offer some indication of prevalence, however. In his study of neurotic women, Coppen (1965:163) reports that 31% had dyspareunia and/or a very distinct aversion to intercourse. His earlier 1959 study of normal women found that only 6% (a surprisingly low figure) placed themselves in the base category, that is, no pleasure but no special aversion to intercourse. Certainly, only a fraction of these 6%, perhaps 1 or 2% of all the normal women, would have dyspareunia. In another study, Kenyon (1968a:136) found that 2% of heterosexual women characterized their sexual intercourse as painful. Although these studies suggest that the prevalence of dyspareunia may fall in the 1–2% range, it is only safe to state that those who specialize in sexual disorders do not consider dyspareunia to be rare.

Discussion

Psychic stress is the single most important cause of coital inability. And, while it persists, coital inability tends to cause infecundity rather than subfecundity. Thus, psychic stress factors that operate through coital inability tend to have a much greater impact on an individual's fecundity than do many conceptive failure and pregnancy loss factors, which may simply lower the probability of conception and successful pregnancy. Moreover, individuals with coital inability tend to delay seeking treatment or not to seek treatment at all. Patients have great difficulty reporting these conditions to physicians (Braiman 1970:739) and rarely volunteer complaints about coital difficulties to them (Golden 1967:54). Thus, the effect that such factors have on fecundity is often unnecessarily prolonged.

The psychosexual disorders discussed in this chapter not only cause coital inability in the individual but also often compound their effect on fecundity by inducing sexual dysfunction in the mate. For example, primary impotence frequently predates vaginismus and orgasmic dysfunction in women (Masters and Johnson 1970:238,251–252), and vaginismus can play an important role in the precipitation of secondary impotence in men (Johnson 1968:47; Masters and Johnson 1970:252,256). Vaginismus and primary impotence are also highly associated, antedating one another with equal frequency. Masters and Johnson (1970:252) state that, if either exists prior to a marriage, consummation of the marriage cannot occur, and sexual dysfunction is likely to appear in the partner. They and other experts emphasize that psychosexual disorders, regardless of whether originally invested in the male or female, are a couple's rather than an individual's problem. Thus, the subfecundity they cause is often difficult to alleviate because it may require the cooperation and successful treatment of both partners.

Many sexologists have made sweeping statements in both the scientific and popular literature about the prevalence of coital inability (Hunt 1974:178). Claims such as the one cited previously that "impotence is epidemic and as prevalent as the common cold" abound. However, a demographic evaluation of the prevalence of coital inability has never been attempted, or, if it has, it has not been reported (Masters and Johnson 1976b). It is particularly hard even for clinicians to offer an informed guess concerning prevalence, since so much of coital inability goes unreported or untreated. It may be possible, however, to estimate a minimum prevalence figure based on impressionistic material in the literature.

Impotence is the most prevalent of the four factors. The estimate here is that about 2% of U.S. men between the ages 20 and 45 suffer from psychic-stress-induced impotence. The combined prevalence of vaginismus and dyspareunia probably amounts to only 1% of similarly aged women. Thus, it is estimated that psychic stress factors probably cause coital inability in about 2–3% of American couples in their reproductive period.

It should be mentioned that this discussion of psychic stress and its prevalence is not as inclusive as it might be. It does not take into consideration, for instance, the impotence caused by pharmacological treatment of various psychic stress disorders (cf. Dubin and Amelar 1971:471; Marshall 1971:656). It is well known, for example, that male patients often avoid medication in order to retain their potency. Another factor having a negative influence on heterosexual coital ability that could have been included under the psychic stress rubric is homosexuality, a condition considered by many authorities to be a neurosis (cf. Wahl 1967:194). Homosexuality, however, is treated in this book as a personality disorder and will be covered later in the chapter on sexual deviations.

If the estimate of the combined prevalence of the three psychic stress factors that have been found to cause coital inability is even remotely accurate, then psychic stress has considerable influence on population fecundity via coital inability. Moreover, since these dysfunctions tend to arise from the social and cultural organization of societies, their prevalence undoubtedly varies substantially by population and over time. Thus, the amount of sub-fecundity produced would vary also from population to population.

This chapter has dealt with the ways in which psychic stress can cause coital inability. It is also worth noting that psychic stress can cause coital inadequacy as well, which technically is not a form of subfecundity. Perhaps the most bizarre example is the couple, complaining of subfecundity, that has never consummated their marriage due to a grossly abnormal lack of sexual knowledge (cf. Amelar *et al.* 1977; Chisholm 1972; Duxon and Dawkins 1964; Friedman 1962; and Oliven 1974). A high proportion of these individuals are psychiatrically abnormal (Mai 1969:31). Stallworthy, in a review of 1000 infecund married couples, found that 5% of the women were virgins (cited in Mai 1969:31). Similarly, Dubin and Amelar (1972:581), in a study of 69 couples with psychosexual problems supposedly leading to infecundity, reported that 2 couples (3%) never had actual coitus; both women had intact hymens. Thus, these couples comprise a small but still significant fraction of couples referred to physicians for fertility problems.

More commonly, psychic stress can cause coital inadequacy by decreasing or obliterating libido (Kleegman and Kaufman 1966:289). Mental fatigue, fears of sexual failure, various worries and preoccupations, and other forms of psychic stress contribute to such a decline quite apart from the conscious will of the individual (Pearlman and Kobashi 1972:300). Psychic stress, on the other hand, can also lead to increased sexual activity, since some individuals use coitus as a way of serving their own neurotic needs (Friederich 1970a:695).

However, none of the above affects fertility via fecundity; they do so through another intermediate variable, the frequency of intercourse. As such, they do not cause coital inability and thus lie outside the subject matter of this study. There is the possibility, however, that decreased libido may impair the quality of coitus when it occurs and, subsequently, may lower the probability of conception (cf. Nag 1962:126).

3

Psychic Stress and Conceptive Failure

In order for conception to take place, a number of male and female processes must function properly. By interfering with these processes, psychic stress can lead to subfecundity via depressed conceptive ability or complete sterility. This chapter discusses the major ways this can occur, beginning first with a discussion of how psychic stress can reduce the capacity of the male to impregnate. This is followed by a review of the role of psychic stress in conceptive failure in women.

Male Infertility

Psychic stress can lower the male's capacity to impregnate by reducing either the quantity or the quality of the sperm available for reproduction. This is accomplished by the effect of psychic stress on either the production or the transmission of sperm and can occur in both mentally healthy and mentally unhealthy individuals (Abse 1966:133).

SPERM PRODUCTION

The production of sperm is called spermatogenesis. Normal conceptive potential requires both the production of a sufficiently high number of sperm and the production of sperm that have the necessary structural and functional characteristics, including normal motility and proper biochemical and genetic makeup. It is generally accepted that psychic stress can affect both sperm quantity and sperm quality (cf. Seward *et al.* 1965:534).

Practically all the research in the literature focuses on the impact of psychic stress on sperm count. However, Oliven (1965:192) has noted that psychic stress may depress male fertility by altering sperm function and structure. Psychic stress, especially conflicts over fatherhood, may, for example, produce enzymatic changes in the sperm. Sperm quantity and motility may be normal, but, if one or more enzyme systems are missing as a result of faulty protein synthesis, the genetic organizer material necessary for normal fertilizing power will not be present. It is recognized that stress disrupts nucleoprotein metabolism and interferes with the sperm's capacity to fertilize. Yet, scant attention has been paid to these kinds of infertility questions (Kroger 1962d:340).

The number of sperm contained in the semen, if not normal, is either deficiently low (oligospermia) or absent altogether (azoospermia). Experts (cf. Amelar *et al.* 1977:74; Kleegman and Kaufman 1966:294; Palti 1969:328) on psychogenic male subfecundity point out that psychic stress can lead to oligospermia and azoospermia. Progressive deterioration of spermatogenesis related to psychic stress is illustrated in the following case (Palti 1969):

> The wife of a healthy man, aged 30, became pregnant soon after the birth of their first child. The pregnancy was interrupted on the insistence of the husband. The first child died soon after the abortion which was accompanied by severe emotional trauma for both parents. Six months after the abortion, they sought help at an infertility clinic. Sperm examinations showed progressing oligospermia and eventually, azoospermia. The couple was informed that they could not have another child, and therefore stopped going to the clinic. Four months later the wife was pregnant, and the man showed normal values in number and motility of spermatozoa [p. 328].

A study by Steve (cited in Palti 1969:328) of men awaiting verdict for having raped women who subsequently became pregnant also demonstrates the relation between psychic stress and sperm count. The fact that the raped women became pregnant suggests that the men had normal spermatogenesis at the time of the crime. Nevertheless, while awaiting their verdict, all subjects were found to have complete spermatogenic arrest. The conclusion was that their anxiety and tension brought about the spermatogenic failure.

Amelar and his associates (1977:74) are also convinced that psychic stress can depress spermatogenesis. They recount one case in which an

individual's sperm count dropped to azoospermic levels after a serious au-
tomobile accident from which he emerged uninjured. The individual's count
remained at this level for 4 months before returning to the level it had been
prior to the accident. They also discuss a study in which severe progressive
disturbances in spermatogenesis were found in prisoners sentenced to death
who were kept waiting a long time before the sentence was executed.

The cases mentioned above all demonstrate a probable causal relationship between psychic stress and azoospermia, the most drastic form of
spermatogenic failure. However, psychic stress can also cause oligospermia,
which is a more common consequence and, hence, more demographically
important. An interesting study done by Milojkovic and associates
(1966:828–830) examines this relationship. Altogether, 1200 men in subfecund marriages were divided into three groups: nonmigrants and two
groups of rural to urban migrants differentiated by whether or not they had
migrated within the previous 3 years. If the stresses of migration and of
adaptation to a radically new way of life have any effect on spermatogenesis,
the migrants, and particularly the recent ones, should exhibit higher percentages of oligospermia than the nonmigrants. And this was indeed the case.
The percentage of each group that were oligospermic are as follows: nonmigrants, 27%; nonrecent migrants, 39%; and recent migrants, 71%. The authors conclude that the oligospermia is more prevalent among the more
recent migrants because they have not had sufficient time to adjust to the
tenor of industrial life, having migrated from relatively peaceful villages. Both
the psychic stress and the resultant spermatogenic disturbances decline as
the migrants gradually adapt to their new way of life.

A causal relationship between psychic stress and spermatogenic failure
is also indicated by the fact that the elimination of the former frequently
results in improved spermatogenesis, judging from clinical reports about
individuals and groups who improve their overall sperm picture concurrent
with a positive change in their psychological condition. Kleegman and Kaufman (1966), for example, report that a group of infertile men under their care
showed a demonstrable improvement in spermatogenesis following a bet-
terment in their psychological state. "This improvement," they observe, "is
often effected by a change in job, which brings with it less physical over-
exertion, increased satisfaction, decreased frustration and anxiety, and better
economic status [p. 294]." But perhaps the most telling evidence supporting
the hypothesis that psychic stress affects spermatogenesis is the finding that
improvement in sperm production not infrequently occurs following the use
of a placebo (cf. Palti 1969:328).

Thus, there is little doubt that psychic stress can cause male subfecundity by impairing sperm production (Palti 1969:328). But does this phenomenon occur often enough to be of demographic significance? The answer is

unknown, and, due to this lack of knowledge, there is predictable disagree-ment among medical experts concerning the importance of psychic stress as a cause of spermatogenic dysfunction. Rutherford (1965:104), for example, believes that psychic stress factors capable of altering spermatogenesis are not prevalent, and Amelar and his associates (1977) agree, stating: "In gen-eral, stress, anxiety, and emotional tension can also have deleterious effects on sperm production. . . . To affect fertility, however, the stress involved must be of extreme proportions, and the ordinary pressures of life and work have not in our experience been sufficient to cause male infertility [p. 74]." On the other hand, Palti (1969:329) suggests that they are common, speculat-ing that many successfully treated cases of spermatogenic dysfunction that were thought to result from various drug therapies might be due to psychological rather than to pharmacological actions of the therapy.

SPERM TRANSMISSION

Psychic stress can also lower the quantity and quality of sperm during the period between spermatogenesis and the time of actual or attempted insemination. In a susceptible individual, psychic stress may interfere with sperm migration by impairing the motility of the vas deferens or by causing a spasm of the urethra (DeWatteville, cited by Mai 1969:33; Kleegman and Kaufman 1966:289). Psychic stress may also cause retrograde ejaculation, the backward expulsion of semen into the urinary bladder during orgasm, and sham ejaculation, in which seminal fluid is almost exclusively composed of prostate secretion (Palti 1969:327). However, not much is known about these kinds of transmission problems other than that they exist. Of perhaps more demographic significance are two psychosexual ejaculatory disorders that can lead to conceptive failure, namely, premature ejaculation and ejaculatory incompetence.

Premature Ejaculation   Premature ejaculation is a disorder in which or-gasm and/or ejaculation persistently occur before or immediately after pene-tration of the female during coitus (Johnson 1968:43). This disorder may be expressed with all female partners or with selected ones (Money 1967:276).

Most authorities agree that premature ejaculation is almost always due to psychic stress (cf. Abse 1966:133; Amelar et al. 1977:205; Johnson 1968:58; Kroger 1962c:396; Oliven 1974:390; Rutherford 1965:104). However, Oliven (1974:390) does note that, although this psychogenic nature is widely recognized, it remains unproven. The idea that premature ejaculation is a learned response arising from the pressures of early prostitute experiences, adolescent sexual encounters in which fear of observation leads to swift ejaculation, etc., is well accepted (Master and Johnson 1970:94). Other authors describe the disorder as a conditioned anxiety response to sexual situations (Johnson 1968:62).

Premature ejaculation can cause subfecundity (Kleegman and Kaufman 1966:289,301). Whether it does or not depends on how premature the ejaculation is. The considerable variation that does exist is described in the following passage by Masters and Johnson (1970):

> Some men simply cannot be touched genitally without ejaculating within a matter of seconds. Others will ejaculate immediately subsequent to observation of an unclothed female body or while reading or looking at pornographic material. Many others ejaculate during varying stages of precoital play. However, most men who ejaculate prematurely do so during an attempt at intromission or during the first few strokes of the penis subsequent to intravaginal containment [p. 96].

Obviously, the earlier the ejaculation routinely occurs, the greater the negative impact on fecundity.

It does not necessarily follow that if the premature ejaculation occurs intravaginally there will be no negative effect on the probability of conception. Some authorities suggest that certain mechanical factors are known to be of great importance. For example, the probability of conception is increased the closer the ejaculate is deposited to the external os of the uterus by means of deep penetration into the vagina (Abse 1966:133; Swyer, cited in Nag 1962:126). Premature ejaculators often do not achieve deep penetration before they ejaculate, thus lowering the chances of conception. There is also the contention that precoital sexual play may increase the chances of conception (cf. Nag 1962:126). If this is valid, the fact that many premature ejaculators must forgo precoital sexual play in order to maximize their opportunity to ejaculate intravaginally is another reason why the disorder can lead to subfecundity.

Premature ejaculation can also depress fecundity by contributing to the development of other psychosexual problems both in the individual and in his mate. For example, premature ejaculation often leads to secondary impotence. Masters and Johnson (1970:101) report that an increasingly large number of men with lack of ejaculatory control move inexorably toward secondary impotence. In fact, they (1970:160) conclude that a prior state of premature ejaculation is the most frequent potentiator of secondary impotence, having found the former in 63 (30%) of 213 men treated for secondary impotence. However, most premature ejaculators probably remain so without ever developing secondary impotence (Masters and Johnson 1970:100). Premature ejaculation can also lead to female sexual dysfunction, especially orgasmic deprivation. Over an 11-year period, Masters and Johnson (1970:229) treated 223 marital units with bilateral partner complaints of sexual inadequacy. In 107 of these marriages, the male sexual inadequacy was premature ejaculation and the female dysfunction was orgasmic deprivation. The relationship between orgasmic deprivation and subfecundity is discussed later in this chapter.

If premature ejaculation does affect an individual's fecundity, the effect may persist for a substantial portion of the reproductive career. Onset is frequently in the teens, and the dysfunction often becomes a stubbornly chronic condition (Oliven 1974:390). Premature ejaculation can be treated successfully, as is evidenced by the fact that only 4 of the 186 men treated for this disorder by Masters and Johnson (1970:113) failed to learn adequate control of ejaculation. But, as with so many other psychosexual problems, few sufferers seek professional help, and those who do usually delay from 5 to 20 years after marriage (Masters and Johnson 1970:96–97). Thus, any effect on subfecundity is usually allowed to persist for long periods of time. Furthermore, some forms of treatment may themselves lead to subfecundity. Money (1967:277) reports, for example, that certain pharmacological treatments, although purportedly lengthening the reaction time of orgasm, may also abolish the seminal discharge but not the feelings and spasms of orgasm.

Aside from its effect on fecundity, premature ejaculation affects fertility through other intermediate variables. Premature ejaculation leads to the partner's sexual frustration and probably increases the likelihood of extramarital affairs and marital disruption (Masters and Johnson 1970:97–100).

Premature ejaculation is one of the two most common ejaculation disorders met in clinical practice (Johnson 1968:57). According to Masters and Johnson (1970:96), probably hundreds of thousands of men in the United States never gain sufficient control over ejaculation to satisfy their partners, regardless of the duration of their unions. Kinsey *et al.* (1948:580) also found premature ejaculation in a considerable number of their research subjects. Unfortunately, there are no demographic statistics on the prevalence of premature ejaculation (Masters and Johnson 1976b). However, Rosen *et al.* (1972:178) consider it the most frequent of all male sexual disturbances. And many clinical series show about the same number of cases of premature ejaculation as impotence, at least up to age 50 (cf. Tuthill 1955:126). Thus, the impression here is that premature ejaculation is at least as common as impotence up to age 50, meaning that the former exists in no less than about 2% of U.S. men aged 15–50. This appraisal is further supported by the observation that most premature ejaculators do not progress to secondary impotence, although a large fraction (30%) of those with secondary impotence were previously premature ejaculators (Masters and Johnson 1970:100,161).

Ejaculatory Incompetence   Ejaculatory incompetence, the clinical opposite of premature ejaculation, is the inability to ejaculate intravaginally in the presence of normal erection and desire (Johnson 1968:43; Masters and Johnson 1970:116). Frequently, this inability to ejaculate occurs with the first coital experience and continues unresolved through subsequent coital encounters. In other cases, there is a history of normal sexual performance until a specific episode of psychic trauma blocks the ability to ejaculate. Thus, the dysfunction can be either primary or secondary (Masters and Johnson 1970:116–117). Ejaculatory incompetence may also be relative, as it is well known, for example, that many men who have this problem with women of their own social background may be able to ejaculate with those they regard as "degraded," such as prostitutes (Braiman 1970:739).

Ejaculatory incompetence is almost always due to psychic stress (Amelar et al. 1977:205; Rutherford 1965:104). In fact, Masters and Johnson (1970:126) list only psychic stress factors as being of major etiological significance. These include the influence of religious orthodoxy, fear of impregnating, and lack of interest in or physical orientation to a particular woman. Less important etiological factors include maternal dominance and homosexual orientation.

Mai et al. (1972) describe the following case of an infertile couple in which the husband's psychological motivation for preventing conception and the psychosomatic mechanism by which this was achieved are apparent:

> An infertile couple, married five years, consisted of a husband, 31, and his wife, 30. Medical, gynecological, and psychiatric examination showed no abnormality. Physical examination of the husband revealed hypertension and a relatively small vas deferens and epididymis. Psychiatric examination of the husband uncovered the fact that he felt irritable on slight provocations, had an urge to be violent and feared that he would lose control, and was very sensitive to criticism and hostility from others. Although he could develop and maintain an erection, only once had he experienced ejaculation and orgasm during intercourse, though he could via masturbation. He had never intentionally tried to inhibit ejaculation during intercourse.
>
> He confided that he was concerned about his "nervous state" and that it would be genetically transmitted to his offspring. He requested that his wife consider artificial insemination or adoption as a means of satisfying her need for a child without making him father it. The husband was diagnosed as manifesting a paranoid personality disorder [pp. 201–202].

It is obvious that ejaculatory incompetence causes infecundity for as long as it persists. Furthermore, some men contending with this dysfunction experience such sexual performance pressures that they develop secondary impotence (Masters and Johnson 1970:116). Ejaculatory incompetence can be successfully treated, as the 82% success rate of Masters and Johnson (1970:367) attests.

Again, there are no prevalence statistics concerning this disorder. Although it is one of the two principal disorders of ejaculation met in clinical practice (Johnson 1968:57), experts tend to agree that it is not very common (cf. Masters and Johnson 1970:117; Money 1967:277). Kinsey *et al.* (1948:237) found only 6 cases among the 4108 men they interviewed.

Female Infertility

Psychic stress can also cause subfecundity by depressing the ability of women to conceive (Ferreira 1965:109; Palti 1969:326). This effect may occur in women with or without psychopathology. The stress may be the result of shock, anxiety, tension, and so forth flowing from external environmental circumstances such as familial problems, or it may be a product of an internal personality disorder. Common personality traits associated with infertility are overdependence, immaturity, and confusion of sexual identity (Kleegman and Kaufman 1966:293). Perhaps the most consistently expressed feature in psychically-induced female infertility, however, is ambivalence toward procreation (Mai 1969:32). Even though a woman may strongly and consciously express a desire for motherhood, this is frequently a cover for a deeper, subconscious wish to avoid pregnancy and all it involves. Descriptive psychological profiles of women most likely to develop conceptive failure as a result of psychic stress can be found in the literature (cf. Mandy and Mandy 1962:347–348).

Psychic stress can cause conceptive failure in a variety of ways. It can suppress oogenesis, reduce the fertility of the ovum, cause dysfunction in tubal transport, alter cervical secretions, and so forth (cf. Kleegman and Kaufman 1966:293; Kroger 1962d:339; Stone 1954:470).[1] Emotional factors, for instance, may result in the production of abnormal cervical secretions that interfere with sperm migration, a process that is reversed concurrent with the alleviation of the emotional stress (Ferreira 1965:109; Kleegman and Kaufman 1966:293). And the fact that the autonomic nervous system is highly instrumental in regulating the contractile patterns of the smooth muscles of the oviduct, contractions that are believed to be important in gamete transport (Blandau *et al.* 1977:133), suggests that stress could alter reproductive ability at this level. Not much is known about these influences, however, especially about their prevalence.

Psychic stress can also depress conceptive ability through ovulatory failure and psychosexual disorders like frigidity. The remainder of this section is devoted to these dysfunctions, since they are considered to be fairly widespread and, therefore, likely candidates for demographic attention.

[1]It is also strongly suspected that psychic stress can delay menarche. Children interned during World War II, for instance, experienced a delay of up to 3 years. Although malnutrition played a part, it was the coexistence of psychic stress that led to the delay. For a discussion of the relationship between psychic stress and age at menarche, see Oliven (1974:101).

ANOVULAR MENSTRUATION

Ovulatory failure refers to the nondischarge of a mature ovum from the ovary. From the standpoint of this study, the two most important expressions of ovulatory failure are anovular menstruation and amenorrhea.

Anovular menstruation is the condition in which ovulation is suppressed even though cyclic uterine bleeding may occur indistinguishable from normal menstruation. This condition is considered normal during early puberty, at the height of lactation, and in premenopausal women. It also normally occurs sporadically in women of childbearing age, about once every 12 cycles (Israel 1967:475).

Anovular cycles are an important cause of subfecundity. According to Israel (1967:475), they are virtually a constant occurrence and the cause of conceptive failure in about 10% of infertile women. Gyongyossy and Szaloczy (1972:589) report that anovular cycles were found to be responsible for periodic functional sterility in 2–3% of otherwise fertile women in Hungary and are involved in 36% of female sterility cases.

Psychic stress can cause anovular cycles (Israel 1967:476), although the proportion due to this cause is unknown. Some experts believe that disturbances in ovarian functioning due to psychic stress are a common occurrence (Kroger 1962e:255). Whatever the prevalence, there is reason to suspect that anovulation increases with modernization and its attendant psychic stress. For instance, according to Gyongyossy and Szaloczy (1972:589), the incidence of anovulatory cycles increased over the last 20 years in Hungary, in association with the increased modernization. They claim that over this period the proportion of infertility cases involving anovulatory cycles climbed from about 6 to 36%, though these figures are not meant to be hard estimates. These authors also note that stressful occupations probably lead to anovulatory cycles, a situation analogous to the relationship between occupational stress and male infertility via spermatogenic failure, as discussed earlier.

AMENORRHEA

Amenorrhea most often denotes a condition in which there is a complete absence of menstruation, although it also includes its temporal cousin, oligomenorrhea, in which menstruations are few (Israel 1967:186). Amenorrhea causes subfecundity, for, as Israel (1967) notes: "Dysfunctional menstrual disorders and sterility merge imperceptibly. Infrequent menstruation . . . implies either an associated infrequency or a total absence of ovulation with a relative reduction in the chances of fertilization [pp. 470–471]."

Numerous studies have established that psychic stress is a major cause of amenorrhea, although the exact proportion is indeterminate (Fries *et al.* 1974:473; Israel 1967:197; Seward *et al.* 1965:533). Rheingold speculates that one psychic stress factor, the fear of or intense longing for pregnancy, is the commonest determinant of amenorrhea (Israel 1967:197). There is no standard classification of the psychogenic causes of amenorrhea, and this discussion chooses to follow a nosology favored by Israel (1967:197–198). Here, the psychogenic causes of amenorrhea are separated into several clinical entities including: (*a*) amenorrhea of emotional disturbance; (*b*) amenorrhea associated with pseudocyesis; (*c*) amenorrhea associated with anorexia nervosa; (*d*) amenorrhea associated with the Chiari-Frommel syndrome; and (*e*) amenorrhea of psychosis. The first four are discussed here, and the fifth is reserved for Chapter 6 on psychoses.

Amenorrhea of Emotional Disturbance Psychic stress and trauma emanating from wartime situations provide perhaps the most convincing evidence of the power of emotional disturbance to induce amenorrhea. It is not uncommon, for example, for women to become amenorrheic simultaneous with their husbands' departure for war (Rutherford 1965:102). This phenomenon is clearly psychogenic, since menstruation generally resumes once a physician assures the women that they are not pregnant and after other anxiety-reducing therapies. In some cases, however, the amenorrhea is not easily reversed.

Emotional disturbance has also been found to lead to amenorrhea among women subjected to the stress of bombing raids and concentration camps (cf. Chodoff 1976:340; Katz 1972:360). Indeed, many reports from various kinds of internment camps during World War II indicate that such amenorrhea was not caused by local factors, nor was it due to malnutrition. It was the result of psychic stress. As Israel (1967) notes:

> These reports, showing an incidence of from 15 to 50 percent of secondary amenorrhea among the internees, have one thing in common: the amenorrhea appeared within the first two months of incarceration when the state of anxiety was most acute. The promptness of the onset of menstrual dysfunction differentiates such psychogenic amenorrhea from that of malnutrition, which eventually caused amenorrhea in as many as 90 percent of the detained women. Moreover, a direct correlation between the incidence of sudden amenorrhea and the degree of fear was demonstrated by the 800 internees studied by Bass. The camp authorities had divided the 800 women into two groups, the temporary internees, acknowledged to be on route to "an unknown destination," and the relatively more secure permanent internees. The incidence of amenorrhea in the former group was 54 percent and among the latter only 25 percent [p. 198].

Many of these women, once repatriated, and despite care, good food, and resumption of their usual protected lives, remained amenorrheic for months (Rutherford 1965:103).

The wartime amenorrhea cases are well known and often quoted because large numbers of women simultaneously experienced the same kinds of emotional disturbances, making obvious the psychogenic etiology of the amenorrhea. This is not to suggest, however, that the emotional disturbances experienced under these dire circumstances do not exist otherwise. Some women experience similar emotional disturbances during daily living (Israel 1967:198), and it is well known that these disturbances do precipitate amenorrhea (Brown 1972:579). Physicians are familiar with amenorrhea due to a wide variety of human affairs and circumstances, such as occupational difficulties, changes in the status quo, courtship, convalescence, mother-in-law troubles, and so forth (Rutherford 1965:103).

There are studies in the literature that examine matched groups of amenorrheic and nonamenorrheic women to see if the former have a higher incidence of stressful life events. Fries *et al.* (1974:473) found this to be so for a random sample of the total female population aged 18–35 in Uppsala County, Sweden. The amenorrheic women displayed a higher incidence of stressful life events, a higher consumption of sedatives and hypnotic drugs, and a higher occurrence of previous menstrual irregularity. Similarly, Brown (1972:579) found that amenorrheic women tend to have undergone stressful experiences just prior to the onset of amenorrhea. This was true of 9 (38%) of the 24 amenorrheic women in the study. Only 1 (6%) of 18 nonamenorrheic controls experienced a stressful event during the same time period. The Brown study also shows that stressful events may produce amenorrhea of long duration; the study women all had the condition for at least 6 months.

Amenorrhea, by its association with ovulatory failure, depresses fecundity. The fact that amenorrhea due to emotional disturbance can occur in normal women means that the entire female population is at risk during their reproductive years. Amenorrhea may be of short or long duration (Israel 1967:186), and every physician has encountered patients in whom emotional difficulties have produced amenorrhea for months or years (Kroger and Freed 1951:207). Thus, amenorrhea due to emotional disturbance has all the necessary requisites to produce subfecundity of demographic proportions.

Amenorrhea Associated with Pseudocyesis   Pseudocyesis is a conversion reaction in which a nonpregnant woman shows the signs and symptoms of pregnancy. Women with this condition typically develop amenorrhea, nausea, vomiting, and some peripheral signs of pregnancy, such as weight gain and breast fullness (Parkes, 1976:137). They may even exhibit weakly positive tests for pregnancy. Brown and Barglow (cf. Karahasanoglu *et al.* 1972:246) believe that infertility and pseudocyesis are really two points on the continuum of disturbances of reproductive functions.

There is little question about the psychogenic nature of pseudocyesis (Grimm 1967:8). This is revealed not only in the remarkable somatic compliance but also in the tenacity with which patients cling to the belief that they are pregnant, even when it is obviously impossible (Israel 1967:200). It is also evident by the usual rapid return to the nonpregnant state once patients are convinced that pregnancy does not exist (Grimm 1967:17).

Pseudocyesis is an obsession of pregnancy occurring in women with a high degree of neurosis (Israel 1967:200). It can simultaneously express the conscious wish for a child and the unconscious fear of begetting one (Bardwick 1971:73). Why so few women exhibit this syndrome when the presence of such conflicts is ubiquitous remains an open question.

Pseudocyesis can seriously depress the fecundity of individual women because it almost always produces amenorrhea (Heiman 1965:494; Oliven 1965:385). Treatment in some cases is very difficult, and women have been known to maintain their pseudocyesis for as long as 18 years. But, because it is uncommon, pseudocyesis probably is of little demographic significance in terms of population fecundity (Millar 1972:433).

There is some reason to believe, however, that pseudocyesis may actually increase fertility. Fully developed cases of pseudocyesis as just described are uncommon, but it is relatively common for women with either a strong desire for or fear of pregnancy to miss, or almost miss, a period and then to experience some of the early symptoms of pregnancy because they assume they have conceived (Heiman 1965:494). Once this assumption is made, contraception is often discontinued, but not sexual intercourse, and the woman then actually does become pregnant. Millar (1972:434) tried to ascertain the frequency of this phenomenon and found that 81 (4%) of 2000 pregnant women missed or had a scanty period *prior* to conception. Although many of these episodes went unexplained, Millar found in at least a quarter of them (1%) clear social and psychological factors that, when taken along with other subjective symptoms of pregnancy, such as nausea and sore breasts, justified a diagnosis of pseudocyesis.

Amenorrhea Associated with Anorexia Nervosa Anorexia nervosa is a serious nervous condition in which the individual loses appetite and systematically takes little food, eventually becoming emaciated. Young women aged 15–30 (Starkey and Lee 1969:376) and with immature personalities are its principal victims; the illness often follows prolonged emotional conflict (Israel 1967:201). Although some experts insist that it is premature to conclude a psychological origin for all cases (Lieb 1975:8–9), most authorities agree that the disease has purely psychological origins (*Time* 1975:July 28, 51). Indeed, anorexia nervosa is believed to be the most dramatic syndrome among the psychogenic illnesses, a multiple system failure bearing witness to the power of psychogenic turmoil to arrest vital functions (Rutherford 1965:103).

Anorexia nervosa produces subfecundity by interfering with menstruation or, in the case of premenstrual women, by delaying it (Mai 1969:34; G. Russell 1972:582). Amenorrhea almost always develops, as can be seen in two clinical series in which 56 of 58 (Starkey and Lee 1969:377) and 12 of 12 (Farquharson and Hyland, cited in Starkey and Lee 1969:376) women with anorexia nervosa became amenorrheic. Amenorrhea is a constant feature, usually beginning early in the disease, after some weight loss has occurred, though it may precede weight loss in some individuals (Marshall and Fraser 1971:590). In one series of 41 cases, for instance, 34 women became amenorrheic concurrent with weight loss, and 7 did so 1–3 years prior to it (Starkey and Lee 1969:376). Although the amenorrhea is psychically induced, the severe malnutrition that accompanies the condition perpetuates it (G. Russell 1972:583).

Prognosis for recovery from anorexia nervosa and, hence, for return of normal menstruation and fecundity is inversely related to the age at onset and to the amount of weight loss. The chances are good if anorexia nervosa presents under age 23 and/or if weight loss does not exceed 30% (Starkey and Lee 1969:378). Combining cases from three clinical series reported in Starkey and Lee (1969:375), it was found that 69 of 92 women with anorexia nervosa accompanied by amenorrhea regained menses. Many of these women became pregnant and had children, although substantial numbers had irregular menses and remained infertile, and others voluntarily did not attempt pregnancy.

For those women who regain menses, it commonly returns with the regain of normal weight, but it may take considerably longer. Starkey and Lee (1969:376) report that 38 of 41 cases experienced the return of normal menses from 3 months to several years after the beginning of weight gain. Frequently, however, it does not occur until the woman is back to her original weight and, occasionally, not for many months or years after an otherwise complete recovery (Starkey and Lee 1969:377). Amenorrhea has been known to persist in women from 18 to 79 months after achievement of normal weight (Marshall and Fraser 1971:590).

Aside from depressing fecundity via amenorrhea, anorexia nervosa may also reduce fertility through abstinence. "Sexual fasting" is typically present in the early stages and is followed by a complete decline of reproductive functions as the condition progresses (Money 1967:270).

The prevalence of anorexia nervosa is unknown. Pflanz (cited in J. Russell 1972:593) estimates an incidence of 15 to 75 per 100,000 population at risk, and Sours (cited in Fries *et al.* 1974:478) found similar figures in a review of the literature. But these figures probably underestimate the true prevalence because, except in adolescent girls with dramatic weight loss, anorexia nervosa is often not recognized and is thus overlooked (Israel 1967:201). It is well known that denial of symptoms is a characteristic feature of the syndrome, and many sufferers, failing to seek remedial treatment, go unreported. In a recent study of amenorrhea, not anorexia nervosa per se, Fries et al. (1974:478) incidentally found the anoxeria nervosa prevalence rate to be a minimum of 1 per 1000 of the female population of Uppsala County, Sweden. And Davis (cf. *Time* 1975:July 28) recently cautioned that the condition "may be more common than we ever thought [p. 50]." There is also a growing consensus that anorexia nervosa has been occurring more frequently in the past decade or two (J. Russell 1972:593) in the United States (*Time* 1975:July 28, 50) and elsewhere (Fries et al. 1974:478).

Amenorrhea Associated with the Chiari-Frommel Syndrome   The Chiari-Frommel syndrome is characterized by amenorrhea, prolonged galactorrhea (excessive and spontaneous milk flow), and moderate obesity and is the result of hypothalamic dysfunction (Oliven 1965:382). In this syndrome, the amenorrhea is associated with marked atrophy of both the uterus and the ovaries. The syndrome may have a purely psychogenic origin, although this is not necessarily the case (Israel 1967:199–200).

The Chiari-Frommel syndrome, seen chiefly in young women, produces subfecundity via amenorrhea. In more than half the patients reported, no pregnancies have ever occurred. The treatment of the syndrome has been difficult, though recently a new treatment has restored ovulatory cycles and has led to subsequent pregnancy (Israel 1967:199–200). No indication of prevalence was immediately available in the literature, but there is no suggestion that the syndrome is anything but rare.

FRIGIDITY

The psychopathology literature is full of different names, definitions, and descriptions for frigidity.[2] In this discussion, frigidity is defined as a female psychosexual disorder characterized by orgasmic incapacity and the inability to abandon the self to sexual participation and pleasure (Money 1967:278). Most clinicians currently believe "that orgasm capacity is an integral part of female sexuality, and that its absence constitutes a significant finding both as a symptom and as a potential pathogen [Oliven 1974:407]."

Frigidity usually occurs in the presence of normal anatomy and gonadal function,[3] organic frigidity being rare (Braiman 1970:738; Kroger 1962j:383). Thus, frigidity is psychogenic in the overwhelming majority of cases and is a

---

[2]For a typical but dated presentation, see Kroger and Freed (1951:294–295). For a more recent discussion, see Oliven (1974:402–410).

[3]However, some authors (e.g., Karahasanoglu et al. 1972:46; Macavei 1973:95) suggest that frigidity and inorgasmy may lead to disorders of ovulation.

symptom of emotional disturbance (Braiman 1970:738; Kroger and Freed 1951:311; Oliven 1974:408; Talkington 1971:27; Taylor 1969:492). A study by Coppen (1965:13) found, for instance, that 50% of neurotics, as compared to only 6% of normal women, were frigid.

The psychic causes of frigidity are almost as varied as the individual women affected (Dreikurs 1962:415). According to Oliven (1974), "Probably the most frequent cause of [frigidity] is chronic unconscious self-inhibition of the capacity to love and let go unreservedly during the sex act. The inhibitants are congealed negative emotions such as fear, shame or hostility, residues of a large variety of past traumata, which have become fused with components of the sexual drive [p. 408]."

Frigidity may be present with all men or with only one specific partner, usually the husband (Dreikurs 1962:415). It can last a lifetime, which often happens, since frigid women seldom seek treatment (Kroger 1962c:389). For those who do, the success of the treatment is variable (Money 1967:278), the cure rate hovering between 30 and 60% (Oliven 1974:410).

Subfecundity Many authors and clinicians have suggested that subfecundity is associated with frigidity (Mai 1969:32). Indeed, there are reports that frigidity can actually cause subfecundity. Frigidity is thought by some (e.g., Kroger and Freed 1951:297) to cause subfecundity through coital inability by frequently leading to vaginismus and dyspareunia. However, most discussions center on the proposition that any subfecundity is caused by conceptive failure resulting from the lack of sexual excitement or inorgasmy. A variety of mechanisms have been advanced (Seward et al. 1965:534).

Nag (1962:126–127) is one of the few population scientists to recognize the potential relationship between frigidity and subfecundity. And though he is skeptical about the importance of frigidity as a population subfecundity cause, he does discuss three hypothetical causal mechanisms which could link the two. The first is that there is secretory activity associated with sexual excitement or orgasm, the absence of which would reduce the probability of conception by adversely affecting the viability or motility of sperm (see also Karahasanoglu et al. 1972:246; Mai 1969:32). The alkaline nature of these secretions is believed to decrease the natural acidity of the vagina, which is hostile to sperm, thereby enhancing sperm survival and the chances for fertilization. Others believe that simply the absence of vaginal lubrication, which is associated with frigidity, may impair sperm migration and lower the chances of conception (cf. Mai 1969:32).

The second hypothesis discussed by Nag is based on two premises, to wit, that sexual excitement leads to deeper coital penetration and that deeper penetration increases the probability of impregnation. If these are valid, Nag believes it is reasonable to assume that a high degree of sexual excitement is generally more favorable to impregnation. He goes on to suggest that this is why precoital sexual play may have some importance in connection with fertilization. It is well known, for instance, that, among many animal species, precoital courtship and the resultant emotional excitement are absolute requirements for fertile mating. But whether this hypothesis and the two premises upon which it is based are, in fact, valid or have any material effect on human fecundity is at best conjectural.

The third hypothesis discussed by Nag is that a woman's chances of conception are slightly increased if she attains orgasm simultaneously with the man, because during orgasm the sucking movement of the uterus tends to assist the progress of sperm toward the ovum. The mechanism involved here has been elaborated upon by Rossi (1977:17,29), who observes that the degree of sexual excitement in the female is directly related to the amount of oxytocin released by the pituitary. Since oxytocin stimulates uterine contractions that propel the sperm toward the oviduct and is present in increasing amounts as sexual excitement increases and reaches even greater levels if orgasm is achieved, frigid women could be at a disadvantage from the view of conceptive ability. However, others (e.g., Chang et al. 1977:436) believe that, although such contractions are necessary for rapid sperm transport, rapid transport is not a prerequisite for conception, since many spermatozoa reach the tubes, albeit more slowly, based on their innate motility. And, indeed, conception will not occur unless the spermatozoa are motile, since motility is necessary for fertilizing ability (Harrison 1977:379). Masters and Johnson (1966:80–88) provide information that orgasm has at least one negative effect on fecundity. In their investigation of the functional role of the vagina in reproduction, they report that semen deposited in the vagina is better retained (and fertility thereby enhanced) if a woman does not go on to the fourth and final phase of sexual response (orgasm) but instead remains at phase three, the "orgasmic platform." During this phase the outer third of the vagina is constricted, creating a stopperlike effect that retains seminal fluid—an effect rapidly lost if a woman continues to orgasm.[4]

In sum, hypotheses associating frigidity with conceptive failure, though they are outwardly attractive because they propose clear-cut physiological explanations for conceptive failure (Mai 1969:32), are vague, speculative, and suspect. And, due to a lack of rigorous research, it is not known conclusively whether frigidity or inorgasmy actually cause infertility (Karahasanoglu et al. 1972:246; Oliven 1965:243). Authorities tend to divide on this issue. On the negative side, for instance, Noyes and Chapnick (1964:555) conclude,

---

[4]In the sexually repressive Victorian era, one justification for the norm that orgasm in women must be avoided was that it interfered with conception by inducing a relaxation and weakness that could lead to subfecundity (Williams 1977:198). Interestingly, this idea is consistent with the finding of Masters and Johnson discussed here.

after reviewing some of the literature, that frigidity does not cause infertility. And Helen Deutsch, who wrote extensively on the psychopathology of subfecundity and to whom many psychogenic subfecundity hypotheses owe their origin, was unable to find a convincing causal connection between frigidity and infertility (Mai 1969:32). However, on the affirmative side, other authors (cf. Mai 1969:32) conclude that many infertile women are frigid, and some workers (e.g., Kleegman and Kaufman 1966:301) consider the frigidity to be a contributing cause.

If frigidity does cause infertility, it probably acts only to delay conception rather than to cause sterility. Most authorities (cf. Kleegman and Kaufman 1966:289; Masters and Johnson 1970:216) concede that elevated levels of female sexual tension or orgasm are not technically necessary for conception. In this connection, Oliven (1965) remarks:

> Experience with artificially inseminated, raped, dyspareunic, and totally frigid women has dispelled the belief in the *absolute* orgasm-dependence of conception; nor has it been shown that highly orgasm-prone women are, as a group, also most fertile; nor has suppression of orgasm been shown to be anticoncipient. The present consensus is that the women's orgasm is *advantageous to conception* but not essential [p. 243; emphasis added].

But, if orgasm is advantageous to conception, it would follow that anything less represents a degree of subfecundity.

It is also possible to argue that frigidity is a cause of subfecundity if the unit of observation is the couple rather than the individual. It is well known, for example, that frigidity can cause impotence in the woman's mate. Johnson (1968) notes:

> Sexual frigidity in the wife may be a cause of impotence in the husband. Fear of inflicting injury upon the female, or shame of revealing arousal to an inhibited wife, may be responsible. Bergler and Eliasberg have written at length on this subject. . . . A psychoanalytical study by Friedman of women with non-consummated marriages has particular relevance to the primary role played by the partner's sexual attitudes in some cases of male impotence. Bergler's warning might well be heeded, that impotence in the husband can be the alibi of a frigid wife [pp. 36–37].

Similarly, Rosen and associates (1972:445) report that frigidity not uncommonly leads to ejaculatory dysfunction in a woman's mate.

Other Intermediate Variables   Frigidity can also affect fertility through intermediate variables other than subfecundity. Authorities on psychosexual dysfunction point out that frigidity increases the incidence of all six Davis–Blake intermediate variables affecting exposure to coitus, particularly those relating to marital stability and coital frequency (cf. Kleegman and Kaufman

1966:289; Kroger 1962c:386). For example, frigidity is a common cause of marital disruption and divorce (Perry and Perry 1976:31).

Coital frequency, however, is probably the most powerful variable affecting the fertility of frigid women. It is likely that this frequency would be lower in unions in which the woman is frigid, perhaps even to the point of indefinite abstinence. The incidence of vaginismus and dyspareunia, being disproportionately high among frigid women, would reinforce this tendency. Frigidity can also reduce coital frequency in a variety of other subtle ways. A frigid woman, for example, may use obesity as a sort of "chastity belt," theorizing that obesity will discourage sexual advances. Psychiatrists are well-acquainted with the married woman who dislikes coitus and overeats to discourage unwanted intercourse (Kroger 1962a:533).[5] Frigidity can also lead to extramarital promiscuity in either or both partners (cf. Kroger 1962c:386; Oliven 1974:287). Hence, the overall coital frequency of individuals in some frigidity-plagued unions may not decline even though the marital frequency does. Although in such instances it is usually the male who is unfaithful, a woman who is frigid only with her husband may also participate in extramarital affairs.

Unfortunately, hypotheses concerning the effect of frigidity on fertility via the intermediate variables have not been carefully tested, and there is no consensus among authorities concerning this relationship. Even though Seward and his associates (1965) observe that "We cannot escape the fact that frigid women have borne children through the ages [p. 534]" and Masters and Johnson (1970) write that "Legions of women conceive and raise families without ever experiencing orgasm and carry coition to the point of male ejaculation with little physical effort and no personal, reactive involvement [p. 159]," such statements do not rule out the possibility that, on the average, frigid women have lower fertility than they would have had otherwise.

Prevalence   There is little more agreement about the prevalence of frigidity than about its impact on fecundity and fertility. Although frigidity is recognized as the most common female psychosexual disorder in any age group (Braiman 1970:738), precise prevalence figures are nonexistent. Prevalence estimates vary widely, depending a great deal on the individual's definition of frigidity and on when the estimates were made. The following passage from Kroger (1962c) illustrates this point: "Most followers of Freud adhere to the vaginal theory of orgasm and label 75 percent of American women

---

[5]Obesity, however, is not associated with reduced libido per se. Indeed, the opposite may be true. In a recent book anthropologist Anne Beller (1977) cites studies showing that obese women are more responsive to erotic stimulation and have greater sexual appetites than do their thinner counterparts. In one Chicago hospital study, obese women outscored their thin sisters by a factor of almost two to one in terms of degree of excitability.

frigid—a figure perfectly correct according to their definition. A disciple of Kinsey or a proponent of the clitoral theory would contend that less than 25 percent of these same women are frigid [p. 387]." Similarly, Braiman (1970:741) reports that some prevalence estimates run as high as 40–50% of all women. Judging from more recent research, however, these high estimates are no longer applicable to the U.S. population, for as Rosenbaum (1976) notes,

> When Masters and Johnson demonstrated that the observable physiological reactions were identical, whether an orgasm was stimulated clitorally or vaginally, they challenged the longheld hypothesis of the two orgasms, postulated by psychoanalytic theory. The dichotomy between the clitoral and vaginal orgasm is slowly receding into mythology—and we are stating with increasing conviction that there is essentially one kind of female orgasm, with both clitoral and vaginal elements [p. 92].

High rates of frigidity were a by-product of this orgasm dichotomy, and they too are following the latter into mythology.

Whatever the prevalence of frigidity now, there seems to be widespread support for the contention that it was greater in the past, particularly toward the end of the nineteenth century. At that time some of the best-informed physicians in Europe and America estimated that frigidity affected up to three-fourths of all women (Hunt 1974:177). Such estimates, based on clinical samples, were only educated guesses, but nonetheless they probably reflected that era's tendency to stifle sexual expression. From that point to the present, estimates of frigidity prevalence have steadily declined (Hunt 1974:209–213). Kinsey et al. (1953:357) offer some data that corroborate this trend, since, in their sample, the proportion of women in successive cohorts who were completely frigid declined over the first half of the twentieth century.

A recent survey (Hunt 1974) indicates that the prevalence of frigidity is still declining. Like the Kinsey study, its basic measure of frigidity is the absence of orgasm in all or almost all coital experiences, a procedure that tends to overestimate frigidity prevalence. Although the data are not strictly comparable, they indicate that since the Kinsey survey there has been an apparent decrease from about 12 to 7% in the proportion of women who nearly always fail to achieve orgasm in their marital coitus (Hunt 1974:212).

ORGASMIC DEPRIVATION

Frigid women are not the only women who experience chronic orgasmic failure. This may also occur in women who are capable of passion and emotional release in sex (Money 1967:13). Unlike frigid women, in whom orgasm capacity is absent, these women have orgasm capacity but are chronically kept from attaining it by adverse circumstances. This phenomenon can be termed orgasm deprivation (Oliven 1974:411). Thus, orgasmic failure includes two phenomena, frigidity and orgasm deprivation. In one study (Coppen 1965:13), 32% of otherwise normal women were inorgasmic, 6% were classifiable as frigid, and the remaining 28% as orgasm deprived.

Oliven (1974:411) lists many causes of orgasm deprivation, including the following: (a) habitually deficient, perfunctory, or overly rapid performance by the mate; (b) habitually practiced coitus interruptus, particularly in cases in which the woman has no confidence in her mate's timing and thus cannot relax; (c) lack of precoital stimulation for many reasons; (d) the naive belief that women have no orgasm; (e) fear of appearing oversexed; and (f) apprehensive or purposeful self-inhibition of orgasm due to phobias, guilt over an extramarital venture, contraceptive superstition, severe maternal indoctrination against orgasm, or an anxious–compulsive personality type who, throughout the act, remains tensely, futilely expectant as to whether orgasm will occur. Obviously, some of these causes are psychopathological whereas others are not.

In the previous section, the relationship between inorgasmy and subfecundity was discussed with respect to frigid women. There is no reason to believe that the effects of the lack of orgasm per se on fecundity are different for women with orgasm deprivation than for frigid women, making it redundant to discuss those effects here. However, Oliven (1974:410) argues that, if a woman with orgasmic capacity is frequently deprived of orgasm, her reactions consolidate eventually into a pattern of chronic tension or psychic stress, and certain other physical and emotional ill effects appear. Among these may be some that decrease fecundity and fertility.

With respect to fecundity, orgasm deprivation can lead to pelvic congestion syndrome, a distressing psychosomatic disorder that, in turn, may result in coital inability through dyspareunia or in conceptive failure as a result of the production of sperm-hostile mucus (Oliven 1974:412–413). The phenomenon of burdensome pregnancy, which may be accompanied by massive psychosomatic symptoms, some of which increase the risk of pregnancy loss, also seems to be particularly common in these women (Oliven 1974:411). Finally, orgasm-deprived women frequently resort to barbiturates and tranquilizers in an effort to calm down, drugs that themselves can affect fecundity (cf. Chapter 10). In fact, as Oliven (1974) notes: "A fair proportion of complaints of insomnia by women of reproductive age, for which no obvious cause can be found, may be related to orgasm deficit. In some cases hypnotics are taken with increasing regularity; at first, only after each unsuccessful intercourse; later, in anticipation of coitus; and eventually, in a way which constitutes barbiturate habituation [p. 412].

As with frigidity, orgasm deprivation may also affect fertility by leading to marital disruption, low coital frequency, abstinence, extramarital promiscuity, and so forth. Oliven (1974:411) points out that the resentment caused by orgasm deprivation not infrequently leads to arbitrary, unmotivated family limitation and even to attempts to have pregnancies interrupted for no apparent rational reason.

Precise prevalence figures for orgasm deprivation are unavailable. But, judging from estimates of total orgasmic failure (which include that due to frigidity), orgasm deprivation undoubtedly affects sizable fractions of some populations. Kinsey et al. (1953:408), for instance, reported that, of U.S. women during their first year of marriage, 25% never achieved orgasm and 36% experienced it in less than one out of three instances of coitus. In the fifth year of marriage, these percentages were 17 and 30, respectively; in the tenth, 14 and 28%; and by the fifteenth, they were 12 and 28%. The more recent Hunt (1974:211) survey found that, irrespective of age or duration of marriage, only 8% virtually never achieved orgasm and only 15% experienced it less than a fourth of the time. Thus, the prevalence of orgasmic failure, like frigidity, has apparently declined substantially in the last 30 years among U.S. women, and, in all probability, so too has that of orgasm deprivation. A major reason for this decline may be increased knowledge about sexuality and a liberalization of sexual mores. Orgasm deprivation is also readily and easily treatable, the more successful programs, such as that of Masters and Johnson, reporting cure rates of about 80%.

Discussion

Psychic stress affecting either partner or the relationship between them may inhibit conception (Seward et al. 1965:534). Though there are fewer reports and hypotheses about the ability of psychic stress to cause male infertility (Mai 1969:32), this is probably because it is culturally more accepted that women are the "nervous sex" and are more vulnerable to psychogenic infertility (Kleegman and Kaufman 1966:294). In this connection, Heiman (1962) notes: "The woman carries the major burden of the reproductive function. From early childhood this function is a greater source of concern and conflict for her than for the man, and so she will more frequently manifest disturbances of fertility as the consequence of these psychologic conflicts [p. 358]." Thus, with the preponderance of research directed at female infertility, it should not be surprising that the psychic stress–infertility relationship is better established and documented in women than in men (Palti 1969:326). However, many authorities are convinced that male psychogenic factors are no less important than female factors as contributors to a couple's infertility (Seward et al. 1965:534).

Any measurement of the effect of psychic stress on fecundity is a long way off. Though rates of psychic stress are known to be high, especially in urban areas, it is not known, for example, how often this psychic stress causes conceptive maladies rather than some other reproductive or nonre-productive dysfunction. Even if the psychic stress does result in conceptive failure, the severity and duration of the dysfunction varies depending upon, among other factors, the nature of the stress and the susceptibility of the individual. For instance, amenorrhea following a single emotional shock is seldom enduring (G. Russell 1972:583), but the infertility due to childbearing conflicts may persist for a lifetime, as the following passage from Bardwick (1971) indicates:

> I suspect that women with psychosomatic dysfunctions start having menstrual problems early in adolescence and that the problems increase as the sexual aspects of dating grow more important. The symptom severity is probably strongest during their twenties and thirties, when the marital pressure for pregnancy is strongest and most threatening. So long as this type of woman can perceive herself as young enough to bear children she will be increasingly anxious, but consciously she will be running from one obstetrician to another looking for the miracle of pregnancy. Menopause is likely to come as a relief and be relatively symptom-free [p. 78].

The possibility that psychic stress has a demographically significant effect on fecundity via conception cannot be readily dismissed. Psychic stress is a feature of everyday life, especially in industrial societies, and does have the power to cause conceptive failure in mentally healthy as well as in mentally unhealthy men and women (cf. Abse 1966:133; Israel 1967:198). Thus, the population as a whole is at risk. Substantial prevalence rates are supported by the fact that psychic stress is a common finding among couples seeking treatment for infertility (Kleegman and Kaufman 1966:300; Platt *et al.* 1973:972), and disturbances due to psychic stress in such conceptive requisites as ovarian functioning are common occurrences (Kroger 1962e:255). Moreover, infertility due to psychic stress is frequently aggravated and allowed to persist because it is often neglected (especially by individuals who want to avoid childbearing) or is treated by those with little psychiatric competence. Few infertile or frigid women, for instance, seek psychiatric treatment (Rommer 1962:372).

This chapter has dealt primarily with a subfecundity intermediate variable, conceptive failure. The reader is again reminded that psychic stress can affect the probability of conception and, hence, fertility in many other ways. It has already been mentioned that psychosexual disorders such as premature ejaculation and frigidity reduce fertility via intermediate variables such as the frequency of intercourse, marital disruption, and so forth. Psychic stress can also reduce the probability of conception through a variety of bizarre behavioral mechanisms. The infertility literature is replete with case reports of men, for example, who refuse to come home during their wives' fertile periods without consciously being aware of the reasons for this abnormal behavior (Rutherford 1965:104). Such behavior is a clear sign that the husband may not really want a child even though he may be voluntarily seeking a cure for "infertility." Similarly, some "infertile" women have been found who are unconsciously aware of ovulation and abstain from coitus at that time (Kroger 1962d:339).

These bizarre behavioral mechanisms may coexist with a psychosomatic mechanism affecting fertility via subfecundity. A woman reported by Mai *et al.* (1972:202) who unconsciously confined intercourse to the time of her menstrual periods and whose anovular cycles were probably psychomatic provides a good example and is summarized as follows:

> A husband 29 and a wife 26 had been married for five years and had had a daughter ten months after marriage. Following the birth, the woman's periods became irregular. Medical examination of both partners was negative, and the sperm count of the husband was normal. However, despite patent tubes, the wife was found not to be ovulating.
>
> The wife had several non-specific psychic and somatic symptoms including tension and irritability. She also exhibited strong negative feelings with respect to both parents, particularly her father, who treated her as a boy during her childhood.
>
> The wife's attitude during the interview was one of helplessness and dependency. She overdressed, wore exaggerated make-up, frequently cried, and showed hostility toward the examiner. It was concluded that she had an hysterical personality disorder.
>
> The husband confirmed the wife's story, and described her as anxious and worrying. He noted that coitus tended to be confined to the time of the wife's periods. The woman was offered treatment but refused, stating that she and her husband were not really anxious for a child at the moment, having come to the clinic for diagnostic purposes only.
>
> This woman demostrated a marked ambivalence toward motherhood. She not only exhibited anovulation of hypothalamic origin, but confined intercourse to the time of her menstrual periods.

Behavior, especially that of neurotics, may result also in an increase in conceptions and fertility. Some women become pregnant as a way of serving their own neurotic needs, and for a fraction this is a repetitive process (Friederich 1970a:694). Many adolescents, for example, become pregnant for neurotic reasons (Daly 1970:716). Unwed mothers seize pregnancy as a way to deal with loneliness and depression or as a way to feel fulfilled and feminine. Other women, emotionally starved and unable to form close relationships with adults, produce babies in order to love and care for them.

Psychic stress may also increase the probability of conception by increasing the likelihood of contraceptive failure. Personality factors must be assessed in determining the likelihood of failure of various forms of contraception and of contraception in general (Braiman 1970:743; Winn 1970:705).

4

Psychic Stress and Pregnancy Loss

Pregnancy is an example par excellence of a condition in which psychology and physiology are inextricably linked. Thus, many aspects of pregnancy and delivery are vulnerable to interference and disruption from psychic stress (Chertok 1972:8). If a woman worries a great deal or has a severe emotional shock, biochemical disturbances due to such stress can alter or disrupt the delicate maternal–placental–fetal relationship (Babson and Benson 1971:12). Psychic stress may also cause pregnancy loss by inducing neuromuscular disorders, such as those of the uterus and cervical sphincter, which lead to expulsion of the fetus (Israel 1967:597). Indeed, psychic stress is recognized as an important cause of pregnancy loss, especially among habitual aborters (Kroger 1962h:133; Seward et al. 1965:535).

Psychic stress capable of precipitating pregnancy loss may be divided into two categories: acute emotional stress and dispositional emotional stress (Tupper and Weil 1968:757).

Acute Emotional Stress

Acute emotional stress, such as a death in the family or a frightening experience, increases the risk of pregnancy loss. Clinicians frequently report that women who experience this kind of stress are more likely to abort, to have a complicated pregnancy or delivery, or to deliver a stillborn child than are women not subjected to such stress (Richardson 1967:viii). In this connection, Heiman (1965) notes: "It is a certainty that psychologic stimuli can bring about the most massive functional and structural changes if they take place very suddenly and are of great intensity, such as overwhelming fear, fright, or shock [p. 498]."

Dispositional Emotional Stress

Psychic stress resulting from certain dispositional characteristics or psychological makeup can also bring about pregnancy loss. Indeed, psychic stress of this nature is thought by many to be the most frequent cause of pregnancy loss among women who repeatedly fail to successfully terminate their pregnancies, the so-called habitual aborters. As the relationship between psychic stress and pregnancy loss is most strikingly illustrated by the habitual aborter, momentarily the discussion will focus on this group. Evidence for this relationship will be presented, namely, the absence of identifiable abortigenic pathology in many habitual aborters, the similar psychological profiles observed in these women, and the success of psychotherapy in terminating the abortion habit.

HABITUAL ABORTERS

Habitual abortion is defined as the premature spontaneous termination of at least three consecutive pregnancies with or without preceding successful confinements (Tupper and Weil 1968:751). In the major studies of hundreds of habitual aborters (cf. Grimm 1967; Mann 1959; Mann and Grimm 1962), the typical finding is that over 80% of these women are free of detectable abortigenic pathology but that they possess definite psychological patterns, suggesting a relationship to their abortions (Ferreira 1965:109). Kroger (1962h:133), for example, found in habitual aborters the relative absence of organic changes in the genital tract, abnormal fetuses in only about 12% of those examined, but substantial hypersensitivity of the uterus to emotional stimuli.

In addition to the finding that a high proportion of habitual aborters are seemingly free of abortigenic pathology, further evidence supporting the primary role of psychic stress as the cause of habitual abortion stems from the facts that a high proportion of such women have marked psychic conflicts (Javert 1962) and that their psychological profiles are markedly similar (cf. Dunbar 1962:137; Grimm 1967:17; Israel 1967:596–597). Tupper and Weil (1968:757), for instance, found that aborters fall mainly into two personality groups: first, the predominantly immature woman, who cannot accept the challenges of mature femininity and the responsibility of motherhood; and, second, the independent, frustrated woman who has adjusted to a man's world and whose main aspirations are beyond socially imposed limits. In a more specific vein, Israel (1967:597) states that a frequent basis for abnormal emotional reactions that lead to repeated abortion lies in the woman's formative years, particularly in her parental relationships. When psychosexual development is arrested at an immature level, this frequently takes the form of dependency, which can find expression in habitual abortion. This dovetails well with James's (1969:824) contention that women who grow up in households from which their biological father is absent experience relatively high rates of perinatal mortality due to the deleterious psychological consequences of his absence. Israel (1967:597) notes, however, that the emotional factor in habitual abortion may not be so deep but may instead arise from superficial fears such as fear of the delivery itself, misgivings in regard to the role of mother, anxiety concerning the effect of the coming baby upon an already insecure marriage, or the fear itself of being a habitual aborter. He also observes that the psychodynamic factors of parental origin are usually more serious than the superficial fears and require psychiatric aid for their resolution.

The importance of psychic stress as a cause of pregnancy loss is further supported by the success of psychotherapy in curtailing habitual abortion (cf. Ferreira 1965:109; Grimm 1967:17; Kistner 1964:514; Tupper and Weil 1968:758). Mann and Grimm (1962:155) treated 150 gynecologically "normal" habitual aborters with psychotherapy alone, and 80% delivered normal full-term infants. And 24 out of 25 habitual aborters similarly treated by Tupper (1962:147) and his associates produced viable babies, although some were premature. Furthermore, it is well-documented that almost any type of treatment for habitual abortion is successful. Thus, a growing number of authorities (cf. Mann and Grimm 1962:154; Tupper 1962:147) believe that the process of cure in many instances quite possibly has less to do with specific curative agents than with the therapist's personality and the witting and unwitting psychotherapeutic use made of it in relating to habitually aborting women.

OCCASIONAL ABORTERS

This discussion of dispositional causes of pregnancy loss has dwelt on habitual aborters because they have been the focus of the bulk of research on the relationship between psychic stress and pregnancy loss. But this does not imply that the same dispositional factors are not present or cannot lead to pregnancy loss in women who are not habitual aborters. All women experience psychic stress of one form or another during pregnancy,[1] as Grimm (1967) indicates in the following passage:

> Regardless of their theoretical framework, virtually all those who have studied emotional reactions in pregnancy agree on two issues—namely, that all women have both positive and negative attitudes toward their pregnancy and that all women experience an increase in anxiety or tension during this time. In many women existing conflicts appear to be exacerbated, and even those women who are emotionally mature and motivated for pregnancy show some anxiety about the unknown. It is even possible that current practices and attitudes in obstetrics contribute to a rise in psychological tension. There are those, such as Bibring, who regard pregnancy as a period of crisis and as a time at which there is a temporary personality disturbance peculiar to pregnancy [pp. 3–4].

Lorimer (1954) discusses in the following passage some of the conflicts faced by most pregnant women:

> Conflicting with the desire for children are other motives. Paramount among these are the wish to avoid pain and suffering. Childbirth is an unpleasant experience. The woman who becomes pregnant finds herself increasingly handicapped and frustrated. She feels that her labor will be painful, that her child will be deformed or stillborn, and that she may die in childbirth. She knows that after her baby is born she must spend a greater proportion of her time attending to its wants [p. 17].

Thus, psychic stress is virtually an omnipresent feature of the pregnancy experience and, if other requisites are present, can lead to random abortion among "normal" women and habitual abortion in abortion-prone women.

Psychic stress is most likely to be experienced when a pregnancy is unplanned or unwanted. In fact, those characteristics are among the most critical factors related to high risk pregnancies. When the pregnancy is unwanted, sufficient maternal stress may interfere with fetal development (Babson and Benson 1971:12). In Heiman's (1965) words: "The woman who didn't want to become pregnant, didn't plan to, and didn't look forward to it, the woman who reacted with a high degree of hostility toward being pregnant, is the woman more likely to show obstetric pathology [p. 497]."

Mechanisms

The mechanisms by which psychic stress causes pregnancy loss are multifarious (cf. Ferreira 1965). Some mechanisms are designated as occur-

[1]For a review of the kinds of anxieties and concerns that preoccupy the pregnant woman, see Asch (1965:465), Biskind (1962:35), or Baker (1967:34).

ring in specific classes of women, such as the habitual aborters. Most, however, are hypothesized mechanisms believed to occur in times of psychic stress without designation to any specific class of women. Almost all these mechanisms are based on the knowledge that the reproductive organs are responsive to hormonal and neurogenic stimuli and that these stimuli can bring about biochemical or mechanical changes in the uterine–tubal environment.

The following three mechanisms have been proposed for two specific classes of women: women suffering severe emotional trauma and the habitual aborters. In women suffering severe emotional trauma, especially if there is emotional instability present, uterine circulation may be disturbed sufficiently to cause placental detachment and abortion (Dunbar 1962:137). Two mechanisms have been proposed for the habitual aborter. It is believed that psychic stress in such women induces hormonal or neurogenic changes that increase the contractility of the uterus when quiescence is instead required, and so the fetus is expelled. Also, hormonal or neurogenic action on the cervical sphincter may cause the cervical os to become "incompetent," that is, unable to contain the products of conception within the uterus (Israel 1967:597–598).

The other mechanisms of pregnancy loss are divided into those occurring early and late in pregnancy. The earliest events in pregnancy, from conception to nidation, may be the most susceptible to psychic stress; at least, this has been the case in animal experiments (Richardson 1967:viii). Psychic stress has been linked to interference with tubal function, which inhibits migration of the conceptus to the uterus (Kleegman and Kaufman 1966:289), as well as to interference with nidation (Asaoka *et al.* 1971:94; Kleegman and Kaufman 1966:293). Early abortion may also result from faulty nourishment of the fertilized ovum due to psychic stress (Kleegman and Kaufman 1966:289). And, in women with uterine defects, psychic stress is particularly likely to cause early abortion (Thomas 1965:50).

Psychic stress may also cause pregnancy loss later in pregnancy by inducing or aggravating obstetric disorders (cf. Bardwick 1971:79), thus constituting a serious problem for many obstetric patients (Babson and Benson 1971:111). Psychic stress has been linked to nausea and vomiting (Asch 1965:465; Biskind 1962:38; Ferreira 1965:110; Grimm 1967:18; Heiman 1965:485; Taylor 1962:117), uterine dysfunction (Grimm 1967:14; Israel 1967:597), cervical problems (Israel 1967:597; Mann and Grimm 1962:153), toxemia of pregnancy (Ferreira 1965:110; Grimm 1967:18; Kroger 1962f:103), prolonged labor (Ferreira 1965:110; Grimm 1967:13), and prematurity (Ferreira 1965:110; Grimm 1967:10).

With respect to prematurity, a leading cause of stillbirth, extensive etiological studies have shown no obstetrical or other medical organic cause in over 50% of cases. Blau *et al.* (1963) make the following observation regarding these findings:

> It does not necessarily follow, of course, that the cause is psychogenic. However, emotional stress as a factor is suggested by the relatively higher incidence in Negroes, primiparas, young women, deprived groups, unwed mothers, and in those who had a previous miscarriage, stillbirth, or premature, and by the fact that, with increasing maturity of the mother, the incidence lessens [p. 202].

Psychoanalysis also provides evidence of a link between psychic stress and prematurity. For instance, Helen Deutsch describes the case of a woman who had four prematures without any apparent obstetric defect. However, after undergoing analysis, she gave birth to a normal-term baby (Blau *et al.* 1963:202). It is also noteworthy that children of women who experienced psychic stress during pregnancy have significantly higher deformity and neonatal mortality rates (Bardwick 1971:79).

Psychic stress has been causally linked to stillbirth in animals. Newton (1972:17), for example, found that disturbed mice gave birth to 54% more dead pups than did the control mice. Although there may be no conclusive evidence that psychic stress leads to stillbirths in humans, there are some indications that it does. James (1969:824) notes, for instance, that illegitimate infants are at a greater risk of being stillborn and that evidence has been adduced that is consistent with the hypothesis that maternal psychic stress is responsible for some of the additional risk.

Discussion

Psychic stress affects pregnancy loss via the psychosomatic mechanism. The criticisms of the research concerning this mechanism's relation to sub-fecundity were reviewed in Chapter 1 in the section entitled "Psychosomatic Subfecundity: An Overview and Critique," and much of the research cited in this chapter is subject to these criticisms. Some of the evidence presented is, for example, associative rather than causative. Nevertheless, few if any authorities would suggest that the role of psychic stress in pregnancy loss is trivial or nil. The evidence suggesting that psychic stress can cause pregnancy loss is, in fact, fairly compelling. It is derived from diverse forms of investigations, including psychoanalysis, psychiatric observations of aborting women, studies of the effectiveness of psychotherapy, and studies of cases in which intense psychic trauma brought about a premature interruption of pregnancy (Tupper and Weil 1968:756–758). These latter case-studies linking acute psychic stress to almost immediate pregnancy loss constitute the clearest evidence that such stress can definitely cause pregnancy loss.

But, although most experts believe that psychic stress can cause pregnancy loss, they are not in agreement about what proportion of pregnancy loss is due to psychic stress. There are some authorities who are convinced that the proportion is very high. Psychoanalyst Helen Deutsch, for example, believes that psychic stress is virtually the sole cause of spontaneous abortion (cf. James 1969:811). Deutsch bases this claim on the impressions she received from the many abortions she has studied, which, according to her analysis, were unmistakably so much influenced by psychogenic factors that the latter could be held responsible for the process (cf. Tupper and Weil 1968:757). Tupper (1962) and his associates tend to agree with Deutsch's conclusion, stating: "In any case, these intriguing similarities between abortion and a collagen disease, fairly well accepted as emotionally produced, in addition to our definite findings of emotional difficulties in so many aborting women and the excellent response they make to purely psychiatric therapy, constrain us to the belief that most spontaneous abortions are emotionally caused [pp. 150–152]."

Nevertheless, a more moderate appraisal of the role of psychic stress in pregnancy loss is in order, especially in the case of the developing world, where diseases known to cause considerable pregnancy loss, such as malaria and syphilis, abound. The role of genetic abnormalities in the etiology of spontaneous abortion must also not be overlooked. One study of abortuses (Szulman 1965:811) found chromosomal aberrations in 50% of specimens studied. Nevertheless, the exact cause of such defects is unknown, and the fact that they may be of endocrine origin (Israel 1967:584) also keeps the door open for psychic stress as an etiological factor in these abortions. In sum, appropriate data that would enable a determination of the role of psychic stress in pregnancy loss are unavailable. The conclusions of Babson and Benson (1971:111) and of Kroger and Freed (1951:142) are, therefore, most appropriate, since they state that psychic stress is not the only cause of pregnancy loss but is still a serious problem for many obstetric patients.

Most authorities do not believe that enough data presently exist upon which to make accurate estimates and decline to speculate about what proportion of pregnancy loss is due to psychic stress. The World Heath Organization (1970) recently concluded the following: "Whilst emotional factors [stress] have often been incriminated in the causation of spontaneous abortion, this relationship must still be regarded as hypothetical and in need of further study [p. 24]." Thus, it is currently not possible to determine the potential for psychic stress to depress population fecundity through pregnancy loss.[2] However, although conclusive evidence is unavailable, there is strong circumstantial evidence that psychic stress causes or contributes to a

---

[2]Hansluwka (1975:208) is one of the few writers in the population literature to hint at the possibility that psychic-stress-induced pregnancy loss may be of demographic significance.

substantial amount of pregnancy loss. And, if this is true, given the high prevalence of psychic stress in many populations and its cultural and temporal variability, the effect of psychic stress on pregnancy loss would be of considerable demographic importance.

Furthermore, psychic stress apparently has the ability to cause subfecundity via pregnancy loss in population subgroups of particular demographic interest. Psychic stress is more often a cause of pregnancy loss in women with multiple spontaneous abortions. Thus, involuntarily childless and low parity women probably have more abortions due to psychic stress than do their high parity counterparts. Psychic stress also increases subfecundity among teenage women, especially those unwed, by increasing obstetric complications and pregnancy loss in general.[3]

Induced Abortion

Although induced abortion is not a form of subfecundity, it is noteworthy that psychic stress is also a frequent reason for such abortions, both therapeutic and nontherapeutic. In societies that restrict abortion, psychic stress and even the prospect of it are among the few admissible reasons for therapeutic abortion (Winn 1970:709). The following passage (*Family Planning Perspectives* 1971) indicates that, prior to the liberalization of U.S. abortion laws, the vast majority of legal terminations in this country were reportedly performed for mental health reasons:

> [A] report to the APHA [American Public Health Association] meeting, surveying abortion practices in ten states . . . found that almost 96 percent of all hospital abortions were performed for mental health reasons,[4] another 2.2 percent were performed to protect the physical health of the woman and only 1.3 percent were performed because of a history of rape or incest, with potential fetal deformity the indication for less than 1 percent [p. 59].

Psychic stress also frequently precedes induced abortion in societies that do not restrict the procedure. Studies have found that, when women seeking abortion are matched against control groups, the former exhibit more emotional disturbance than the latter (e.g., Jacobsson *et al.* 1976:15). It may be that an unplanned and unwanted pregnancy often is itself a symptom of psychological instability (Potts *et al.* 1977:226). In any case, many women who desire not to continue with an unwanted pregnancy are emotionally

---

[3]For a discussion of the importance of such incremental teenage subfecundity in terms of lifelong fertility, see Masnick and McFalls (1976:226).

[4]The 96% figure must be viewed as an inflated one, since many mentally healthy women undoubtedly obtained abortions that were falsely justified on these grounds.

distressed, and often desperately so (Fleck 1970:48). Thus, an above-average number of pregnancies that were deliberately aborted may have spontaneously aborted anyway.

Interestingly, it is not just the case that psychic stress leads to induced abortion; it has long been thought that the reverse is also true—that induced abortion causes psychic stress. This was thought to be particularly true for illegal abortions, which were usually performed under furtive and squalid conditions by incompetent and disreputable individuals. Knowledge of such an abortion often subjected the woman to social condemnation. It would not be surprising, therefore, if induced abortion did precipitate serious emotional problems under such conditions (Horton and Leslie 1978:203). However, though the psychological complications of induced abortion are difficult to assess, the current consensus is that the risk of psychological damage subsequent to both illegal and legal abortion is slight (cf. Horton and Leslie 1978:205; Potts *et al.* 1977:224–227, 529). Addressing this point, Potts and his associates (1977) note:

> A fact often overlooked is that long-term psychiatric disturbances after illegal abortions are rare, although the guilt and emotional trauma associated with such an abortion must be far greater than when the operation is done openly and legally. In Gebhard's series, only four percent of women admitting to criminal abortions reported adverse emotional consequences. Legal abortion, when done on a large scale and for social reasons, is also free of psychological complications. For example, in Hungary, where legal abortions are more frequent than births, it is almost impossible to find an admission to psychiatric inpatient care precipitated by a termination. Of course, like all operations, abortion may be a relevant incident, among a complex of other factors, in the evolution of a woman's psychiatric condition and, like sterilization or mastectomy, it may be the subject of regret, but it does not seem to carry the emotional penalties imagined of it [pp. 226–227].

And, it should be noted, for some women an induced abortion brings genuine relief and a reduction of psychic stress (Potts *et al.* 1977:227).

5

Psychic Stress and Population Subfecundity: Conclusion and Discussion

There is no doubt that psychic stress causes enough subfecundity to be of demographic significance. The fact that it is responsible for up to 90% of impotence, the single most important form of coital inability, would be basis enough for this judgment without even considering its many other links to coital inability and to conceptive failure and pregnancy loss as well. However, there currently is no way to determine just how important a role psychic stress plays in population subfecundity, because too many facts remain unknown, including the following. First, the proportion of any population undergoing psychic stress cannot be estimated accurately given the present level of development of psychiatric epidemiology (cf. Kramer *et al.* 1972:1; Mechanic 1970:5–7). Second, even if this proportion could be satisfactorily estimated, the proportion of those undergoing psychic stress who would experience psychosomatic reactions is presently indeterminable. For a variety of reasons, some individuals tend to be more susceptible to the operation of psychosomatic mechanisms than are others (Grimm 1967:18; Israel 1967:197). Third, assuming these first two problems were solved, the proportion of those who react psychosomatically with a reproductive dysfunction would still be unknown. The target organ, for instance, could be the stomach instead of the uterus or the fallopian tubes. It is important to recognize that these three proportions—those subject to psychic stress, those experiencing a psychosomatic response, and those undergoing psychosomatic reproductive dysfunction—all vary among populations and their subgroups. Finally, any effort to estimate the importance of the role psychic stress plays in population subfecundity is hampered by the lack of knowledge concerning the impact of psychic stress on individual fecundity. Thus, the relationship between psychic stress and reproductive dysfunction is complex (Grimm 1967:19) and awaits further research to determine its nature. For these and other reasons, no estimates of the amount of population subfecundity due to psychic stress are available (Veevers 1972:268) or can be made at the present time.

Reasons Supporting a Causal Relationship between Psychic Stress and Subfecundity

There are, however, a number of reasons that support the proposition that psychic stress is an important, even one of the most important, causes of population subfecundity. Each of these reasons is reviewed in turn.

UBIQUITY

First, although the prevalence of psychic stress is unknown, there is no doubt that it is widespread. Although estimates of its prevalence differ depending on the criteria used to define these disorders, they are usually shockingly high.[1] For instance, estimates for just one element of psychic stress, neuroses, run as high as 40% of the U.S. adult population (Clinard 1968:447). The high estimates tend to include a greater proportion of the less severe forms of psychic stress, and some authorities (cf. Grimm 1967:43) suggest that these less severe forms may not play much of a role in causing reproductive dysfunction. If so, it would follow that the high prevalence estimates would tend to exaggerate the potential importance of psychic stress as a subfecundity factor. But this suggestion is presently only a hypothesis, and a counterhypothesis could be based on the observation that many of the studies linking psychic stress to fecundity impairment were

[1]A preliminary report of the President's Commission on Mental Health states that at any given time one-fourth of the U.S. population are experiencing psychic stress that produces varying degrees of depression and anxiety (Shearer 1977:12). Other data come from Fries *et al.* (1974:477), who cite a "reliable" epidemiological study in which the estimated cumulative risk of contracting a mild to severe mental illness was reported to be 43% in women 20 to 29 years of age. In their own random sample of 18–35-year-old women in a Swedish county, they report that 44% of the amenorrheic women and 34% of the rest of the female population had nervous symptoms or illness in the last year. For a summary of the prevalence statistics from 16 other studies, see Horton and Leslie (1978:535).

investigations of women who were not suffering from obvious and severe psychic stress syndromes (Bardwick 1971:79). Wherever the truth lies, the fact remains that psychic stress is ubiquitous and thus cannot be easily dismissed as an important subfecundity factor on the basis of insufficient prevalence.

MANY REPRODUCTIVE DYSFUNCTIONS

Second, the fact that psychic stress has been implicated as a significant factor in the etiology of coital inability, conceptive failure, and pregnancy loss also suggests that it may be an important population subfecundity cause. The preceding discussion has reviewed studies linking psychic stress to impotence, male and female dyspareunia, vaginismus, oligospermia, azoo-spermia, deficient sperm motility and form, retrograde ejaculation, sham ejaculation, premature ejaculation, ejaculatory incompetence, ova abnor-malities, tubal and cervical dysfunctions, anovular menstruation, amenorrhea, pseudocyesis, anorexia nervosa, the Chiari–Frommel syn-drome, frigidity, inorgasmy, spontaneous abortion, stillbirth, prematurity, obstetric disorders, and a variety of other reproductive dysfunctions. Moreover, psychic stress is thought to play a part in menarche and menopause (Seward et al. 1965:533), neonatal and infant mortality, lactation and breastfeeding (Bardwick 1971:70,80; Simmel 1945:172), and other phenomena related to fecundity. Thus, one of the reasons psychic stress may be influential is that it can affect fecundity in many different ways. Heiman (1965) recognizes this versatility in the following passage:

> The tug of war between giving life and not allowing, or at least interfering with, life may find its individual expression by one woman abhoring intercourse, a second being frigid, a third having hostile cervical mucus, a fourth experiencing habitual abortion, a fifth hyperemesis, a sixth premature delivery, a seventh toxemia, and an eighth postpartum depression with repressed destructive ten-dencies toward the newborn [p. 495].

Though psychic stress has been linked to subfecundity in many ways, its importance with respect to the psychosexual disorders (impotence, vaginis-mus, dyspareunia, frigidity, inorgasmy, premature ejaculation, ejaculatory incompetence, etc.) should receive special note. Psychic stress is undoubt-edly the number one cause of these disorders, and, specifically, the neuroses are particularly important etiological factors. As West (1968) re-marks: "Impotence, sexual frigidity, guilt feelings, and general [sexual awk-wardness] are the prime features of neurosis [p. 175]."

In addition, psychosexual problems are ubiquitous. According to Wahl

(1967:xi), almost all people experience some problems concerning their sexual lives at one time or another. Masters and Johnson (1976b) also feel that sexual problems are present in an appalling number of marriages. And clinicians note that psychosexual problems are a major cause of subfecundity. Amelar and his associates (1977), for instance, conclude the following about male sexual dysfunction:

> Male sexual dysfunction may now be the primary causative factor or an important contributing factor in almost 10 percent of involuntarily infertile marriages, especially when it is remembered that a number of men have sexual problems as well as oligospermia. Thus, the sexual and psychological problems of infertility are highly important. Even in those cases in which there is a clear-cut organic cause, psychological repercussions are inevitable by the mere revelation of the existence of infertility in the male. Furthermore, the diagnostic tests and treatments themselves may create psychological difficulties [p. 203].

However, a demographic evaluation of the prevalence of psychosexual problems has never been attempted or, at least, has never been reported.

INDIRECT EFFECTS

Third, the effect of psychic stress on fecundity is not restricted to the direct effects just mentioned and fully discussed in Chapters 2–4. Psychic stress can influence subfecundity factors yet to be discussed in this book, for example, personality disorders such as alcoholism (see Chapter 8). It can also influence the onset, duration, and severity of diseases detrimental to fecundity, including brucellosis, influenza, tuberculosis, diabetes, hypertension, and other acute and chronic illnesses (Foa 1962:556; Greenfield and Alexander 1965:205–206; Kroger 1962a:549; Suinn 1970:261).

MULTIPLE EFFECTS

The fourth reason supporting the proposition that psychic stress is an important cause of population subfecundity is the tendency for many of the negative reproductive effects of psychic stress themselves to cause other reproductive dysfunctions in the individual or the partner, thereby increasing the existing subfecundity. Thus, habitual aborters tend to be frigid, a woman with dyspareunia may eventually develop vaginismus, and a premature ejaculator often develops secondary impotence. In couples with psychosexual disorders, it is not unusual for the woman's vaginismus to be the result of her husband's primary impotence, and so forth. In fact, some authorities (cf. Abse 1966:133) conclude that psychic stress generally alters the fecundity of both partners in subfecund unions.

AGE AND DURATION ASPECTS

The fifth reason supporting the proposition that psychic stress is an important cause of population subfecundity is the fact that it is prevalent at all the reproductive ages.[2] In addition, the psychic stress can persist for a substantial portion of an individual's reproductive life. Neuroses can last for years and can even be lifelong. The psychophysiologic disorders may also be chronic. Everyday stress may also be a persistent feature. However, many persons in stressful situations are able successfully to adapt. And some stressful conditions are themselves of a transitory nature, such as stress experienced by recent migrants. In the Milojkovic *et al.* (1966) study, for example, rural to urban migrants were able to adapt after approximately 3 years (see Chapter 3).

TREATMENT SITUATION

Another reason pointing to psychic stress as a major subfecundity factor is that many of its dysfunctional reproductive effects are either not treated or are treated ineffectively, often with counterproductive results, thus perpetuating the subfecundity. It has already been noted that those suffering from various psychic stress-induced dysfunctions, such as psychosexual disorders and anorexia nervosa, deny the presence of the condition, wait many years before seeking treatment, or never seek treatment at all. The tendency to seek treatment is undoubtedly inversely proportional to parity, since childless and low parity women comprise the bulk of those seeking remedial therapy. It is probably a fair assumption that many high parity individuals who become subfecund or infecund from psychic stress (or from other causes) do not want any more children and do not seek treatment.

But even those who do seek treatment for psychogenic subfecundity often fail to receive the proper therapy, for several reasons. First, individuals suffering from many of these psychic-stress-induced forms of reproductive dysfunction, particularly the psychosexual disorders, actually conceal the problem from the physician, hoping the physician will be able to diagnose the problem independently. Lidberg (1972), for instance, notes: "The symptoms presented to the practitioner are often diffuse and unspecific, e.g., fatigue and weakness. Patients often request a 'general checkup' or ask for vitamins or a tonic. Despite enduring or increasing distress, the first contact with a doctor is often drastically broken off after one single consultation [p. 136]."

Second, individuals may seek help from careless or incompetent professionals, including lay analysts, clergymen, and so forth. Even physicians tend

[2]For rough age distributions for the components of psychic stress, see USNIMH (1967:20–21).

to be ignorant in the area of human sexual behavior (Castelnuovo-Tedesco 1967:238; Chez 1967:2; Wahl 1967:x), and many do not have enough psychiatric training to recognize the role of psychic stress in their patients' reproductive disorders or to administer effective psychotherapy (cf. Taylor 1962:120). Again, in the words of Lidberg (1972): "When patients openly discuss their symptoms from the beginning, they often receive only brief, clumsy, superficial therapy, even from doctors trained in psychiatry. This reflection of medical uncertainty and ignorance often leads to an unfortunate termination of consultations [p. 136]." Thus, even medical consultations often fail to help and may, in many instances, aggravate a problem. Such iatrogenic factors are, for example, a fairly common cause of secondary impotence. Moreover, it is only rarely that a subfecund couple is referred for a psychiatric opinion (Mai 1969:31). This is partially because it has been virtually impossible in recent years to obtain psychiatric consultation except for overt problems (Taylor 1962:120). Finally, individuals suffering from various forms of psychic stress are frequently treated with drugs (Suinn 1970:226), many of which are themselves prejudicial to fecundity (Dubin and Amelar 1971:471).

EXPERT ESTIMATES

The seventh reason supporting the proposition that psychic stress is an important cause of population subfecundity is that psychic stress is involved in the reproductive dysfunction of a substantial fraction of those who seek treatment for subfecundity. It is almost impossible to define that fraction of reproductive dysfunction that is due to psychic stress (Lubke 1972:482), and very few authors have been willing to commit themselves to an estimate (Mandy and Mandy 1962:343). But those clinicians that do estimate the proportion of subfecundity caused or contributed to by psychic stress typically give figures that fall in the 18–30% range (cf. Babson and Benson 1971:111; Bos and Cleghorn, cited in Mandy and Mandy 1962:343; Dimic *et al.* 1972:475; Kleegman and Kaufman 1966:293; Stone 1954:740). There are, however, higher (cf. Ford *et al.*, cited in Mandy and Mandy 1962:343) and lower (cf. Karahasanoglu *et al.* 1972:241; Mai 1971:513) estimates in the literature. Karahasanoglu and his associates, proponents of lower estimates, argue that recent advances have been made in discovering the organic causes of subfecundity and that this evidence indicates that no organic cause can be found in only 5–10% of all subfecundity cases. Nevertheless, a higher estimate in the 18–30% range remains modal.

Heiman (1962:355–358) suggests that these 18–30% estimates may even underrate the role of psychic stress in subfecundity. In an effort to assess the status of subfecundity research, he analyzed 16 pertinent papers that were in his view a fair cross-section of the psychic stress–subfecundity literature. These papers were written by gynecologists, by gynecologists and psychiatrists jointly, by psychoanalysts, by psychologists, by physiologists, or by general practitioners. Collectively, the papers dealt with 652 infertile couples, both members of which were given adequate study insofar as the physiologic aspects of subfecundity were concerned. Two findings support the proposition that psychic stress may be underrated as a subfecundity factor.

First, not a single study reported a psychiatric evaluation of the husband. It is as if it were tacitly assumed that male fecundity belongs solely to the realm of organic physiology and is unaltered by psychological factors. Second, the probability that the wife's psychological evaluation would find evidence of emotional disturbance varied directly with the quality of that evaluation. The gynecologist, whom many women consult for fertility problems, found psychic conflicts in only 1% of his conferees, a shockingly low figure. However, of those women seen by a psychiatrist, 67% were said to have "emotional dynamics characteristic of functional infertility."

Although this latter figure is somewhat high, the overall impression, and Heiman's conclusion, is that if both husband and wife receive competent psychological evaluation the proportion of subfecundity that has a psychic basis would be found to be substantial, perhaps even higher than the usual 18–30% estimates.

SUCCESS OF PSYCHOTHERAPY

The importance of psychic stress is also indicated by the apparent success of direct and indirect psychotherapy in alleviating the subfecundity of clinic patients. Note, for example, the extraordinary success rates Masters and Johnson (1970:364–369) have achieved with respect to coital inability and psychosexual disorders in general. And Kroger (1962d:340) reports that about 35% of women experiencing conceptive failure get pregnant soon after treatment of any form is begun. Often, the enthusiasm with which the woman is investigated is itself the therapeutic agent. Finally, as discussed earlier, psychotherapy alone has achieved success rates of 80% in helping habitual aborters give birth to full-term babies.

SUMMARY

This discussion has pointed to eight reasons that tend to support the proposition that psychic stress is an important cause of population subfecundity, namely: (a) the ubiquity of psychic stress; (b) the evidence linking psychic stress to many forms of reproductive disorder in both sexes; (c) the ability of psychic stress to cause or aggravate other factors that themselves adversely affect fecundity; (d) the tendency for the negative reproductive effects of psychic stress to themselves cause other reproductive dysfunctions; (e) the fact that psychic stress and its effects on fecundity can persist for a sizable fraction of the reproductive period; (f) the fact that many psychically-induced reproductive dysfunctions are either ignored or are treated ineffectively, thus perpetuating themselves; (g) the opinion of specialists that psychic stress causes or contributes to reproductive dysfunction in from 18 to 30% of those who seek treatment for subfecundity; and (h) the success of psychotherapy in alleviating subfecundity in these patients. Any judgment as to the impact of psychic stress on population fecundity must take these factors into consideration, but they are not sufficient in themselves to permit an estimate.

Any appraisal of the potential effect of psychic stress on population fecundity is bound to be uncertain and only as good as the assumptions upon which it must be made. It should be clear to the reader that no one really knows how important psychic stress is—not authorities on the relationship between psychic stress and individual fecundity, not social scientists, not demographers. There is, however, strong evidence that the impact of psychic stress on population fecundity is demographically significant.

Psychic-Stress-Induced Subfecundity as a Population Variable

There is every reason to believe that the subfecundity caused by psychic stress varies in importance from population to population and over time, thus giving rise to fecundity differentials and possibly to fertility differentials. There is, for instance, much speculation in the literature that the effects of psychic stress on fecundity are more substantial in advanced as opposed to primitive populations (cf. Kroger 1962g:115). Toxemia of pregnancy may serve as a good example of a psychic-stress-related cause of subfecundity that varies widely in prevalence between advanced and primitive societies.

Toxemia is a symptom-complex unique to pregnant women and includes hypertension, generalized edema, and proteinuria. It is generally diagnosed after the twenty-fourth week of pregnancy or during the puerperium. Toxemia of pregnancy becomes eclampsia when convulsions or coma complicate the disorder (Babson and Benson 1971:63). Toxemia and eclampsia lower fecundity by causing pregnancy loss. The perinatal mortality rate is two to three times the normal in toxemia and amounts to 20% of births in eclampsia (Babson and Benson 1971:64). Though the cause of these disorders remains unknown and, as such, constitutes one of the most important unsolved problems in the field of human reproduction, many workers believe that psychic stress is the principal or at least a major contributing cause (cf. Soichet 1959:1072). Of interest here is the fact that the prevalence of these disorders varies widely between advanced and primitive societies, being much more common in the former than in the latter. In the United States, for example, between 3 and 20% of pregnant women develop toxemia, the percentage varying inversely with access to quality medical care. On the other hand, these conditions are rare in less developed populations, such as African blacks, Eskimos, and tribes in the South Pacific. Thus, there seems to be a "nontoxemic world" scattered about the globe, leading some workers to conclude that toxemia is a disorder of Western civilization, probably due to stress and to other characteristics of industrialism (Soichet 1959:1065).

There is also speculation that the effects of psychic stress on fecundity are increasing over time, especially in advanced societies, due to the increasing complexity and stressfulness of the social and cultural organization (cf. Braiman 1970:739). The prevalence of psychosexual disorders may be particularly responsive to social change. Ginsberg et al. (1972), for instance, believe that impotence is currently on the rise. In their words: "We report on one aspect of our changing culture: the effect of increased sexual freedom of women on their male partners. Clinical observations are cited which suggest that this culture shift is resulting in an increase in complaints of impotence among younger men [p. 218]." Although this view is held by still other authorities (cf. Hunt 1974:186), some researchers (e.g., Lief, cited in Knight 1978:18) do not concur. However, there is little disagreement about the changing prevalence of female inorgasmy. The following passage (Hunt 1974) reflects consensus opinion on this matter:

> Frequent female orgasm failure has diminished over a period of several generations, even as all those broad social changes were taking place that elevated women from their socially inferior status, made contemporary marriage a partnership and intimate friendship of equals, and liberated men and women sexually and gave them a greater capacity for guilt-free pleasure. . . . The fact is that orgasm regularity has increased almost in direct ratio to the progress of the twin liberations—the sexual and the female—over a period of three generations [p. 209].

In sum, the amount of subfecundity produced by psychic stress probably varies from population to population and, within a population, over time.

Other Intermediate Variables

The reader is also reminded that psychic stress can influence fertility through other intermediate variables besides fecundity. Coital frequency and mate exposure are of particular importance as variables. When psychic stress affects coital frequency, it is usually through a decrease in sexual activity, though there certainly are neurotic forms of hypersexuality (Pumper-Mindlin 1967:167). The relationship between psychic stress and coital frequency has already been discussed in Chapter 2.

Psychic stress can reduce mate exposure by decreasing the chances of entering and/or remaining in a union. For instance, impotence is a cause of divorce (Perry and Perry 1976:31) and has always been regarded as invalidating a marriage if the wife chooses to petition for annulment (Johnson 1968:3). Moreover, it is among the highly fecund younger age groups that psychic stress, particularly psychosexual disorders, is the greatest threat to marital stability (Cooper 1972:552). Slater *et al.* (1971:S64,S67) provide figures on the number of years in the 25-year period between ages 20 and 44 that normal persons and neurotics, in whom psychosexual disorders are commonplace, spend in the marital state. For males in the general population, the number was 17.8 years; for obsessional neurotics, 13.0; and for other neurotics, 15.7. For females in the general population, the number was 20.1; for obsessional neurotics, 18.7; and for other neurotics, 18.4 (cf. Table 11.3). Finally, there is evidence that psychic stress is a particularly important cause of repetitive marital disruption, since most cases of serial divorce occur among basically maladjusted persons (Horton and Leslie 1978:223).

Some workers argue that psychic stress may not only cause involuntary childlessness through subfecundity but may also be a cause of voluntary childlessness. Pohlman (1970), for instance, states:

> We hypothesize that, when the culture has severe pressures against childlessness, a higher proportion of intentionally childless spouses are either somewhat maladjusted or strongly individualistic, or both, although not all should be so classified. When pressures against childlessness are relaxed, a higher proportion of spouses choosing it are simply average people. . . . If there is a correlation between childlessness and maladjustment, it is not because childlessness produces maladjustment, but because the maladjusted, such as women rejecting the feminine role, more often than others opt for childlessness [p. 9].

Thus, psychic stress has a variety of ways of affecting fertility other than through subfecundity.

It is worth reemphasizing that psychic stress may be the result as well as the cause of intermediate variables such as marital disruption, coital frequency, and subfecundity. In the previous chapter, for instance, the possibility that induced abortion may cause psychic stress was discussed. Horton and Leslie (1978) describe how another intermediate variable, marital disruption, can also lead to psychic stress:

> Divorce is also known to create temporary deviancy in some otherwise well-adjusted persons. Even though it may be anticipated for months or years, the experience of divorce frequently is traumatic. Habit patterns and personal rela-

tionships of long duration are suddenly uprooted. The person must finally face up to having failed in marriage and having been rejected by the partner. Extreme bitterness and despair often follow. To assuage the hurt and to cope with the frustrations of suddenly being unmarried again, the individual may enter a more or less promiscuous series of sex relationships. Gradually, as reorientation occurs, these symptoms of deviancy are replaced by a more conventional pattern. Some persons, of course, never completely recover from divorce, and divorce may be expected to remain at least temporarily disorganizing in the foreseeable future [p. 223].

Often the relationship between psychic stress and an intermediate variable may be circular. For example, psychic stress due to interpersonal conflicts within a marriage can lead to sexual difficulties, such as impotence. The sexual difficulties may then lead to additional marital problems and stress, which in turn may result in marital disruption and further stress (cf. Knight 1978:8). Thus, a simple cause-and-effect relationship is, in many cases, difficult to establish.

Adoption and Subfecundity

Before moving on to the next chapter, a few comments on the relationship between adoption and subfecundity may be of interest. The long-standing belief that adoption or even the decision to adopt will often alleviate a couple's subfecundity is cited often in the medical literature (cf. Ferreira 1965:109; Pohlman 1970:10; Siegler 1944:42; Taylor et al. 1958:115) and has even found its way into the population literature (cf. Flapan 1976:45; Kiser 1964:4929; Nag 1962:128). This quasi-magical effect of adoption on subfecundity has usually been explained in terms of hypothetical changes, such as improved ovulation, reduction of tubal spasm, reduced frigidity, increased sexual activity, or, more generally, the resolution of conflicts that had been inhibiting conception (Humphrey 1969:354; Kroger 1962b:632; Mai 1971:509). Although many authors argue in favor of this relationship (e.g., Benedek et al. 1953; Blum 1959; Bos and Cleghorn 1956; Orr 1941; and Schellen and Sassen 1967), many others deny its validity (e.g., Banks 1962; Banks et al. 1961; Hanson and Rock 1950; Raymont et al. 1969; Rock et al. 1965; Tyler et al. 1960). In general, however, the more rigorous studies have yielded negative results (Humphrey 1972:491), and most authorities now consider the supporting evidence to be simply anecdotal (cf. Amelar et al. 1977:75; Noyes and Chapnick 1964:555).

It should be noted, however, that, although the validity of this relationship has been investigated with regularity over the last 30 years, apparently no one has been able to devise and execute a study that cannot be faulted methodologically. Thus, at least one author (Mai 1971:514) contends that the relationship between adoption and conception remains an open question.

6

Psychoses

Psychoses are conditions characterized by profound disturbance and disability; they often entail loss of contact with reality and sensory distortions and may exist without the patient's being aware of the nature and severity of the disturbance (Suinn 1970:43). In terms of personal suffering, health care demands, and overall social and economic costs, psychoses may represent the number one public health problem in the United States and elsewhere (Bellack 1969:3). Moreover, psychoses have been causally linked to the atypically low fertility observed in psychotic individuals. This chapter explores the relationship between psychoses and subfecundity in order to gain at least a rudimentary understanding of its demographic significance.

As noted in Chapter 1, this discussion focuses only on psychopathology of psychogenic origin. Thus, psychoses associated with organic brain disease or injury are not considered here. Among the psychoses of psychogenic origin, only two groups, schizophrenia and manic-depressive psychoses, are both capable of affecting fecundity and common enough to be of potential demographic importance.[1] This discussion will focus on these two groups of psychoses.

---

[1]Paranoid disorders, along with schizophrenia and affective disorders (which include manic-depressive psychoses), represent the three major groupings of psychogenic psychoses. Paranoid disorders are ignored here because they are not very common. Paranoia, for example, is extremely rare, there being only 3 authentic cases in one investigation of 5,000 successive hospital admis-

Schizophrenia is the most common group of psychoses (Kendler 1963:506). It includes disorders characteristically manifested by disturbances in thinking, mood, and behavior. Disturbances in thinking are distinguished by concept-formation alterations that can lead to misinterpretation of reality, delusions, and hallucinations. Corollary mood variations may include ambivalent, constricted, and inappropriate emotional responsiveness and lack of empathy with other individuals. Withdrawn, regressive, and bizarre behavior may exist (APA 1968:33).

Manic-depressive psychoses, the principal affective disorders, are the second most prevalent group of psychoses (Kendler 1963:510). They are characterized by either extreme depression or elation or both, in circular fashion. They rule over the individual's mental life and cause loss of contact with the environment. These disorders are marked by severe mood swings and a tendency to remit and recur. Manic-depressive psychoses, which are dominated by a mood disorder, are to be differentiated from schizophrenia, in which the mental state is due chiefly to a thought disorder (APA 1968:33).

Psychoses and Subfecundity

A century ago, medical experts were convinced that psychoses had an adverse effect on fecundity. This notion was propounded as part of the then popular "degeneration theory" by, among others, Morel and Maudsley. Stevens (1969) summarizes Morel's position as follows:

> Morel considered that degeneration was the moral depravities of the parents being transmitted to the offspring; the first generation would thus contain a high proportion of neurotics . . ., the second generation would involve more insane [psychotics] and mental defectives until finally defects would be so severe as to produce sterility [p. 2].

Similarly, Maudsley (cited in Lewis, 1958) states:

> Such is the benevolent purpose of Nature that no efforts whatsoever can perpetuate a morbid human type; for although the offspring of degenerate parents is a further degeneration, the evil soon corrects itself; and long before man has descended to the animal level, there comes an incapability of producing offspring, and the morbid type dies out. Insanity . . . is but a step in the descent towards sterile idiocy. . . . It is almost impossible to avoid expressing a grateful

---

sions. Paranoid states are relatively more common, but even these disorders are not seen frequently. Some texts, in fact, no longer include discussions on paranoid disorders (Suinn 1970:371). Many other psychoses typically occur too late in life to materially affect fecundity. For example, involutional melancholia is a disorder that occurs during the climacteric.

admiration of the wise, sure and merciful provision of Nature by which the degenerate mind is so quickly blotted out [p. 92].

Thus, psychoses were viewed, due to their associated subfecundity, as the terminal stages of a degeneration process. Though the degeneration theory was eventually discredited, its postulate that psychoses are accompanied by an abnormal amount of subfecundity apparently remains valid.

Curiously, however, the relationship between psychoses and fecundity has not been developed in the medical literature. Eugenicists, who have a keen interest in the relatively low fertility of psychotics, have exhibited little interest in their fecundity, particularly in the last several decades. Perhaps this is because they are distracted by the obvious explanatory importance of such other Davis–Blake (1956:212) intermediate variables as involuntary abstinence (hospitalization) and low marital rates. Likewise, subfecundity specialists, many of whom stress the importance of less severe forms of psychopathology as causes of subfecundity, seldom discuss the possibility that psychoses may have similar effects. This may be symptomatic of an underlying conviction that any subfecundity among psychotics is a blessing in disguise and ought to be the subject of benign neglect. Indeed, subfecundity specialists not infrequently raise the question of whether or not it is prudent to relieve the subfecundity of individuals subject to various forms of psychopathology, especially psychoses (cf. Kroger 1962i:361; Mandy and Mandy 1962:346). Whatever the reasons, no systematic studies or reviews were found in the literature dealing with the relationships between psychoses and either coital inability, conceptive failure, or pregnancy loss. The following discussion collates pieces of information on these subjects gleaned from sources dealing with these relationships obliquely.

COITAL INABILITY

Coital inability is relatively frequent among male psychotics. In 1841, Smyth (cited in Johnson 1968:72) noted that psychotics were frequently impotent and concluded that all psychotics were at some time impotent. Similarly, Bleuler (1950:168) observed more recently that schizophrenics are often impotent, and Mayer-Gross et al. (1969:162) and Cooper (1972:550) note impotence in schizophrenics and psychotic depressives as well. In fact, Hastings (1960:431) comments that impotence is often the first symptom to appear in individuals becoming depressed and is often the last to depart once the depression has subsided. He believes such impotence is due to the overwhelming loss of interest "that descends like a black cloud on every aspect of life [p. 431]." Oliven (1974) expresses a similar view in the following passage:

Loss of libido, followed shortly by impotence, may be among the earliest symptoms of a major depression. These men, especially at the height of the illness, have no interest in sex, as they have lost interest in virtually everything else. . . . The patient, or his wife, says that he became depressed because he could not perform intercourse any longer, that he worried himself into wanting to die because he thought he was sexually neglecting and hurting his wife, breaking his marriage vows, going against his religion, breaking the law, driving her into someone else's arms or similar delusional self-accusations. However, the sequence of events here is thoroughly misrecognized by patient and wife alike. *One finds almost invariably, that onset of the depression preceded the sexual difficulty* [pp. 386–387; emphasis added].

It is the contention of Amelar and his associates (1977) that the sexologic, urologic, and gynecologic literature "strikingly underplays the role of depression [p. 205]" as a cause of impotence. In their view, depression rarely exists without some form of impotence.

In addition, homosexuality is reported to be a common preoccupation of schizophrenics during some stages of the illness (cf. Lidz 1973:210; Sullivan 1962:207). Socarides (1968), for instance, notes: "A large number of paranoic schizophrenics, paranoiacs, psuedo-neurotic schizophrenics or latent schizophrenics have a concomitant homosexual conflict and many manifest homosexual behavior [p. 92]." As will be discussed in Chapter 7, on sexual deviance, homosexuality is associated with coital inability and various other forms of subfecundity.

Schizophrenia and manic-depressive psychoses may also lead to coital inability in women because, according to Siegler (1944:27), they may cause vaginismus and dyspareunia. In his study, Coppen (1965:163) classified 15% of schizophrenics and 14% of women with affective disorders as suffering from dyspareunia or a very distinct aversion to intercourse, as compared to an unknown figure, but one less than 6%, for a group of normal women.[2]

Attempts were made to obtain more specific information about the relationship between these psychoses and coital inability, but these efforts were unproductive. As Johnson (1968) observes, "The description and assessment of disorder of sexual function in the major psychiatric syndromes has been grossly neglected [p. 74]." Of particular interest would be data on the proportion of individuals with various psychoses who experience coital inability and on the average duration that the inability persists.

---

[2]This figure was arrived at by deduction. Data on the normal women were not as detailed as those on the psychotic women. No figure was given for the percentage of normal women with dyspareunia or extreme aversion to intercourse, though these women were, by definition, included in a larger category into which were placed women whose sexual relations were of the lowest quality. The value for this category was 6%.

CONCEPTIVE FAILURE

Psychoses can also lessen the chances of conception and may even prevent conception entirely (Karahasanoglu et al. 1972:246–247; Ossofsky 1972:747; Stone 1954:740). Shader (1970:65–68), Arieti (1967:233), and Brill (1969:123), in similar discussions of the relationship between schizophrenia and male infertility, cite several early studies[3] of biopsy material that found an abnormal amount of infertility-causing pathology in the reproductive organs of schizophrenic males. Mott (1919), for example, reported atrophy of the testicles of hospitalized schizophrenics, as well as a complete arrest of spermatogenesis. Shader and his associates also found infertility among schizophrenic men. He (1970) states:

> The presence of oligospermia in several schizophrenic males and the subsequent finding that urinary FSH levels were low to absent in schizophrenic males who had shown early or preadolescent schizophrenic symptomatology suggest that there may be nondrug factors involved which would connect schizophrenia to abnormalities in fertility or reproductive mechanisms [p. 65].

In addition, Oliven (1965:192) reports that psychotic syndromes have a downgrading effect on the structure and function of sperm. Some authors (Morse, cited in Arieti 1967:233; Tourney et al. 1953) caution that this infertility may not be due to the psychoses per se but to common sequelae, such as malnutrition. However, Shader (1970:66–67) reports that the subjects he and his co-workers studied were adequately nourished, as were those of some of the other workers who found infertility among male psychotics.

Data on the prevalence of infertility among male schizophrenics are unavailable.

Psychoses have a more pervasive influence on the conceptive ability of women than on that of men. They have been linked to puberty delays (Katz 1972:360), to a variety of menstrual and ovarian dysfunctions throughout the reproductive period (Brill 1969:122; Israel 1967:325; Kroger 1962e:256; Siegler 1944:27), and to premature termination of the reproductive period (Arieti 1967:233). Puberty delays, however, are probably germane only to those women who experience severe psychic disturbance prior to puberty. A study by Coppen (1965:157) of women suffering from schizophrenia and affective disorders whose onset of illness occurred mostly in adult life supports this contention. He found that their average age of menarche, 13.8

---

[3]Included are the studies of Mott (1919) and of Hemphill and Reiss (1948). At least one study (Blair 1952), however, failed to confirm this finding.

years for both groups, was higher than that of a pertinent general population (13.4) but that this difference was small and statistically insignificant.

Amenorrhea, a frequent occurrence in women with schizophrenia and manic-depressive psychoses (Mayer-Gross *et al.* 1969:371), is probably the most important cause of conceptive failure in psychotics. Bleuler (1950:168) and Gregory (cf. Bellak and Loeb 1969:122) report that amenorrhea following an acute episode of the disease is a very common event among schizophrenics. And under chronic conditions menstruation may cease for years (Bleuler 1950:168). Although schizophrenics of the simple, hebephrenic, and paranoid types may avoid amenorrhea in the early stage of the illness, menstruation may cease as the illness progresses (Mayer-Gross *et al.* 1969:371).

Similarly, amenorrhea is a common feature of manic-depressive psychoses. (Ossofsky 1972:747). Although there is typically no interruption of menses during manic phases (Allen, cited in Bellak 1952:93), menstruation not infrequently ceases during depressive phases (Mandy and Mandy 1962:345; Mayer-Gross *et al.* 1969:211). In fact, Ossofsky (1972:747) concludes that gross menstrual irregularities, including amenorrhea, in otherwise healthy women are almost specifically distinctive of depression. In addition, anorexia nervosa, a syndrome that almost always includes amenorrhea, is often seen in manic-depressive psychoses and may be an indication of the impending outbreak of this illness (Kroger and Freed 1951:359).

The enormous impact that psychoses may have on an individual's fecundity can be seen in the case history of a manic-depressive woman described by Ossofsky (1972:744–746), which is condensed and paraphrased as follows:

> This woman's initials are H.C. For H.C., menarche occurred at age 12 and appeared normal, but after a year menses became irregular, occurring approximately six or eight times annually. Shortly after her marriage at 19 the menstrual periods ceased, but she was not pregnant. At age 24, following five years of amenorrhea and infertility of unknown cause, a physical examination revealed no abnormalities. At age 28, nine months after the onset of psychotherapy, H.C. experienced her first menstrual cycle in nine years. Continued treatment led to menstrual periods occurring regularly every 28 days and a normal intrauterine pregnancy.

Some workers (Fries *et al.* 1974:477; Mayer-Gross *et al.* 1969:371) reckon that amenorrhea is far more common in schizophrenia than in the affective psychoses. Whether this is true or not, the reader may note from the following estimates that amenorrhea is a common feature of both forms of psychoses. For instance, Israel (1967:203) states that amenorrhea is experienced by about one-third of those suffering from either schizophrenia or the depressive phase of manic-depressive psychoses. Siegler's (1944:41) estimate of this proportion is similar, 30–40% of both groups. Coppen (1965:160) reports percentages of 39 for schizophrenia and 29 for the affective psychoses, and Cahane and Cahane found a 50% incidence of amenorrhea in their manic-depressive patients (Bellak 1952:69). Finally, Shader *et al.* (1970) relate the following:

> Hanse reported in 1923 that amenorrhea was present in the majority of his female patients (62.5 percent in catatonia, 50.0 percent for paranoia and hebephrenia, 60 percent for melancholia, and 45 percent for mania). These figures are clearly in the extreme range and may reflect the additional contribution of factors such as chronicity and diet. In a careful, more recent predrug era study of menstrual irregularities in women of childbearing age, who had been diagnosed as schizophrenic (N = 144), depressed (N = 81), and elated (N = 26), Ripley and Papanicolaou found amenorrhea to be present in 18, 14, and 12 percent respectively. Long cycles (35–59 days) were reported for 31, 33, and 19 percent, respectively. Thus, disregarding diagnostic category, 68 (31 percent) patients had delayed or prolonged cycles, and 34 (15 percent) reported amenorrhea (a delay beyond 60 days) [p. 10].

Some authors contend that frigidity and inorgasmy increase conceptive failure (cf. Chapter 3). If this is true, psychotic women may experience elevated levels of conceptive failure due to their relatively high rates of frigidity and inorgasmy. Coppen (1965:163) found 51% of the schizophrenics in his study to be inorgasmic and 28% to be frigid. Similar figures for women with affective disorders were 39% inorgasmic and 29% frigid. By comparison, only 32% of the normal women he cites were inorgasmic, and only 6% were classified as frigid. Zilboorg reports that in his experience about 60% of schizophrenic and manic-depressive women have a history of frigidity (Bellak, 1952:209), a figure substantially higher than Coppen's.

PREGNANCY LOSS

Some women who are not actively psychotic at the time of conception develop psychotic reactions during pregnancy and the puerperium. The emotional stress of pregnancy can bring out these psychoses, just as any marginally compensated psychopathology can become manifest under sufficient stress. Statistically, however, overt gestational psychoses are rare; only about 1 occurs in every 300–750 pregnancies (cf. Asch 1965:466–467). Of more demographic interest, therefore, are already psychotic women who become pregnant, the subject of this section.

It is unclear whether or not psychotics have higher-than-normal rates of pregnancy loss. Evidence concerning this possibility is both scarce and conflicting. Rasidakis (1972:2) observes that schizophrenics spontaneously abort more frequently than the general population, and Rieder and his associates (1975:200) report a significantly greater number of fetal deaths among offspring of schizophrenic mothers as compared to those of nonpsychotic controls. In addition, Bliss (1976:50), citing the work of others, notes that schizophrenics have a high incidence of perinatal mortality. However, Niswander and Gordon (1972:261–265) failed to corroborate these findings. They found no increased risk of stillbirth or perinatal death among the offspring of psychotic women who were studied prospectively as part of the Collaborative Perinatal Project.

Studies of the relationship between psychoses and pregnancy complications[4] can not be used to infer the probable relation between psychoses and pregnancy loss, since they too offer conflicting results. On the one hand, studies by Sameroff and Zax (1973), Mednick and Schulsinger (1968), Paffenbarger and McCabe (1966), Paffenbarger et al. (1961), and Woerner et al. (1973) have reported a greater number of pregnancy complications among psychotic (usually schizophrenic) mothers than among controls. However, studies by Maura (1971), McNeil and Kaij (1973, 1974), Cohler et al. (1975), and subsequent research by Mednick et al. (1971, 1973) have shown little relationship between maternal mental illness and pregnancy complications.

The relationship between maternal psychoses and the birth weight of offspring is also unclear. Mednick et al. (1971, 1973), Niswander and Gordon (1972), Kallman (1938), Sobel (1961), and Paffenbarger and McCabe (1966) have all reported that the birth weight of children born to psychotics, usually schizophrenics, is lower than that of controls. Mednick et al. (1973:111), for example, found the average birth weight for the psychotics' offspring to be 3053 grams, 210 grams below that of the infants of the normal women. However, other studies (cf. Lane and Albee 1970, McNeil and Kaij 1973) report no such group differences.

In sum, judging from the literature, there is no strong evidence that psychotics have substantially higher rates of pregnancy loss than do nonpsychotic women or that, in fact, their rates are higher at all. If psychoses were simply more severe forms of psychic stress, this apparent lack of a relationship between psychoses and pregnancy loss would cast doubt on the validity of the hypothesis, held by many investigators, that psychic stress

---

[4]These studies were undertaken primarily to determine which prenatal events are associated with the development of psychoses in the offspring. As such, many focus on mother–child pairs and retrospectively investigate the circumstances surrounding the offspring's gestation and birth. Thus, pregnancies resulting in fetal, neonatal, or infant mortality are excluded. Since these pregnancies are subject to higher rates of complication, their exclusion tends to bias downward the proportion of pregnancies that were complicated for both psychotic and nonpsychotic women. Nevertheless, these studies are still useful for inferences concerning the relative frequency of complications in the pregnancies of psychotic women as compared to those of normal women.

increases pregnancy loss (see Chapter 3). But the assumption that psychoses are merely a more severe form of psychic stress is erroneous. And there is no reason to believe that the two groups of disorders would have the same effects on pregnancy. Soichet (1959:1070–1071) raises the possibility that nonpsychotic women who are subjected to psychic stress during a pregnancy (sometimes as a result of the pregnancy itself) tend to react psychosomatically. If this is true, such women would probably show, for example, high rates of toxemia of pregnancy. However, Soichet suggests that psychotic women do not need to resort to somatic defense mechanisms because the psychoses have self-contained mental defenses against stress. To test this hypothesis, a study of schizophrenic pregnant women was made to determine the frequency of toxemia of pregnancy. The results were supportive, since only two cases (0.26%) were found among 767 pregnancies; yet, toxemia of pregnancy usually complicates about 7% of all gestations (Soichet 1959:1065). This hypothesis is further corroborated by observations that women suffering from schizophrenia have higher rates of toxemia prior to the onset of the disease and after its remission (Soichet 1959:1071; Wiedorn 1954:8). However, if it is true that psychotics do not have high rates of pregnancy loss because they do not need to resort to somatic defense mechanisms because psychoses themselves are defense mechanisms, how are the high rates of coital inability and conceptive failure explained?

DISCUSSION

Not all psychotic individuals are subfecund, as some extremely ill ones appear to have no difficulties in childbearing (Grimm 1967:19). But there is no doubt that psychotics as a whole are less fecund than the general population. Schizophrenics and manic-depressives were found to have relatively high rates of coital inability and conceptive failure, although no increased rate of pregnancy loss was established. Due to its high prevalence, amenorrhea is probably the most important cause of subfecundity. It is also worth noting that certain drugs commonly used to treat psychoses may also decrease fecundity via impotence (Amelar et al. 1977:93b; Bellack 1958:494; Dubin and Amelar 1971:471) and menstrual irregularities (Bellak 1958:494). Indeed, some psychotics have been known to avoid medication because of the impotence side-effect (Marshall 1971:656). In addition, other types of treatment for psychoses can increase the risk of pregnancy loss (Asch 1965:466–467).

It is impossible to estimate the amount of subfecundity produced by psychoses, for, since this topic is seldom raised, much about it remains unknown. This precludes any determination of the effect of psychoses-induced subfecundity on fertility. However, two features of schizophrenia and manic-depressive psychoses suggest that the effect of subfecundity on the fertility of many psychotics may be substantial.

First, both these illnesses often occur early in the reproductive period.[5] This is particularly true of schizophrenia (Odegard 1960:27), which frequently requires hospital admission well before completion of the reproductive period (Erlenmeyer-Kimling *et al*. 1969:917), since it develops primarily between the ages of 15 and 30 (Clinard 1968:454; Suinn 1970:3). Although manic-depressive psychoses tend to develop more often toward middle life (Baker 1967:82), they often occur early in the reproductive period, too. Dube and Kumar (1973:691) report that in their study population the maximum number of manic-depressive breakdowns occurred in females aged 15–34 and in males aged 35–54. Thus, both illnesses can get an early start at limiting lifetime fertility via subfecundity.

Second, both schizophrenia and manic-depressive psychoses can persist for long periods of time. In the event of early onset, these illnesses (and associated subfecundity) can be coincident with substantial portions of the reproductive period. Again, this is particularly true for schizophrenia, which may begin at an early age and continue uncured for the remainder of the individual's life (Odegard 1960:27; Suinn 1970:381). The average length of hospitalization, 13 years (Suinn 1970:381), indicates that schizophrenia persists for long periods.

Manic-depressive psychoses can also affect individuals for many years. The subfecundity reported earlier pertains mostly to the depressive phases, which run their course in about 9 months. Between depressions, the individual usually leads an undisturbed, essentially normal life. The depressive phases vary in frequency, from patients with widely interspersed attacks to those with almost annual depressions (Suinn 1970:356–357). Thus, the proportion of the reproductive period during which an individual is in depression can vary from zero to about 75%, depending on age at onset and the number of depressive phases experienced.

Although schizophrenia and manic-depressive psychoses can affect the fecundity of individuals, are they prevalent enough to affect that of populations? Perhaps. Though these illnesses are not widespread, they are by no means rare. As many as 2% of some populations succumb to them (Kellett 1973:860). The prevalence of schizophrenia in developed countries has been frequently placed at about 1% (cf. Erlenmeyer-Kimling *et al*. 1969:916; Moran 1972:299; Stevens, 1969:22; Wender 1973:1383[6]). The recent preliminary

[5]For age distributions of first admissions to state and county mental hospitals for schizophrenia and manic-depressive psychoses, see USNIMH (1967:19).

[6]Although Wender states here that the risk of developing schizophrenia is 1%, he notes that, though exact statistics are not available, various studies suggest that borderline schizophrenia is present in about 5% of the population.

report of the President's Commission on Mental Health states that about two million Americans (1%) have been or would be diagnosed as schizophrenics (Shearer 1977:12). Another study (Shields and Slater 1967:579) reports a pooled estimate of .86% derived from 19 studies carried out throughout the world. However, there are other studies reporting prevalence figures higher and lower than 1% (cf. Hare 1967:9–24; Sanua 1969:269–290; Yolles and Kramer 1969:69–79). The following comment by Ketty (1976) shows just how firm this 1% estimate is:

> I think we have to be very cautious in drawing any conclusions at all from prevalence rates of schizophrenia. One is not dealing with an element which has an objective, definable criterion, and the truth of the matter is that the prevalence rates or the lifetime incidence which have been recorded in Europe and Japan are still showing a wide spread. In Germany during the thirties the incidence was reported as .5%. There was one study in Switzerland where it was 1.25% and there are studies in between, and we oversimplify that by saying, "Well the incidence is about 1%" [p. 37].

Yolles and Kramer (1969) report the following about the future prevalence of schizophrenia in the United States:

> On the basis of data derived from incidence studies done in the United States, which determined the number of persons diagnosed as schizophrenic who have had a first contact with one of a broad network of psychiatric facilities per year, it is estimated that at a minimum two percent of the persons born in 1960 would have an attack of schizophrenia some time during their subsequent lifetime. Under certain conditions the maximum could be as high as six percent. The precise figure depends on the levels of the age specific incidence rates, the demographic and social structure of the community and other related factors [p. 104].

Estimates of the prevalance of manic-depressive psychoses are lower than those for schizophrenia, ranging from .05 to .5 percent of the population (cf. Dube and Kumar 1973:695–696; Rawnsley 1968:27–36; Silverman 1968:43). But the recent preliminary report of the President's Commission on Mental Health found that at least 1% of the population of the United States suffers from profound depressive disorders (Shearer 1977:12), which suggests that depressive psychoses can be more prevalent than commonly thought.

Rates of schizophrenia and manic-depressive psychoses may vary; cultural, temporal, racial, social class, urban–rural, and many other differentials have been reported. There is much conflict in the literature, however, concerning the existence or degree of variation (cf. Eaton and Weil 1955:74–97; Hammer 1972:423–450; Hare 1967:269–290; Mechanic 1970:7,17; Sanua

1969:269–290; and Wolf and Berle 1976:34–39). Although some authors claim that psychoses occur at different rates in different populations, others believe that rates are about equal. Similarly, there is disagreement as to whether or not psychoses are common in primitive societies, though the contention that psychoses are almost nonexistent among primitives no longer has adherents today (Sanua 1969:290–291).

The observed differential rates are ascribed at least in part to theoretical and methodological problems. Various theories have been forwarded, for example, to explain observed class and urban–rural differentials in the rates of psychoses. The well-documented association of schizophrenia and social class (cf. Hollingshead and Redlich 1958) has been explained by two alternate theories. It has been proposed that the increased incidence in the lower classes is due to some factor in their environment and/or that schizophrenic or preschizophrenic middle- and upper-class individuals drift into the lower classes because of their mental problems. Similarly, rural areas may have lower rates of psychoses than urban areas; this may be because the rural environment is more conducive to mental health and/or because emotionally unstable people tend to move frequently and gradually to drift into the socially disorganized inner city.

Differential rates may also be due in part to methodological problems. The development of an adequate vital statistics or descriptive epidemiology of psychoses has been impeded by a variety of problems, and these problems become doubly troublesome when comparisons are made between study populations or between population subgroups within and between studies. These problems include lack of comparability in diagnostic and classification criteria and methods, varying definitions of a case and differences in case-finding methods, difficulties arising from the selection of the population used in the computation of rates, differences in the composition of the study population by age and other demographic characteristics, and differences in the types of rates computed (cf. Hare 1967:9–24; Mechanic 1970:3–17; Sanua 1969:269–290; Silverman 1968:37–53; Yolles and Kramer 1969:69–79). Because of these and other difficulties, all the prevalence figures discussed in this chapter, if not in this entire book, must be considered problematic.

Nevertheless, despite the above theoretical and methodological considerations, it is probable that populations and population subgroups do have different rates of psychoses and, therefore, different rates of subfecundity due to these illnesses.

In sum, a substantial fraction of those suffering from schizophrenia and manic-depressive psychoses are subfecund for at least part of their reproductive period. In these individuals, psychoses-induced subfecundity may affect their fertility, especially if the age of onset is early. These psychoses may also contribute to population subfecundity, even if only in a minor way. However, such minor effects should not be considered negligible and consequently ignored, because the potential importance of the collective effect of many such factors on population fecundity might then be overlooked.

Psychoses and Fertility

Researchers have traditionally been interested in the fertility of psychotics relative to that of the general population. Historically, the fertility of psychotics was regarded mainly from the eugenic point of view, as one of the factors capable of increasing the population frequency of mental disorders. But this concern decreased with the accumulation of studies showing that psychotics have relatively low reproduction rates (Odegard 1960:25). Now, the fertility of psychotics is being studied for a variety of genetic and social psychiatric purposes (Odegard 1960:25; Price et al. 1971:S74).

Many authors report that psychotics have lower fertility than does the population as a whole (cf. Erlenmeyer-Kimling et al. 1966:259, 1969:916; Hammer 1972:437; Kellett 1973:860; Kroger and Freed 1951:283; Larson and Nyman 1973:273; Mandy and Mandy 1962:345; Odegard 1960:25; Reed et al. 1973:117; Slater et al. 1971:S73; Stevens 1969:169). Some authors find that schizophrenics have lower fertility than manic-depressives, and others report opposite results (cf. Lewis 1958:105; Odegard 1960:28). Overall, at least in developed countries, the fertility differential between the general population and psychotics has been lessening, probably due to the joint effects of the secular fertility decline in the former and the impact of community care on the latter (Stevens 1969:159,169).

The observation that psychotics generally have lower fertility than the general population is plausible, considering the serious and deviant symptoms of psychoses—hallucinations, delusions, loose associations, fragmented and incoherent speech, prolonged melancholy or elation, isolation, and withdrawal from others (Buss 1966:32)—symptoms that often represent significant social obstacles that psychotics must overcome in order to reproduce. Researchers typically explain the relatively low fertility of psychotics by describing the relationship between these symptoms and various Davis–Blake (1956:212) intermediate variables, particularly those affecting exposure to intercourse. The following is a brief review of the fertility-inhibiting relationship between psychoses and specific intermediate variables.

MARITAL RATES

The high proportion of schizophrenic and manic-depressive individuals never entering sexual unions is perhaps the most important reason for their depressed fertility. Authors reporting reduced marital rates include Odegard (1960:27), Price *et al.* (1971:S93), Lewis (1959:131), Larson and Nyman (1973:279), Erlenmeyer-Kimling *et al.* (1969:916), and Slater *et al.* (1971:S73). Odegard (1960:27), for instance, reports relatively low marriage rates for both schizophrenics and manic-depressives. Using the marriage rates of Norway as an index of 100, the marriage rate index of male schizophrenics was found to be 38, for female schizophrenics, 57, and for either male or female manic-depressives, about 91. Some studies (cf. Slater *et al.* 1971:S73) have also found that psychotics who marry tend to do so relatively late, though there is counterevidence (cf. Odegard 1960:28).

Such differences in marriage rates give rise to marital status differentials. It has long been observed that unmarried persons are disproportionately found in mental institutions. Scandinavian figures show that the schizophrenia rate for single men is 5 times higher than that for married men; for women, the rate is 3 times higher. English data show similar differentials; for example, first admission rates for schizophrenia were 6 times higher among single men. The corresponding differentials for manic-depressive psychoses are in the same direction, although they are of less than half the magnitude of the schizophrenia differentials (Lewis 1958:98).

The most probable explanation for the relatively low marriage rates and the overrepresentation of singles among psychotic persons is that psychotic personality traits select against marriage, and this may occur even before the onset of manifest psychoses. Essen-Moller, for example, found that before illness marriage was half as prevalent in schizophrenics as in normal people of the same age and was only about one-sixth of the normal rate after illness in those who had been single at the time of first hospitalization (Lewis 1958:99). Similarly, Stevens (1969:169) concluded that the basic difference between schizophrenics and normal women in her study was their considerable reduction in marriage probability to 75% of normal before illness and to 33% of normal afterwards. It is also noteworthy that in some places, such as certain U.S. states, marriage is prohibited to psychotic persons (Oliven 1965:222).

MARITAL DISRUPTION

The low fertility of psychotics is also attributed to higher rates of marital disruption (Odegard 1960:27; Slater *et al.* 1971:S73). Stevens (1969:130) found that schizophrenics in her study, in comparison with normal women, had higher rates of separation and divorce; this was the case both before and after their illness. Manic-depressives also had higher marital disruption rates, but only before their illness. In addition, marriage entered into by psychotics is generally void or voidable (Oliven 1965:222). The chances of marital disruption are particularly high if the psychotic requires indefinite hospitalization, in which case, Oliven (1965:279) observes, the prognosis as to marital stability is almost uniformly poor.

A good indication of the total effect of these marital status variables on fertility potential is given by Slater *et al.* (1971:S64, S67). They compared the number of years in the 25-year period between the ages of 20 and 44 inclusive that the general population of Britain and the two psychotic groups spent in the married state. The married state was defined to include periods of separation and to exclude time spent after the death of a spouse or a divorce. Their results reveal substantial differences between psychotics and the general population (cf. Table 11.3). Whereas males and females in the general population spent 17.8 and 20.1 years, respectively, in a marital union, comparable figures for schizophrenics were only 7.5 and 12.1 and, for manic-depressives, 13.9 and 17.6.

INVOLUNTARY ABSTINENCE

The lower fertility of psychotics is also partly attributed to another intermediate variable, involuntary abstinence, which results from required hospitalization (Erlenmeyer-Kimling *et al.* 1969:917; Money 1967:268; Reed *et al.* 1973:117; and Stevens 1969:164). Though psychotics tend to marry less (cf. Stevens 1969:169), have relatively low marital fertility (cf. Odegard 1960:27), and high rates of marital disruption (cf. Stevens 1970:149) even prior to their first hospital admission, these differentials are increased by custodial isolation, which deprives them of the usual opportunities of finding a mate, keeps them apart from their regular sexual partner (Money 1967:268), and heightens their probability of separation or divorce (Stevens 1970:149). Thus, Reed *et al.* (1973) note: "Our data are in agreement with other investigators in demonstrating a lower fertility of schizophrenic persons than either their unaffected siblings or a control population. It could hardly be otherwise in view of the prolonged hospitalization of many of the schizophrenics [p. 117]."

However, two current trends have decreased the negative effect of hospitalization on the fertility of psychotics. The first is the trend away from hospitalization itself. In the United States, for example, the percentage of hospital beds occupied by mental patients declined from about 50 to 37% in the decade ending in 1974 (Horton and Leslie 1974:528). Over roughly the same period, the population of state mental institutions declined by almost half (*Time* 1973:74). These declines do not signify a decrease in the prevalence of psychoses, since outpatient treatment has increased more than inpatient treatment has declined. Rather, this trend is due largely to the development of psychoactive drugs, such as tranquilizers and antidepressants, which enable the mentally ill to remain more in the community.

Although chemotherapy cuts down the number of psychotics in hospitals, its cure rate is low. A three year follow-up study of hospital discharged patients, for instance, showed that only 11% of schizophrenics remained symptom-free over this period of time, whereas 72% showed sufficient return or exacerbation of their symptoms to require rehospitalization (Suinn 1970:395).

The second trend that is decreasing the impact of hospitalization on the fertility of psychotics is one toward shorter hospital stays (cf. Erlenmeyer-Kimling et al. 1969:916). The length of these stays has been substantially shortened as a result of advances in medical technology and drug therapy, liberalization of hospital administrative policies, and growing interest in the rights and welfare of the mentally ill (Erlenmeyer-Kimling et al. 1969:916; Mauss 1975:324). Moreover, even extended hospital stays have less impact on fertility than formerly because such patients now have frequent periods of leave during which they can initiate a pregnancy (Slater et al. 1971:S61).

COITAL FREQUENCY

The relatively low fertility of psychotics may be partly the result of another intermediate variable, coital frequency, Many authors have reported that schizophrenics and depressives tend to have relatively low libido, which probably leads to reduced coital frequency (e.g., Arieti 1967:228; Cassidy et al. 1957:1538; Johnson 1968:72,73; Jones 1973:690; Lewis 1959:130; Mayer-Gross et al. 1969:162,211; Money 1967:270; Oliven 1974:403; Pearlman and Kobashi 1972:300; Stevens 1969:8; and Suinn 1970:356). Arieti (1967:228–233) contends that a large fraction of schizophrenics have one or more psychosexual problems that can lead to a reluctance to indulge in heterosexual relations. These problems include the inability to establish a stable sex identity, sexual indifference, a feeling of inadequacy as a sexual partner, and a feeling of inadequacy as a sexual object. According to Arieti, the first-mentioned of these problems, the inability to establish a stable sex identity, is the most prevalent of the four, affecting about 15% of schizo-phrenics. Considering these psychosexual problems, the inability to relate to people, and the general withdrawal from social situations (Schafer et al. 1975:69), the schizophrenic's inability to maintain a regular sexual relation-ship would seem likely. It is also likely that psychotics have less frequent coitus due to a reluctance on the part of their nonpsychotic partners to have children (Odegard 1960:27) and to the libido-repressive effect of some com-monly used psychotherapeutic drugs (Stevens 1969:32,40).

It should also be noted, however, that manics and schizophrenics with certain features may have for a time an increased sexual drive (cf. Arieti 1967:235–236; Lukianowicz 1963:250; Mayer-Gross et al. 1969:162,281;

Mednick *et al.* 1971:S109; Oliven 1974:426,430; Reed *et al.* 1973:133; and Suinn 1970:356).

BIRTH CONTROL

Three other intermediate variables that could affect the fertility of psychotics are contraception, sterilization, and induced abortion, all forms of birth control. Due to the potential problems involved in raising children when one parent is psychotic, it seems reasonable that psychotics and their partners would rely on birth control to limit their fertility. However, since surprisingly little attention has been devoted in the literature to the use of birth control among psychotics, the extent to which they or their partners practice it is unknown (Stevens 1969:31–32). The fact that it is rarely considered in fertility studies of psychotics, studies that do focus on other intermediate variables, implies that most authors believe that birth control is not a significant factor. Moreover, because the twentieth-century fertility decline in Western nations, a decline that was facilitated by the spread of birth control, may have lessened the fertility differential between the general population and psychotics (cf. Stevens 1969:31,159), it might be inferred that psychotics and their partners have actually been slower than the general population to adopt birth control.

The literature suggests that manic-depressives are probably more likely than schizophrenics to practice birth control. Odegard (1960:29), for instance, observes that manic-depressives, unlike schizophrenics, are often very concerned about their condition, and requests for sterilization are far from rare. It might also be expected that psychotics would make relatively frequent use of therapeutic abortion, since psychiatric indications are the most common grounds for this procedure, especially in areas that do not have liberalized abortion laws (cf. Heath 1971:55; Mayer-Gross *et al.* 1969:376). However, there is some indication in the literature that sterilization and therapeutic abortion do not contribute to the relatively low fertility of psychotics, for, as in nonpsychotic women, sterilization and perhaps even therapeutic abortion tend to be employed by psychotics who already have high fertility (cf. Stevens 1969:101).

SUBFECUNDITY

Another intermediate variable typically ignored in explanations of the relatively low fertility of psychotics is subfecundity. Odegard (1960) even states that "biological fertility per se is unlikely to be affected either by schizophrenia or by manic-depressive psychoses [p. 29]." This dismissal of subfecundity as a potential fertility factor flies in the face of the evidence reported earlier in this section, particularly that pointing to the high preva-lence of amenorrhea among psychotics. This may be due to the fact that such subfecundity-producing conditions in psychotics are frequently overlooked (Ossofsky 1972:746–747). It is fair to say about schizophrenia and manic-depressive psychoses what Silverman (1968) concludes about the latter, to wit, "Nothing is known of the relative contribution of involuntary and volun-tary influences on fertility [p. 90]."

7

Sexual Deviations

Sexual deviation is behavior in which gratification of sexual impulses is obtained by practices other than intercourse with a legally consenting, genitally mature person of the opposite sex.[1] The aberrant behavior may involve a deviation in the choice of the sexual object, in the sexual act, or in the degree of sexual desire. Deviations in object choice, in which the individual becomes sexually aroused and engages in intercourse with a deviant sexual object, include such disorders as homosexuality, excessive masturbation, pedophilia, zoophilia, fetishism, and necrophilia. Sadism, masochism, exhibitionism, voyeurism, and coprolalia are examples of deviations in the sexual act whereby the individual becomes sexually gratified through acts other than those involving genital stimulation. Deviations in degree of sexual desire are conditions in which the sexual urge is either impaired or exaggerated, examples of which are frigidity, impotence, nymphomania, and satyriasis (Suinn 1970:311, 313).

Sexual deviations tend to lower fertility via many of the Davis–Blake (1956) intermediate variables. Thus, Nag (1972) notes: "It should be remem-

[1]For a discussion of sexual deviation in terms of psychopathology, see Suinn (1970:3ll–318), Buss (1966:453–464), Oliven (1965:511–582), and Rosen *et al.* (1972:273–298). For a discussion of sexual deviation as a social problem, see Clinard (1968:343–387), Perry and Perry (1976:455–477), and Schafer *et al.* (1975:51–65).

bered that homosexual and other types of sexual perversions may, in some cases have *indirect* effects on fertility [p. 231; emphasis added]." The word indirect in this statement is significant, because by using it Nag is referring to intermediate variables other than subfecundity, such as coital frequency, the proportion marrying, and marital disruption. Nag is essentially overlooking subfecundity, apparently a common practice. Few studies have examined the relationship between various sexual deviations and subfecundity, and therefore little is known about it.

Though there are no indications in the literature that sexual deviations are associated with abnormally high rates of pregnancy loss, there are scattered references suggesting that they do increase rates of coital inability and conceptive failure, particularly in men (cf. Johnson 1968:36, 75–77). Romm (1967:222) details the relationship between one deviation, fetishism, and sexual potency. Mayer-Gross and his associates (1969:161) observe that many of the sexual deviations may lead to impotence. As Cooper (1972) notes: "Sexual deviations of one sort or another including homosexuality, fetishism, and excessive autosexuality may be associated with sexual aversion manifesting as heterosexual impotence [p. 549]." Johnson (1968) offers the view that "a fully developed sexual deviation and normal potency are by definition mutually exclusive [p. 76]" and notes that "sexual deviations have long been recognized to manifest themselves by a disorder of heterosexual potency [p. 75]." Included in his discussion are the coital inability factor, impotence, and the conceptive failure factors, ejaculatory incompetence and premature ejaculation.

Thus, in the absence of a specific abnormal stimulus, one that a mate may be unable or unwilling to provide, men with certain sexual deviations may be subfecund (Dubin and Amelar 1972:582). Sexual deviations may also lower fecundity in ways other than through psychosexual disorders. For instance, as will be discussed shortly, certain sexual deviations, such as homosexuality, may be accompanied by endocrine abnormalities that influence fecundity.

It is also noteworthy that women with sexual deviations may experience coital inability and conceptive failure, though probably not as frequently as do sexually deviant men. Nymphomaniacs, for example, are generally inorgasmic (cf. Pumper-Mindlin 1967:168), a condition that may cause subfecundity (see Chapter 3). And most prostitutes, if they can be considered to be sexual deviates, are subfecund for a variety of reasons (cf. Oliven 1974:452–453).

In view of their prevalence and ability to produce subfecundity on the individual level, only three of the sexual deviations, homosexuality, frigidity, and impotence, seem potentially capable of significantly influencing population fecundity.[2] Since the latter two have already been discussed in Chapters 2 and 3 as psychosomatic responses to psychic stress, this section will confine itself to homosexuality.

Homosexuality and Subfecundity

Homosexuality, as the term is employed here, refers to a persistent, conscious, sexual attraction to members of the same sex (Wahl 1967:194).[3] Homosexuality and heterosexuality do not represent a clear-cut dichotomy. Rather, the two are extremes on a continuum, with many individuals occupying intermediate positions. Kinsey and his associates (1948:638–641) grouped the population into seven categories on this continuum. This rating scale ranges from category 0, the exclusively heterosexual, to category 6, the exclusively homosexual. This discussion is primarily interested in individuals who are more or less exclusively homosexual, which, in terms of Kinsey's scale, includes categories 5 and 6, because only this group probably differs significantly from the general population in terms of fecundity.

Although there is a large and growing literature on homosexuality, the etiology and many other aspects of this condition are still poorly understood, and this is particularly true of female homosexuality (cf. Trimmer 1972:384). One area about which there is hardly any specific information is that concerning the fecundity of homosexuals. Not a single paper was found in the literature that dealt with this topic, though general statements concerning the physiological characteristics of homosexuals abound.[4] Evidently, as with

[2]One of the few allusions to the possible effect of sexual deviations on population fecundity is reported by Nag (1962) in a discussion of the causes of depopulation on Yap. Nag mentions that "Price (1936) states that abnormal sex practices among the Yapese make men impotent and women sterile, but he gives no further details [p. 35]."

[3]The traditional view of the American Psychiatric Association has been that homosexuality is a form of mental illness (cf. APA 1952, 1968). However, in December 1973 the APA board of trustees voted to remove homosexuality per se from the list of mental illnesses, although some homosexuals could still be diagnosed as ill under a new category called "sexual orientation disturbance." Although disagreement existed among the members, the board's decision was endorsed by a vote of the APA membership in the Spring of 1974. However, the issue of whether or not homosexuality is a mental illness has not been settled. Recently, the journal *Medical Aspects of Human Sexuality* sent questionnaires to 10,000 members of the APA and compiled the first 2500 responses. Of those answering, 69% said that homosexuality is usually a pathological adaptation, as opposed to a normal variation; 18% disagreed; and 13% were uncertain (*Time* 1978a:102). Provision has also been made for listing homosexuality, at least in some forms, in the APA's *Diagnostic and Statistical Manual of Mental Disorders,* 3rd ed., which is currently being drafted. Because of the current uncertainty, this discussion adopts the traditional view that homosexuality is a form of psychopathology. For an excellent and brief discussion of the reasons why some experts believe that homosexuality should not be considered a mental illness, see Williams (1977:233).

[4]Most authors agree that homosexuals do not have outwardly distinctive physical traits (cf.

many other forms of psychopathology, those who study homosexuality must consider its effect on fecundity to be of little interest. The following statement by Oliven (1974) is characteristic of the prevailing disinterest in homosexual fecundity: "Among those [lesbians] who have tried to conceive, many have succeeded [p. 527]." Though Oliven uses this statement to support the contention that there are no physiological differences related to fecundity between homosexual and heterosexual women, it does not, in fact, preclude a conceptive failure differential and thus throws little light on the question of whether lesbians are less fecund than heterosexual women.

The following discussion splices together pieces of fecundity-related information found in the literature in an effort to gain at least a rudimentary perspective on the relationship between homosexuality and both coital inability and conceptive failure.

COITAL INABILITY

Male   Many sexual deviations, but especially homosexuality, can lead to impotence (Hastings 1960:429; Johnson 1968:35–36; Kaufman 1967:144; Mayer-Gross et al. 1969:161; Oliven 1974:392). A male homosexual may be able to function in homosexual relationships but may fail to achieve erection in normal heterosexual relationships (Braiman 1970:739).[5] This is plausible given the fact that some homosexual males have an aversion to females as sexual partners (Freund 1974:46). Even those who do not feel any heterosexual aversion or any attraction may be impotent, for, as Hastings (1960) notes, "Neurotic impotence describes the situation wherein psychologic potency never fully developed. The problem posed by homosexuality can be used to illustrate this group. If a man has little or no fundamental interest in the opposite sex, he is not apt to be potent [p. 432]." In one study (Saghir et al. 1969:224) of homosexuals, the majority (63%) reported an absence of heterosexual arousal during adult life. Although the literature provides no estimate of the proportion of homosexuals who are heterosexually impotent, it is undoubtedly much higher than that of heterosexual men.

Masters and Johnson (1970:140–141, 179–183) emphasize the importance of a homosexual influence as an etiological factor in both primary and

---

Oliven 1965:579; West 1968:69,160). Dickenson, however, thought it possible to diagnose female homosexuals on the basis of various genital features (cited in Kroger and Freed 1951:397), but few adhere to this view today.

[5]It should be noted that "coital ability," as the term is used in this study, refers only to heterosexual intravaginal intercourse between two humans. The ability to perform homosexual or heterosexual anal intercourse, intercourse with animals, and so forth does not enter into the determination of coital ability. It is, of course, possible for homosexuals to be impotent in homosexual relations as well (Talkington 1971:26). Indeed, as Williams (1977) notes, "homosexual couples are now appearing for sex therapy with the same kinds of problems that heterosexual couples have [p. 235]."

secondary impotence. With respect to the former, they report that a commitment to an overt pattern of homosexual response during the early to middle teenage years was a major etiological factor in failed coital connection during initial and all subsequent heterosexual exposures for 6 (19%) of the 32 primarily impotent men they treated. This suggests that perhaps a substantial minority of primarily impotent men are homosexual or have homosexual orientations, assuming that this study group is fairly representative of all primarily impotent men.

If homosexual performance has been recorded and enjoyed before significant heterosexual exposure has been experienced, secondary impotence may develop (Masters and Johnson 1970:179–183). Although relatively little if any difficulty in heterosexual functioning may be experienced during courtship or in the initial years of marriage, the secondary impotence surfaces at a later date. Typical histories report that an overwhelming drive to return to homosexual functioning develops somewhere between 5 and 20 years after marriage. Once acknowledged, the revived demand for homosexual behavior is consuming. These men temporarily try to pursue both homosexual and heterosexual lives, but often their ability to function bisexually diminishes. When actively oriented to homosexuality, they usually lose what little interest they may have developed in heterosexual coitus. Finally, they fail to attain erection, primarily because heterosexual functioning is devoid of psychosocial interest and provides little or no physical stimulation. As Masters and Johnson (1970) note: "once an episode of erective failure has occurred, the homosexually oriented male usually cannot consistently attain and/or maintain an erection quality sufficient for effective coitus. His sexual value system is no longer attuned to heterosexual influence [p. 182]."

Of a total of 213 men treated by Masters and Johnson for secondary impotence, 21 found heterosexual functioning objectionable, repulsive, or impossible after making a marital commitment. Making the liberal assumption that these 213 men are fairly representative of all secondarily impotent married men, then homosexuality would account for about 10% of the secondary impotence among married men. But, since most exclusively homosexual males are not married and would not be expected to seek treatment for heterosexual impotence as frequently as would heterosexual men, the proportion of all homosexual men who would be impotent heterosexually is undoubtedly much higher. Perhaps this proportion is close to that of heterosexual men incapable of homosexual functioning during adult life.

Female Lesbians can and often do experiment heterosexually even though they have few spontaneous feelings toward men (West 1968:68). However, lesbians probably do have more coital inability than do other women because lesbianism may cause vaginismus and dyspareunia (Oliven 1974:420,270). Masters and Johnson (1970:252) report that a prior homosexual identification is the fourth most frequent etiological factor in vaginismus. And, in some women, vaginismus may actually be the extreme manifestation of bisexual conflict and the resulting sexual fear (Kroger and Freed 1951:316). Lesbianism can also lead to insufficient spontaneous lubrication, a common cause of dyspareunia (Oliven 1974:270). Though many of these women attempt regular coitus for socioeconomic and other reasons, they frequently do not lubricate well during heterosexual activity even though there usually is ample lubrication during their homosexual activity (Masters and Johnson 1970:276).

The proportion of lesbians who suffer from vaginismus or dyspareunia is unknown. However, one study (Kenyon 1968a:1346) found that 14% of lesbians as compared to only 2% of heterosexual women characterized their sexual intercourse as painful.

CONCEPTIVE FAILURE

Many authors seem to take for granted the assumption that homosexuals are equally able to impregnate or to conceive as are heterosexuals because some homosexuals are known to have children (e.g., Oliven 1974:527). However, the probability of conception for couples with at least one homosexual member has never been studied, at least to this writer's knowledge. Thus, the possiblity exists that homosexuals are relatively infertile. Indeed some indications that this might be the case were found in the literature in studies that do not deal with subfecundity per se.

Male The previous section discussed the fact that homosexual males may experience relatively high rates of impotence due in part to their disinterest in or aversion toward heterosexual intercourse. For the same reason it may also be true that homosexuals who do achieve coital connection may experience higher rates of psychosexual disorders that interfere with conception. Masters and Johnson (1966:219), for example, found positive homosexual histories in two of five men with ejaculatory incompetence, although a later report (1970:120) on an expanded series mentioned a homosexual orientation in only 1 of 17 cases. This case (cf. Masters and Johnson 1970:120–121) provides a glimpse of how homosexuality might produce psychosexual disorders and subfecundity, and, therefore, it is presented here in a condensed form:

> This man offered dislike, rejection, or open enmity for his wife as sufficient reason for failure to ejaculate intravaginally. He married a distant relative, whom he found totally objectionable physically, primarily for monetary reasons and

social support. Though his sexual commitment was of homosexual orientation, he was able to function coitally with his wife from an erective point of view. But after penetration he was repulsed rather than stimulated by his wife's demanding pelvic thrusting and delighted in denying to her the ejaculatory experience. After 6 years of marriage and continuation of his homosexual activities, the man thought that children should be a part of his marriage's image to the community. However the pattern of voluntary restraint was so strong that he could not ejaculate and after 3 years of involuntary ejaculatory constriction, the man and his wife sought treatment.

Homosexuality has also been linked to spermatogenic deficiencies due to endocrine dysfunction. In the past, studies of hormonal differences between homosexuals and heterosexuals have generally yielded negative findings, though it was commonly thought that as research methods became more sophisticated significant relationships would be discovered at least for some groups of homosexuals (Horton and Leslie 1974:569). Perhaps that time has already arrived, since recent urinary and plasma studies have found measurable differences in the levels of certain hormones between homosexual and heterosexual men (Brodie *et al.* 1974:82; Oliven 1974:507). Investigators who have found evidence of endocrine dysfunction or differentials include Loraine *et al.* (1970:406, 1971:552), Margolese (1970:151), Kolodny *et al.* (1971:1170, 1972:18), Evans (1972:146), Pillard *et al.* (1974:453), and Doerr *et al.* (1976:611).

Kolodny and his associates (1971, 1972), for example, found significantly lower levels of plasma testosterone and higher levels of luteinising hormone, follicle-stimulating hormone, and prolactin in a group of exclusively homosexual males than in a group of heterosexual males. But what makes these two studies particularly valuable sources for this discussion's effort to shed light on the relationship between homosexuality and conceptive failure is the fact that they explicitly studied and report differences between homosexuals and heterosexuals in sperm count and sperm quality. For the sake of simplicity, the following discussion will be confined to the 1971 study.

Kolodny and his associates interviewed 30 male homosexual students between the ages of 18 and 24 and classified them according to degree of homosexuality, using the scale devised by Kinsey and his associates. Of the 30 homosexuals in the study, 15 were judged to be exclusively or almost exclusively homosexual. Physical examinations including plasma testosterone determinations and semen examinations were performed. They found that the plasma testosterone levels in the 15 exclusively and almost exclusively homosexual males were significantly below those of a control group of heterosexual males. The most startling finding, from a subfecundity standpoint, was that 9 of these 15 had abnormally low sperm counts, 4 being azoospermic and 5 oligospermic. Moreover, impaired sperm motility was found in 7 of the 9 men with low sperm counts. The youth of this sample and their excellent health record make these findings of spermatogenic dysfunction even more striking, since they cannot be readily attributed to another health factor.

Kolodny and his associates note that their work in this area must be interpreted with caution because of the size and nature of the study population. However, they contend that their studies support the idea of a direct reciprocal relationship between spermatogenesis and hormone levels and emphasize that endocrine dysfunction must be considered in association with homosexuality. Their view is that endocrine and spermatogenic dysfunctions are unlikely to be found in most men with a history of homosexual involvement. But they suggest that these dysfunctions may be quite common in men with a predominantly or exclusively homosexual behavior pattern (Kolodny 1972:20), the type of homosexual who is the subject of this discussion.

However, it is important to note that a number of studies have failed to replicate the finding of subnormal plasma testosterone levels in exclusively homosexual men (cf. Barlow et al. 1974; Birk et al. 1973; Brodie et al. 1974; Doerr 1973; Parks et al. 1974; and Tourney and Hatfield 1973). Because of failures to replicate the Kolodny findings, Brecher (1975) believes that "it is now generally agreed that no difference exists between homosexual and heterosexual testosterone levels [p. 149]."

Female As was the case with male homosexuals, it is plausible that lesbians would tend to have above-average rates of psychosexual disorders in conjunction with heterosexual activity. In particular, lesbians tend to be more frigid and inorgasmic, two psychosexual disorders that may affect the probability of conception (see Chapter 3). As Oliven (1974) notes: "More often, the true lesbian has no erotic interest in men; she is indifferent to a man's sexual attentions, irritated by them, repulsed, or occasionally even frightened. The more passive homosexual woman who marries a normal man for convenience or social protection, remains sexually frigid and incapable of genuine love for her husband [p. 530]."

Many investigators (cf. Oliven 1974:403) point to a relationship between lesbianism and frigidity. In one study, Kenyon (1972:380) reports that 6 of 7 married female homosexuals were frigid, and, in another of his studies (1968a:1346), 34% of the lesbians could be characterized as frigid, in comparison to only 2% of the controls. In a review of female homosexuality, Kenyon (1974) also notes that one of the psychodynamic explanations frequently brought forward to explain frigidity is latent homosexuality, and he quotes the following statement by Gluckman (1966): "Frigidity in the female is frequently a defense against unconscious lesbian drives. The female homosexual can get by fairly well in marriage by passive acceptance of her status, especially if there are phantasies that are emotionally satisfying in association with coitus or auto-erotic expression [p. 104]." However, Kenyon adds a note of caution about the concept of latent homosexuality, suggesting that the term is loose, widely abused, and needs to be validated.

Lesbians may also tend to be less orgasmic than heterosexual women. In one study, for instance, Kenyon (1968a:1346) found that 53% of the lesbians were inorgasmic, as compared to only 12% of the heterosexual controls. Masters and Johnson (1970:244) observe that a homophile orientation is a major etiological factor in heterosexual orgasmic dysfunction for many women. They note that there are many women with significant homosexual experience during adolescence who gradually withdraw from this orientation to live socially heterosexual lives. However, many remain subject to orgasmic dysfunction by the prior imprinting of homosexual influence upon their sexual responsiveness.

Little if any evidence exists indicating that lesbians are physiologically different from heterosexual women. Lesbians are of ordinary physique, with menstruation and other indications of female development all present and normal (Oliven 1974:527; West 1968:69). Though one study (Loraine et al. 1971:552) did demonstrate raised levels of urinary luteinising hormone in four homosexual women, on the whole there is no solid evidence that there are hormonal differences between lesbians and heterosexual women. Lesbians apparently are no more anovular or amenorrheic than are heterosexual women. Kenyon (1968b:487), in a study of 100 lesbians who were not psychiatric patients, did find more amenorrhea in the lesbians (15%) than in the controls (10%), but the difference was not statistically significant. Kenyon did express surprise at this overall finding that menstrual irregularities were not more common in lesbians than in heterosexuals. However, it has been suggested by others that lesbians probably have relatively fewer gynecological dysfunctions due to less sexual intercourse and fewer pregnancies (Kroger and Freed 1951:395).

VENEREAL DISEASE

Homosexuals as a group may be relatively subfecund due to venereal disease. The two most common venereal diseases, gonorrhea and syphilis, are powerful causes of subfecundity. Gonorrhea is an important cause of male and female sterility, and syphilis is a cause of abortion and stillbirth. Although the exact extent of the problem is unknown, venereal disease (VD) is rampant among homosexual men (Gluckman et al. 1974:2210; King 1974:188–192). Though homosexuals constitute a small minority of the male population, they are disproportionately represented among VD patients (cf. British Journal of Venereal Disease 1973:329; King 1974:188–192; Racz

1970:117; Schafer *et al.* 1975:52), since they have many more sexual contacts than heterosexual men and, once infected, they tend to delay seeking medical help or to seek it less (Davis 1976:257; Maurer 1975:127, 129; Ritchey and Leff 1975:509). As Davis (1976) observes: "In the 1920's homosexual behavior was a minor source of venereal infection, but by the late 1960's it had become a major factor, with countries reporting anywhere from 10 to 90 percent of venereal cases as homosexual in origin. In surveys in Los Angeles, from 1959 to 1961, from 50 to 77 percent of infected males named purely homosexual contacts; in some districts the percentage was as high as 86 percent [p. 257]." Homosexuals comprised about 25% of all VD sufferers in the United States during 1968 (Webster 1970:406). Although the proportion of male homosexuals who have VD is unknown, one study (Ritchey and Leff 1975:510) found 10 cases among 118 homosexuals.

Venereal disease resulting from homosexual practices is almost exclusive to males and is seldom found in female homosexuals (Kroger and Freed 1951:395). Lesbians seem to run no special risks, though infection is occasionally acquired by contact between two females (King 1974:187). Webster (1970:406) reports that female to female contact accounted for only about 2% of venereal disease cases in women in the United States during 1968.

PREVALENCE

Exact or even reliable statistics on homosexuality are understandably difficult to compile (Oliven 1974:498; Socarides 1970:1199). Assessing the amount of homosexual behavior in a society is no less complicated than is measuring the prevalence of other widely disapproved-of sexual behavior. If anything, it is more problematic, and not solely for the obvious reason that so much of it is concealed (cf. Mauss 1975:362–363). Thus, prevalence estimates are based, to date, on largely inadequate and unrepresentative data (Clinard 1968:356). Many authors (cf. Oliven 1965:549; Schur 1965:75) note that reliable prevalence figures simply do not exist.

Nevertheless, homosexuality, the most frequent and certainly the most important form of deviant sexual behavior (Kroger and Freed 1951:391), is undoubtedly a disorder of considerable magnitude (Wahl 1967:192). Socarides (1970:1199) notes that it is a disorder of epidemic proportions, whose prevalence surpasses that of the recognized major illnesses in developed nations.

Studies have found that large minorities of both men and women have had homosexual experiences during their lives. Kinsey and his associates (1953:474–475), for instance, report that nearly 37% of the white male population and 13% of the white female population in their study had engaged in a homosexual experience to the point of orgasm at least once. However, it is recognized that those who are more or less exclusively homosexual represent a much smaller minority. It is of course this latter group that is the concern of this discussion. Estimates of the proportion of the population in developed nations that is exclusively homosexual range from 2 to 8% for men[6] and about half this for women (cf. Cooper 1974:20; Ford and Beach 1951:125–143; Gebhard 1972:22–29; Horton and Leslie 1974:569; Hunt 1974:310; Levin 1975:190; Linder 1963:61; Magee 1966:43–46; Oliven 1974:498; Renshaw 1974:172; Rosen et al. 1972:283; Trimmer 1972:384; West 1968:33–42; and Williams 1977:234). Kinsey's findings, that about 4% of males and half to a third as many females were exclusively homosexual, have not been seriously disputed (West 1968:35–41), despite the methodological flaws of those studies (cf. Hunt 1974:306–309). These figures have been replicated in other studies (e.g., Magee 1966) and even receive support from gender-identity studies among children. For instance, Green (1967:92) reports that about 4% of the 5–11-year-old boys in his study responded with an unequivocally feminine orientation. In sum, though not problem-free, the Kinsey figures are still the most often cited and are widely considered to be as good as any available to date (cf. Horton and Leslie 1974:568; Oliven 1965:549; and West 1968:35–41).

Whatever the exact prevalence, it is clear that homosexuality is prevalent enough among both men and women to be included in this review of subfecundity factors of possible demographic significance. It should also be noted that homosexuality rates vary from population to population. Ford and Beach (1951:125–143) surveyed studies of sexual behavior in 190 societies and found that ethnographic accounts of homosexual activities were available for only 76. This means that, in at least some populations, the prevalence of homosexuality is nil or almost nil. The other end of the spectrum is probably occupied by developed countries, such as the United States. It is probably a fair guess that the proportion of males who are exclusively homosexual ranges from nil up to 5% among adult populations.

Homosexuality rates also vary within populations, as temporal, cultural, social class, and other differentials have been reported by many studies (cf. Ford and Beach 1951; Gebhard 1972; Hooker 1972; Pomeroy 1969; and West 1968). However, at least a portion of these differentials within populations (and also between them) is due to a variety of theoretical and methodological considerations. Consider temporal variation within the United States as an

---

[6]According to Time (1975b:32), a conservative estimate of U.S. men who were exclusively homosexual in 1975 is 5 million, but homosexual spokesmen claim that the figure is closer to 20 million, most of these still "in the closet."

example. Some authorities (cf. Hooker 1972:11; Hunt 1974:303) contend that the prevalence of homosexuality has not increased since 1950, whereas others (cf. Cooper 1974:20; Oliven 1965:549) hold the opposite view. It is widely recognized, however, that at least a portion of any time differential may be simply apparent and due to the permissive, liberal atmosphere of recent times, which makes it more likely that individuals would admit their homosexuality today than 30 years ago.

DISCUSSION

Given the current state of knowledge, it is impossible to determine the potential importance of homosexuality as a population fecundity factor. Though there is no doubt that it is prevalent enough, the extent of its effect on individual fecundity is unknown. The findings reported in this section indicate that there is a good possibility that homosexuals are substantially less fecund than heterosexuals,[7] but they by no means prove it. If for no other reason, studies of homosexuals, like those on most forms of deviance, tend to be biased by the fact that samples known to medical authorities are often not altogether typical. And many of the studies reported here are based on small samples.

Based on the preceding discussion it is probable that exclusively homosexual males are less fecund than lesbians because the factors associated with male homosexuality, such as impotence and spermatogenic failure, are strong subfecundity agents. Moreover, homosexual men have high rates of venereal disease. Even if VD does not affect their fecundity, they most certainly would pass it on to their regular female partner, if any, thus jeopardizing their joint fecundity. Lesbians, on the other hand, rarely contract VD. And the subfecundity factors that characterize them are limited to an assortment of psychosexual disorders that, except for vaginismus, are not powerful fecundity depressants. Furthermore, there is no suggestion in the literature of a relationship between lesbianism and pregnancy loss.

Any subfecundity produced by homosexuality is likely to be lifelong, since few actively seek reversal of this orientation, and, for those who do, the treatment is unsuccessful more often than not (Oliven 1974:520–521). Moreover, many of the subfecundity factors just discussed are especially difficult to treat in the homosexual population. For instance, Masters and Johnson (1970:213, 217) report that the psychosexual disorders, impotence and dyspareunia, are subject to some of the highest rates of treatment failure when they occur in homosexually oriented individuals.

[7]Although the subject was not discussed above, homosexuals may have relatively high levels of psychic stress, especially neuroses, for a variety of reasons (cf. Rosen et al. 1972:275). This psychic stress could also contribute to subfecundity (cf. Chapters 2–5).

Sexual Deviations and Fertility

In addition to effects on fecundity, sexual deviations can lower fertility through other intermediate variables. For instance, certain deviations can be viewed as means of contraception (cf. Davis and Blake 1956:212). The most important intermediate variables, however, are undoubtedly celibacy, marriage, marital disruption, and coital frequency.

CELIBACY

Individuals with sexual deviations, especially homosexuality, have high rates of celibacy, as is evidenced by many studies. Saghir et al. (1969:224), for example, found that, of 89 homosexual men ranging in age from 19 to 70, 52% had never had sexual intercourse and another 17% had had it less than 5 times. Saghir and Robins (1969:194), in a study of 57 lesbians ranging in age from 20 to 55, report that 21% were virgins. In other studies of lesbians, Hedblom (1973:329) and Kenyon (1968a:1345, 1972:380) found 42–52% to be virgins.

MARRIAGE

Studies also indicate that homosexuals tend to marry less than do heterosexuals. In many cases, this is due to their own inclinations and preferences, and, in others it results from the fact that their deviant behavior makes them less competitive as marital candidates. Of the 89 homosexual men studied by Saghir et al. (1969:219), 82% had never been married and only 2% were currently married. In a study of overt lesbians, Kenyon (1970:200) reports that only 7% had been married. In another group of lesbians, Kenyon (1972:380) found that only 7 (26%) of 27 had ever married

Thus, homosexuals tend to be found in the nonmarried ranks. Gebhard (1972), citing the Kinsey material on white college-educated male homosexuals, reports: "Married adults are seen to have at any age roughly 1 to 1.5 percent predominantly homosexual members while the unmarried have a steadily increasing proportion of predominantly homosexual individuals ranging from about 12 percent at age 25 up to nearly one-third by age 35 [p.27]."

MARITAL DISRUPTION

Once married, sexually deviant individuals experience high rates of marital disruption. The revelation of deviations such as sadomasochism, transvestitism, or nymphomania is often sufficient cause in itself for disruption.

Homosexuals, in particular, have a difficult time keeping their heterosexual unions intact, since homosexuality is a personality trait fundamentally incompatible with marriage (Oliven 1974:524, 1965:279). Many homosexuals marry in an attempt to prove they can be heterosexual or because it is a prescribed societal norm. Such marriages usually do not succeed (Friederich 1970b:697). Statistics on marital disruption among homosexuals are not abundant, but the study of Saghir and his associates (1969:219) found that, of 16 ever-married homosexual men, only 2 (13%) were currently married at the time of interview. Interestingly, Imielinski (1969:127) discovered that the probability of marital disruption among homosexuals is directly related to their Kinsey number. Thus, exclusively or almost exclusively homosexual individuals, the focus of this review, have the highest rates of marital disruption.

Marriages involving lesbians are usually followed quickly by a divorce (Oliven 1974:529). Latent homosexual women, however, are sometimes married for years before they "come out." The psychoanalyst Socarides observes that such lesbians are particularly liable to enter into unsatisfying unions and to persist in them to the detriment of all concerned. He believes that lesbianism is a frequent cause of frigidity but that it is difficult to determine how many marriages founder from this cause, since women may deceive themselves as to the reasons for their difficulties and complain of depression or other symptoms apparently unrelated to homosexuality (West 1968:160). A recent survey (Levin 1975:190) of 100,000 women found that lesbian activities were much more frequent among a group of separated, divorced, and widowed women as compared to the participants as a whole. Sexual encounters with other women were reported by 10% of the former group but by only 4% of the latter group.

COITAL FREQUENCY

In those marriages of sexual deviates that do persist, coital frequency becomes the key intermediate variable affecting fertility. Obviously, homosexuals probably have a below-average frequency of intercourse. And individuals with other forms of sexual deviation, such as transvestitism, tend with uncommon frequency to be low-powered in genitopelvic eroticism (Money 1967:285). Also, excessive masturbation can have the same negative effect on fertility as too frequent coitus because of its tendency to reduce the quantity and quality of sperm available for conceptive purposes (Dubin and Amelar 1971:471). Finally, some of the male deviations are treated with drugs that, as a side effect, diminish libido.

Coital frequency is also related to the marital partner's attitude toward the other's sexual deviation. For example, if a husband requires some form of sexual ritual to achieve potency, coital frequency and fertility may well depend on whether the wife can tolerate and/or participate in the ritual (Johnson 1968:78). If she can, coital frequency may not be a fertility-depressing factor. Indeed, Dubin and Amelar (1972:582) described one such couple in which the husband could only have sexual intercourse if his wife were wearing riding breeches and boots prior to the act. The wife obliged him and the couple easily achieved pregnancy. However, if the partner cannot accept the ritual, coital frequency will probably be low, and abstinence may even ensue.

Where artificial insemination is available, the negative effect on fertility of sexual deviation can be moderated. Again, Dubin and Amelar (1972) provide an example. In their words: "One couple . . . is of interest as the husband was a homosexual and the wife a lesbian. Neither desired nor could tolerate sex with the other; yet they desired children. They requested homologous artificial insemination and they had a child [p. 582]."

In sum, sexual deviations can lower the fertility of individuals through a variety of intermediate variables other than, and probably more important than, subfecundity. The influence of these factors is best documented for homosexuals, a group known to have abnormally low fertility (cf. Baker 1967:94; Davis 1976:255; Oliven 1965:564). In one study of 123 lesbians, for example, Kenyon (1968a:1345) found that only 24 (19.5%) had ever been pregnant. Just what effect sexual deviations can have on population fertility has never been estimated, though the few social scientists who mention the possibility generally discount it immediately, apparently without much consideration (cf. Nag 1962:35; Petersen 1975:200; Thomlinson 1976:173). Nevertheless, on the basis of the material presented in this discussion, it is clear that sexual deviations can lower the fertility of a minor proportion of the population, at least of developed nations such as the United States, by depressing the fecundity of affected persons and, probably more importantly, by reducing the pool of eligible reproducers. The evidence presented here on homosexuality alone, a condition shared by probably 2—4% of the U.S. reproductive population, appears sufficient to justify this conclusion.

8

Alcoholism

Alcoholism is a chronic behavioral disorder manifested by repeated drinking of alcoholic beverages in excess of the dietary and social uses of the community and to an extent that interferes with the drinker's health or his social or economic functioning.[1] The American Psychiatric Association views alcoholism as a personality disorder when alcohol intake is great enough to damage physical health or personal or social functioning or when it has become a prerequisite to normal functioning (APA 1968:45). The American Medical Association also classifies alcoholism as a psychological illness, to wit, a personality disorder of the sociopathic variety (Kessel 1966:131).

Alcoholism is treated in this study under the personality-disorder heading and the drug-abuse subheading. The following statement by Goode (1973) indicates why this is an appropriate classification:

> In terms of medical pathology, alcohol is the most dangerous drug consumed routinely by a large number of people. It is more dangerous, by far, than heroin, for instance. Alcohol is addictive if taken in large quantities over a prolonged period of time, and the withdrawal symptoms, known as delerium tremens, or the "DTs," are characterized by nausea, vomiting, tremors, convulsions, de-

[1]This is the World Health Organization's definition of alcoholism. But alcoholism has a wide range of definitions. Ward (1975:375) notes there are well over 200 definitions of the condition, some of them conflicting. For a discussion of some of the more popular definitions, see Mauss (1975:282–284).

lerium, sometimes hallucinations and coma, and occasionally, death. The effects of the alcohol abstinence syndrome are more severe and life threatening than is true for the narcotics withdrawal, but is similar in all significant respects to that produced by barbiturate dependence [p. 19].

The Relationships between Alcoholism and Subfecundity

To date, systematic research on the fecundity of alcoholics is nonexistent. Knowledge concerning the fecundity of female alcoholics is particularly lacking because, as Linbeck (1972:567) notes, the female alcoholic has been the stepchild in this field of research, and, though references to her problems are abundant, concentrated focus on her is comparatively rare. Nevertheless, there is much in the literature that indicates that many alcoholics, male and female, are subfecund. These persons were either (a) subfecund prior to becoming alcoholic, or the subfecundity (b) is a direct result of the alcohol itself, or (c) arises from pathological states that are the direct (e.g., liver cirrhosis) or indirect (e.g., malnutrition) result of excessive alcohol consumption, or (d) is due to some other subfecundity-producing condition (e.g., psychic stress) that also causes the alcoholism, or (e) is the result of various combinations of the above. Each of the first four relationships, which have been schematically portrayed in Figure 1.1, will be discussed in turn.

REVERSE CAUSAL

In some alcoholics, the drinking problem is precipitated by a life crisis. And many of those who become alcoholic, according to psychoanalysts, do so because of sexual and reproductive problems (Levine 1955:675). Indeed, the onset of alcoholism in both men and women is often preceded by a variety of reproductive dysfunctions. Masters and Johnson (1970:149–150), for example, describe the case of a man who became alcoholic because he was unable to face the psychosocial pressures of his sexual dysfunction.

In women, frigidity and inorgasmy, two psychosexual disorders common among alcoholics that may cause subfecundity (cf. Chapter 3), often precede the onset of alcoholism (cf. Beckman 1975:809; Blane 1968:116; Kinsey 1966:10–11; Linbeck 1972:571; Mayer-Gross et al. 1969:162; and Sherfey 1955:24,32,36). In one study (Levine 1955:677) of 16 alcoholic women, virtually all were characterized as inorgasmic and frigid; in another (Kinsey 1966:180), 33 of 44 alcoholic women were frigid prior to becoming alcoholic. Menstrual dysfunctions are also linked to the onset of alcoholism (Beckman 1975:809), as are abortions (Blane 1968:115). In all, Kinsey

(1966:180) found that 13 of 44 alcoholic women linked infertility to the onset of their alcoholism. Linbeck (1972) sums it up nicely as follows:

> Alcohol is used as a solution to problems long before it becomes their cause. The reasons women give for their chronic, excessive use of alcohol are premenstrual tension, dysmenorrhea, menopause, hysterectomy, infertility, abortion, post-partum depression, miscarriage, frigidity, death, desertion, divorce, the demands of small children, marital troubles, and boredom. There is a high incidence of surgical operations on the uterus and ovaries [pp. 570–571].

Thus, subfecund individuals, in comparison to the general population, probably have a relatively high risk of becoming alcoholic.

DIRECT CAUSAL

Recent research has shown that alcohol may affect fecundity directly, without intermediate pathology such as liver cirrhosis. For example, alcohol may interfere with the metabolism of hormones necessary for the maintenance of potency (Rubin *et al.* 1976:563). It may also interfere with spermatogenesis by a toxic action on the germinal epithelium of the testes (*British Medical Journal* 1955:1170). These mechanisms will be detailed in later discussions of the effect of alcoholism on coital inability and conceptive failure.

INTERVENING CAUSAL

Alcoholism in men and women has long been associated with a wide variety of morbid states (Medhus 1974:5), shortening life expectancy by 10–12 years (USDHEW 1973:112). Whether the observed pathology is due to the toxic effects of alcohol itself or, more likely, to a combination of excessive alcohol consumption and poor diet (Burns 1974:749) is hard to disentangle. Whatever the exact etiology, alcoholism may culminate in a variety of clinical problems, including several types of liver disease, chronic relapsing peptic ulcer and its complications, chronic diarrhea, acute and chronic pancreatitis, cardiomyopathy, a wide variety of acute and chronic brain syndromes, peripheral neuropathy, skeletal myopathy, disorders of the haematopoietic system, chronic bronchitis and cancer of larynx and bronchi, as well as many other disorders (Burns 1974:749; Rosen *et al.* 1972:305). For the interested reader, detailed discussion of the illnesses associated with alcholism can be found in Wallgren and Barry (1970:721–725) and in the report of the National Commission on Marihuana and Drug Abuse (1973:194–196).

German's study (1973:662–665) of 122 chronic alcoholic men admitted to an alcoholic detoxification ward provides a good example of the extent of medical problems among alcoholics. Of 122 patients, 119 had one or more medical problems in addition to alcoholism, most of which were directly or indirectly related to their addiction. The nature of these problems and the percentage frequency in the group are as follows: liver, 81%; neurological, 67%; gastrointestinal, 62%; cardiac, 47%; trauma, 30%; anemia, 25%; and infections, 43%. Infections, for example, were present in 52 patients, 19 of whom had more than one. Ten patients had a recent history of active tuberculosis; 13 had pneumonia; 27 had a miscellaneous group of infections such as orchitis, epididymitis, gonorrhea, and so forth. German notes that the medical disorders related to and stemming from alcoholism are being recognized as increasingly complex and severe.

Thus, alcoholics have high rates of physical illness, and among these are some that are known to adversely affect fecundity, namely, malnutrition, liver cirrhosis, tuberculosis, venereal disease, and trauma. The relationship between each of these disorders and alcoholism will be discussed in turn, though discussion of the mechanism by which they alter fecundity will be reserved for the following section (unless otherwise noted).

Malnutrition Clinical experience with humans and experimental studies on animals both indicate that many of the pathological effects attributed to alcohol are caused by alcohol only indirectly, through the nutritional deficiency that is a consequence of prolonged, excessive drinking (Clinard 1968:396; Wallgren and Barry 1970:806). Alcoholics usually have weak appetites because the large amounts of alcohol consumed provide much of their energy requirement. However, alcohol has little nutritive value, and the consequent restriction of food intake creates risk of malnutrition. This risk is increased in most alcoholics because of the poor quality of the food that is usually eaten (Wallgren and Barry 1970:490). Moreover, alcohol also interferes with the body's ability to utilize the nutrients that are consumed. Indeed, Iber (cited in Green 1974:715) contends that virtually all alcoholics are apt to become malnourished, if for no other reason than the small intestine's reduced ability to absorb proteins, fats, and vitamins (cf. also Wallgren and Barry 1970:183, 806). Thus, a condition of suboptimal nutrition is the rule among alcoholics even when overt deficiencies are not yet apparent (Wallgren and Barry 1970:490).

Some important diseases associated with defective nutrition in alcoholic persons are liver damage, polyneuropathy (associated with deficiency of vitamin B1), pellegra (due to deficiency of niacin and other fractions of the Vitamin B complex), anemia (due to deficiency of iron and cobalamin), and scurvy (due to deficiency of Vitamin C) (USDHEW 1973:135–136).

The effect of poor nutrition on fecundity has received considerable attention in the literature (cf. Mosley 1977).

Liver Cirrhosis Another subfecundity producing disorder common among alcoholics is liver cirrhosis. This is a disease marked by progressive destruction of liver cells, with resulting fibrosis (*Dorland's* 1965:310). Though one of the best-known consequences of heavy drinking, it is caused primarily by nutritional deficiencies and only secondarily by excessive alcohol consumption (Wallgren and Barry 1970:721, 807). Many workers are convinced that adequate nutrition provides effective protection against cirrhosis even in heavy drinkers (USNIMH, n.d.:22). But others (Isselbacher and Greenberger 1964; Lieber and Davidson 1962; Rubin and Lieber 1968) have shown that large amounts of alcohol may cause liver damage even in well-fed individuals.

Although liver cirrhosis is found in moderate drinkers and in abstainers, alcoholism greatly increases the risk (Wallgren and Barry 1970:721). Indeed, alcoholics account for a high proportion of liver cirrhosis cases (Lippincott 1966:52). Estimates by Lelbach (1966, cited in Wallgren and Barry 1970:722) of the percentage of cirrhosis cases attributable at least in part to alcoholism are as follows: North and South America, 25–87%; France, 65–83%; Switzerland, 49–88%; England, 4–55%; and Germany 6–46%.

The exact proportion of alcoholics who have liver cirrhosis is uncertain, though most authorities believe that it must be fairly large (cf. Wallgren and Barry 1970:722). Van Thiel and Lester (1974:252) and Van Thiel *et al.* (1974a:941) conclude that about 10% of alcoholics ultimately develop cirrhosis. Lellbach (1966) found liver cirrhosis in 39 (12%) of 320 alcoholics, and Leevy and tenHove (1967) observed it in 20% of 3000 randomly selected alcoholic patients (cf. Wallgren and Barry 1970:721). Wilkinson and associates (1971:1217) report that 10% of their 1000 alcoholic patients had cirrhosis, and Fox (1966:506) found that 15% of his alcoholic patients showed signs of liver involvement. Judging from the results of these studies, the proportion of alcoholics who have liver cirrhosis probably falls within the 10–20% range.

Tuberculosis Tuberculosis (TB) is another subfecundity-producing disease with a much higher incidence among alcoholics than in the general population (Fox 1966:508; Pincock 1964:851). Wallgren and Barry (1970:724) note that the occurrence of tuberculosis is strongly associated with heavy drinking in France, and Seixas (1971:51) reports that the incidence of alcoholism today in U.S. tuberculosis hospitals runs from 50 to 60%.

Genital tuberculosis is a well-identified, though little considered, cause of subfecundity. In women, tuberculous salpingitis is an important cause of infertility. Since it is usually asymptomatic, difficult to diagnose, and treatment will not restore fecundity, it is a potential population fecundity factor where TB is a prevalent disease.

Venereal Disease Alcoholics also tend to have high rates of another subfecundity-producing disorder, venereal disease (cf. Medhus 1975:29). This is particularly true of female alcoholics, many of whom become promiscuous when their need for money to purchase alcohol becomes sufficiently great (Gebhard 1965:485). Indeed, it has been noted that many prostitutes are alcoholics (Oliven 1974:452). An increase in sexual activity with assorted partners is invariably associated with venereal disease. In one series of 71 female alcoholics, Medhus (1975:29) found that 25 had a history of gonorrhea and 5 had a history of syphilis. Altogether, there were 53 cases reported by 28 women, a rate reportedly about 8 times that of the general population. Another study (Hagnell and Tunving 1972:81) found venereal disease to be 5 times as frequent among a group of alcoholics as among controls. And, in a study of 80 patients with cirrhosis at a hospital in Uganda, syphilis was established in 63% of the 19 alcoholics but in only 10% of the 61 nonalcoholics (Sadikali 1975:69). A Russian study (Bondarevskii 1974; cf. *Journal of Studies of Alcohol* 1976:1104) of women VD patients reports that many of these women were alcoholic and concludes that alcoholic VD patients represent the main source of infection in the country.

The effect of syphilis and gonorrhea on population fecundity has already been discussed by the present author (McFalls 1973).

Trauma Fox (1966:502) and Sclare (1970:103) have noted high rates of traumatic injuries among alcoholics. In one series of 1000 alcoholics, Wilkinson *et al.* (1971:1217) found that 11.6% had had major traumatic injuries, mostly the result of road traffic accidents. Alcoholics typically leave even serious injuries untreated for long periods of time. Subfecundity may result from many traumatic injuries, especially if these involve the head and spine.

SPURIOUS CAUSAL

Finally, the subfecundity observed in alcoholics may be due to some other subfecundity-producing condition that also caused the alcoholism. Paramount among such conditions are the various other types of psychopathology. Indeed, alcoholics tend to have high rates of those types of psychopathology discussed elsewhere in this book (USDHEW 1973:110). Simple psychic stress may be at the root of both problems, for, as Kaufman (1967) notes, "A man who drinks heavily and also has precarious potency may just be reflecting a basic emotional tension in two separate symptoms [p. 137]." Often the mental disturbance is more serious, however; Wallgren and Barry (1970:725) have noted a high incidence among alcoholics of schizophrenia, depression, and psychopathic personality.

Homosexuality may also be more prevalent among alcoholics than in the general population, though certainly there is some disagreement on this point (cf. Kinsey 1966:6–7, 38). In one study (Kinsey 1968:1464), homosexuality was linked to the onset of alcoholism in 3 of 36 women. Saghir *et al.* (1970, cited in Beckman 1975:809) report that lesbians are more likely to be alcoholics than are heterosexual women. However, Beckman (1975:809) cautions that the higher proportion of alcoholics found by Saghir *et al.* may be due to a variety of factors that were not controlled in their research. It appears that the relationship between alcoholism and homosexuality is not a simple one; rather, as discussed by Wallgren and Barry (1970):

> Strong homosexual drives, repressed from conscious awareness, have been attributed to male alcoholics (Lorland, 1945). Contrary to the suggestion of repression of this tendency is a report by McCord *et al.* (1959, 1960), that two of six homosexual boys (33%) became alcoholic compared with 27 (16%) of 166 normally masculine boys and only one (4%) of 24 feminine boys. Gibbins and Walters (1960) reported that male alcoholics were intermediate between male homosexuals and normal men in their reactions to verbal and pictorial symbols of male and female sexuality. This finding is consistent with Menninger's (1938) suggestion of inadequate development of mature sexuality in alcoholics [pp. 737–738].

Another form of psychopathology, not yet discussed, that has a negative effect on fecundity is excessive smoking, and alcoholics tend to be heavy smokers (cf. Dreher and Fraser 1967:259, 1968:65; Fox 1966:507; USPHS 1971:5; Walton 1972:1455). To wit, Burns (1974) observes: "As though committed to a policy of self-destruction, the alcoholic subjects his respiratory system to an almost continuous barrage of cigarette smoke throughout his waking hours [p. 749]." Walton (1972:1456), having found that 123 of 130 alcoholics smoked at least one pack per day, in contrast to only 46 of 100 nonalcoholics, suggests that heavy smoking constitutes part of the syndrome of alcohol addiction. The relationship between smoking and fecundity is discussed at length in Chapter 9.

The above discussion clearly illustrates that alcoholics have high rates of physical and psychiatric illnesses (Wallgren and Barry 1970:725), many of which are capable of adversely affecting fecundity. Whether these relationships are causal (and, if so, the direction of the causality) or merely associative is often difficult to discern. The same difficulties will be encountered in the next section, in the discussion of the effects of alcoholism on coital inability, conceptive failure, and pregnancy loss. Is the impotence observed in a given alcoholic due to temporary or permanent alcohol-induced damage to neurological tissue, or to the direct interference by alcohol with normal testosterone metabolism, or to liver cirrhosis, or to malnutrition? All these possibilities and more are discussed; but, as the designation of causality is a painstaking process with each individual, for an entire study population it is nearly impossible. Thus, many cited studies are able only to show a correlation between specific types of reproductive dysfunction and alcoholism, without reference to etiology.

Mechanisms by Which Alcoholism Causes Subfecundity

COITAL INABILITY

[Alcohol] . . . it provokes desire but it takes away performance.

As this oft-quoted passage in Shakespeare's *Macbeth* demonstrates, it has long been recognized that excessive use of alcohol can lead to coital inability in men. Currently, the medical literature on male alcoholics is replete with references to their high risk of impotence (cf. Amelar *et al.* 1977:205; Burns 1974:749; Cooper 1972:549; Farkas and Rosen 1976:271; Ford and Beach 1951:238; Hastings 1960:430; Johnson 1968:32–33, 36; Kaufman 1967:137; Kessel 1966:133; Leavitt 1974:314; Masters and Johnson 1970:184; Mayer-Gross *et al.* 1969:162; Neshkov 1969:769; Oliven 1974:382, 447; Pearlman and Kobashi 1972:300; Rubin *et al.* 1976:563; Seixas 1971:49; Sherfey 1955:23, 30, 34, 37; Stewart 1975:42; Strecker and Chambers 1949:107; and Talkington 1971:27).

Oliven (1974) describes the sexual life of male alcoholics as follows:

> The chronic alcoholic is often impotent. When he is on a spree he has "no time" for females; if anything, he prefers the company of men to drink, talk and feel good with. When he is on the wagon his marital or love relationship most often turns platonic after a few months and for the next 2 or 3 years he often fares better for a long period if no great sexual obligations confront him. Both organic and psychologic explanations have been advanced to explain this, but the cause remains largely unknown. The malnourished chronic drinker with peripheral neuropathy is very frequently impotent. This applies also to most alcoholic derelicts [p.382].

Similarly, Talkington (1971) observes:

> A large amount of alcohol has a great deterrent effect on sexual performance. The emotional factors which result in chronic alcoholism may or may not produce impotence: alcoholism does produce impotence. Perhaps all heavy drinkers have some degree of impotence. The evidence is that there is much hidden alcoholism in patients who complain of impotence. This may be one of the most frequently missed points in diagnostic history [p.27].

Van Thiel and Lester (1974:252) note that alcoholism is almost certainly the most common cause of nonfunctional impotence in the United States.

Alcohol can produce impotence in several ways. It is a depressant, and large amounts can act on the central nervous system to diminish normal functioning (Cross 1973:2); it may temporarily depress the sexual reflexes to the point of abolishing them (Oliven 1965:434). Moreover, the chronic abuse of alcohol can cause neurological damage. Smith *et al.* (1972:523) and Lemere and Smith (1973:212) contend that much of the impotence found in alcoholic men is due to alcohol-induced damage to structures involved in sexual functioning or what they term the neurologic reflex arc that subserves erection. Theoretically, this arc includes: "1) the cerebral cortex, from where sexual thoughts arise, 2) the anterior portion of the temporal lobe, which determines intensity of libido, 3) perhaps the hypothalamus, 4) the spinal cord reflex center for erection, and 5) the peripheral nerves that convey sensory and vasomotor impulses to and from the genital organs [Lemere and Smith 1973:212]." Smith and his associates (1972:523), in support of their own view, cite the work of Segal *et al.* (1970), who emphasize the damage produced to deep brain structures by prolonged excessive use of alcohol and who report that decreased potency is regularly noted among patients with such damage.

The chronic abuse of alcohol may also cause impotence by upsetting the hormonal balance of the body. Prolonged drinking of alcohol, for instance, can stimulate the liver to drastically increase destruction of the male sex hormone, testosterone, which is essential for the maintenance of normal masculine characteristics, such as potency. Up to 5 times the normal amount of the liver enzyme that breaks down testosterone may be produced, and the human body apparently does not produce more testosterone to make up for the inordinate loss after prolonged drinking (Rubin *et al.* 1976:563). Others have hypothesized that testosterone synthesis would be reduced in the presence of excessive levels of alcohol (Van Thiel and Lester 1974:253). As liver disease is not a prerequisite for such effects, a large number of alcoholics probably experience decreased testosterone levels and diminished potency.

The temporary impotence induced by excessive alcohol ingestion is also a cause of both primary and secondary psychogenic impotence. Steward (1975) notes "that many patients with primary impotence first develop difficulty after a bout of drinking [p.42]." Similarly, Masters and Johnson (1970:143) discuss two cases of men who failed in their first attempts at intercourse while drunk and became primarily impotent. Also, in 35 of 213 secondarily impotent men referred to them (1970:164), there was a specific history of onset of impotence as a direct result of acute ingestion of alcohol. In fact, according to Masters and Johnson (1970), "The second most frequent factor in onset of secondary impotence can be directly related to a specific incident of acute ingestion of alcohol or to a pattern of excessive alcohol intake per se [p.160]." Thus, alcoholic impotence may begin as a temporary organic problem but often continues and is reinforced due to psychological problems. A vicious circle may then develop, as described by Melchiode (1976):"A very common example is the man who has had too much alcohol to drink. The alcohol then interferes with his ability to function [impotence]. The man reacts to this with anxiety and may try to deal with the anxiety by calming himself with alcohol which, of course, perpetuates the problem [p.98]." Similarly, Van Thiel and Lester (1974:252) point out that sexual inadequacy further disturbs the already alcoholic individual, perhaps exacerbating the need for alcohol and creating a vicious circle.

Impotence may also be due to liver damage, which excessive drinking produces in a substantial minority of alcoholics (cf. Cross 1973:7; Gonick 1976:192; Kaufman 1967:137; Kent et al. 1973:111; and Lloyd and Williams 1948:35). Sherlock (1955, cited in Johnson 1968:29) states that 70% of men with hepatic cirrhosis have reduced sexual potency due to associated testicular atrophy. A study by Van Thiel and his associates (1974b) of 40 male alcoholics with liver disease found testicular atrophy in 50% and impotence in 85%. Earlier studies hypothesized that the hypogonadism and impotence were caused by abnormal metabolism of sex hormones in a severely damaged liver (Lloyd and Williams 1948:325). But recent findings (Rubin et al. 1976:563; Van Thiel and Lester 1974:252) have cast some doubt on this hypothesis, since they found hypogonadism in mild as well as severe cases of liver disease.

For the sake of convenience, the relationship between hypogonadism and impotence in alcoholics both with and without liver disease is discussed again briefly in the conceptive failure section in conjunction with a discussion of spermatogenic failure.

Impotence in alcoholic men may also be due to malnutrition, a common feature of alcoholism (cf. Johnson 1968:32). Alcoholics also tend to have extraordinarily high rates of trauma, usually as a result of accidents they have while intoxicated. Impotence is likely to be the outcome of a portion of this trauma, particularly in conditions such as paraplegia or head trauma (Gonick 1976:192). Incidently, chronic alcoholism can also be a direct cause of paraplegia. This form of paraplegia is probably dependent upon peripheral neuritis (Dorland's 1965:1099).

Although the literature is full of sources that point to a relationship between alcoholism and impotence and some that suggest that impotence is regularly found in alcoholics (cf. Hastings 1960:430; Mayer-Gross et al. 1969:162; Talkington 1971:27; and Van Thiel and Lester 1974:252), there are few scientific studies of the sexual behavior of alcoholics (Johnson 1968:32) and none, to this author's knowledge, that offer an estimate of the prevalence of impotence among alcoholics. There is, however, an estimate of the proportion of alcoholics who experience impotence once they are completely detoxified (Lemere and Smith 1973:212; Smith *et al.* 1972:523). Smith and his associates found that 8% of the 17,000 alcoholic patients treated at Shadel Hospital over a 35-year period complained of impotence after detoxification. In approximately 50% of these cases, impotence persisted even after years of sobriety. These authors did not report, and perhaps did not ascertain, what proportion of these men were impotent prior to detoxification. Unfortunately, it is proportions such as this that are necessary for estimation of the fecundity of alcoholics.

Despite the widespread use of alcohol, it is a fair assessment that its effects on coital ability have not been adequately or extensively studied. Aside from its relationship to impotence (reported above), there is little else in the literature. In particular, there are no reports on the impact of alcohol or alcoholism on the coital ability of women (Merari *et al.* 1973:1075). Blane (1968:116) does report that investigations repeatedly reveal that sexual inhibition is a common factor in alcoholic women and that they find sexual relations painful. At least part of this pain may by due to dyspareunia or vaginismus. In any event, Blane notes that sexual activity is minimal, sometimes nonexistent, among alcoholic women. Lemere and Smith (1973:213) found, however, that few of their female alcoholic patients complained of sexual inadequacy from drinking.

CONCEPTIVE FAILURE

In men, alcoholism is associated with hypogonadism, two manifestations of which are feminization marked by loss of libido and impotence, as previously described, and spermatogenic failure. These are commonly seen in men with advanced liver disease, including 50–75% of male alcoholics with liver cirrhosis (cf. Amelar 1966:19; Behrman and Kistner 1968:5; Galvao-Teles *et al.* 1973:174; Gordon *et al.* 1976:793; Kent *et al.* 1973:111; Lippincott 1963:44; Lloyd and Williams 1948:315; Rubin *et al.* 1976:563; Van Thiel and Lester 1974:252; and Van Thiel *et al.* 1974a:941). Earlier workers thought that these abnormalities resulted from elevated estrogen levels because the damaged liver was unable to inactivate or dispose of these hormones (Van Thiel *et al.* 1974b:1188–1189). But recent investigators have shown, first, that steroidal estrogens are not elevated in men with liver insufficiency (Van Thiel *et al.* 1974b:1189) and, second, that hypogonadism in male alcoholics occurs in persons whose liver functions and histology range from near normal to severely deranged (Rubin *et al.* 1976:563; Van Thiel and Lester 1974:252).

The possibility thus arises that hypogonadism, with its associated sterility (and impotence), may be a direct result of the alcohol and not of alcohol-
induced liver disease. If this is true, many more alcoholics, not just the 10%
who develop cirrhosis, could be expected to experience sterility (and impotence) (Van Thiel and Lester 1974:252).

Support for this hypothesis comes from many corners. Alcohol is known,
for example, to suppress the secretion of pituitary hormones. Thus, spermatogenesis, which is stimulated by a pituitary hormone (and testosterone
secretion, which is also controlled by a pituitary hormone and which is
responsible primarily for maintenance of the secondary sexual characteristics and potency), could be altered (Van Thiel et al. 1974b:1196). Also spermatogenesis may be altered directly by two other routes. First, alcohol could
be directly toxic to the germinal epithelium of the testes (British Medical
Journal 1955:1170); second, it might interfere with conversion of Vitamin A
to retinal, a compound necessary for spermatogenesis (Van Thiel et al.
1974:941).

In a study by Van Thiel et al. (1974b), an attempt was made to examine
the semen of 22 male alcoholics who were hospitalized with liver diseases
ranging from slight fibrosis to end-stage cirrhosis. Since 18 of these men
were impotent, only 4 were able to produce specimens. Two of those men
were consistently azoospermic and another was oligospermic. Thus, 3 of the
4 alcoholic men able to produce an ejaculate showed evidence of spermatogenic failure. It is likely that a similar proportion of the total sample was
also so affected.

In addition to depressing sperm count, alcoholism has a downgrading
effect on the structure and function of sperm (Oliven 1965:192). Thus, not only
are there often fewer sperm available for impregnation, but their fertilizing
ability may also be diminished. Moreover, Molnar and Papp (1973:105) conclude that prolonged alcohol consumption irritates the prostatic tissue, which
then produces mucous semen. After ejaculation, sperm trapped in such
semen have a reduced opportunity to migrate successfully to the egg. This is
yet another cause of infertility.

Finally, male alcoholism may also be associated with two sperm transport
problems, premature ejaculation and ejaculatory incompetence, for, contrary
to popular notion, alcohol has a deleterious effect on orgasm (cf. Merari et al.
1973:1095). Of 16 alcoholic men who engaged in frequent coitus, Levine
(1955:677) found that 2 (13%) were premature ejaculators. And Oliven
(1974:446) has suggested that excessive amounts of alcohol can even abolish
ejaculation.

Female alcoholics also have high rates of infertility (Beckman 1975:810;
Linbeck 1972:570–571; Wilsnack 1973:79). One of the reasons, as discussed
earlier, is that many women become alcoholics because of conceptive failure.

But aside from selecting for infertile women, alcoholism itself causes conceptive failure through the effect of excessive amounts of alcohol per se and the
effects of associated disorders, such as malnutrition and cirrhosis.

Amenorrhea is a not infrequent disorder in alcoholic women. According
to Oliven (1965), "The female cyclic functions tend to suspend themselves
during episodic exacerbations in chronic alcoholism [p.384]." Amenorrhea
and other menstrual problems may be related to the damage alcohol inflicts
on the endocrine glands, especially the thyroid and ovary (Rosen *et al.*
1972:305). And an early source (*British Medical Journal* 1955:1170) suggests
that amenorrhea is most likely caused by an alcohol-induced disturbance in
the pituitary–ovarian relationship.

Women whose alcoholism is complicated by cirrhosis of the liver have
particularly high rates of conceptive failure (Block 1972:143; Lloyd and Williams 1948:315; Whelpton and Sherlock 1968:996). Amenorrhea and irregular menstrual cycles are so common in such women that pregnancy rarely
occurs (Shaltuck and Spellacy 1965:171; Slaughter and Krantz 1963:1060).
Green and Rubin (1959) summarize the findings of other studies concerning
the prevalence of amenorrhea among women with liver disease as follows:

> Patek found that return to a normal menstrual cycle was a sign of recovery of
> liver function in chronic liver disease. He notes other reports of amenorrhea
> associated with chronic liver disease. In Eppinger's series 25 percent had scanty,
> irregular menstrual periods as an early symptom of liver disease, and in Rolles-
> ton's series metrorrhagia was an early symptom followed later by amenorrhea.
> Armas-Cruz noted amenorrhea in 59 percent of women of menstruating age
> with chronic liver disease, and similar findings are recorded by Bearn and
> associates, 15 of whose 23 patients had amenorrhea prior to or coincidentally
> with onset of other symptoms. Lloyd and Williams found that 50 percent of their
> patients, and Ratnoff and Patek 40 percent of theirs, had amenorrhea [p.144].

Green and Rubin (1959:141) also note that chronic liver disease may addi-
tionally cause premature menopause.

PREGNANCY LOSS

The proposition that excessive drinking has a negative effect on offspring during pregnancy has a long history. In an historical survey of the
American and British literature, Warner and Rosett (1975) show, for example,
that this topic was of major concern to eighteenth, nineteenth, and early
twentieth century clinicians and researchers. However, they found that
"because of the moralistic tone of medical temperance writing, America and
Britain chose in the latter half of the twentieth century, after Prohibition, to
discount or forget the previous work on parental drinking [pp. 1395–1396]."

Although relatively little is known today concerning the effect of alcoholism on the developing fetus (Gilder 1974:903; Green 1974:713), interest in this topic has recently been revived as researchers are recognizing the deleterious effect of chronic alcoholism on the fetus (cf. Ulleland 1972:169).

It is difficult to determine how these negative effects come about, for, as already stressed in this discussion, alcoholism is usually complicated by other health problems that adversely affect reproduction. Important among these are malnutrition and liver cirrhosis. It has been difficult to assess the effects of the latter on pregnancy loss because, as noted earlier, few women with liver cirrhosis become pregnant, and the literature is understandably thin. But one study does report excessive pregnancy loss. Whelpton and Sherlock (1968:996) found that 7 of 15 pregnancies in women with liver disease were spontaneously aborted or stillborn; another resulted in neonatal death of a malformed child. Other authors (Block 1972:143; Shaltuck and Spellacy 1965:172; Slaughter and Krantz 1963:1066) tend to discount the proposition that such women have increased pregnancy loss. However, the extent of pregnancy loss from this cause remains uncertain due to lack of data.

There is mounting evidence from more than 100 studies that alcohol itself, even in small amounts, is harmful to the fetus (*Intercom* 1977a:3; Jones *et al.* 1973:1267; Little *et al.* 1976:379).[2] This observation has important demographic implications, for, as Forfar and Nelson (1973:634) report, 31% of pregnant women consume alcohol regularly and another 14% can be considered heavy drinkers. The National Institute on Alcohol Abuse and Alcoholism and the National Council on Alcoholism advise pregnant women to abstain from drinking altogether. These institutions note that the risk of fetal damage increases with the quantity of alcohol consumed. The risk is estimated to be 10% if 2–4 ounces are consumed daily and 74% if 10 ounces are consumed. The Council calculates that 250,000 of the 3.1 million live births projected for 1977 in the United States will have birth abnormalities due to alcohol consumed by their mothers (cf. *Intercom* 1977a:3).

Alcohol can endanger the developing fetus because alcohol readily crosses the placenta and travels through the bloodstream of the fetus in the same concentration as that of the mother. However, the developing organs of the fetus cannot process alcohol nearly as well as can those of its adult mother. For example, the undeveloped liver of the fetus can metabolize alcohol less

[2] A study by Little *et al.* (1976:375,379) found that pregnant women reported a decreased use of alcohol during pregnancy, often citing adverse physiological effects as a reason for the decline. The authors speculate that alcohol may be an embryotoxin and that the rejection may be based on the biological regulation to avoid substances that may be noxious to the fetus. Alcoholic women may not be able to heed this warning.

than half as fast as an adult liver can. As a result, alcohol remains in the fetal system longer than in the adult, giving it more time to produce deleterious effects (National Institute on Alcohol Abuse and Alcoholism 1978:4–5).

Whatever the mechanism (or mechanisms) involved, it is certain that alcoholic women often bear children with a host of birth defects. Current research suggests that the risk of serious problems in the developing fetus in an actively alcoholic woman is at least 30–50% (Gilder 1974:903; Hanson 1976:1458), and possibly higher. Typical defects include skull, face, and limb deformations, defects in the cardiovascular system, and mental and physical retardation. This pattern of defects has been labeled the "fetal alcohol syndrome" (cf. Gilder 1974; Jones et al. 1973, 1974; Jones and Smith 1973; Lemoine et al. 1968; Palmer et al. 1974; Smith et al. 1973; Smithells 1976; Tenbrinck and Buchin 1975; and Ulleland 1972).

Maternal alcoholism can also be fatal to the offspring both pre- and postnatally. In a study of pregnancy outcome in 23 alcoholic women and 46 matched controls, all participants in the Collaborative Perinatal Project, Jones et al. (1974:1076) report a perinatal mortality rate of 17% for offspring of alcoholic women as opposed to only 2% for the offspring of controls. Of the perinatal mortality in the former, half occurred prior to birth. It is noteworthy that participants in the Collaborative Perinatal Project had some degree of prenatal medical supervision and delivered in excellent medical hospitals. As prenatal care is suspect in alcoholic women (Green 1974:715), most would experience less favorable health care circumstances than those in the Collaborative Perinatal Project, and higher rates of perinatal mortality would likely ensue.

Finally, it should be noted that alcoholic women may be prone to pregnancy loss irrespective of their addiction. As has already been discussed, women subject to abortions are more likely than are successful reproducers to become alcoholic (Linbeck 1972:570; Wilsnack 1973:79).

There are also indications that male alcoholism may cause pregnancy loss (Babson and Benson 1971 :19; *Revue de Alcoolisme* 1975:xvii). Recent experiments with mice (cf. Badr and Badr 1975) have suggested that a male's heavy drinking might lead to spontaneous abortion, presumably by damaging the genetic material in the spermatozoa. A recent pilot study (cf. *Science News* 1975:116) tentatively confirms a relationship in humans between male alcoholism and spontaneous abortions and birth defects. In this study at St. Vincent's Hospital in Worcester, Mass., scientists studied 52 men who consumed at least four drinks a night during the six weeks prior to conception; a number of spontaneous abortions and infants with birth defects were noted in their offspring. The results of this study should be viewed with some caution, say the investigators, since no controls were used and other causative factors such as emotional stress were not ruled out. But suggestive evidence such as this underlines the need for more research to determine if alcoholism in the male can affect his germ plasm and ultimately his offspring.

Prevalence

At a recent United Nations Conference on drug abuse, the misuse of alcohol was judged to be the number one addiction in developed countries (McNall 1975:204). In the United States, alcohol is the most widely used and most abused drug (Horton and Leslie 1974:524; Mauss 1975:240). As a chronic illness, alcoholism is outranked in prevalence only by heart disease, cancer, and mental illness (not including alcoholism) (McNall 1975:205). The exact prevalence of alcoholism in the United States is almost impossible to measure (Mayer-Gross *et al.* 1969:389), and estimates vary substantially from about 5 to 10 million individuals. The most pessimistic writers claim that 9 to 10 million Americans are alcoholic, with millions more close to becoming so (cf. Galton 1978:10; Knowles 1976:62). The National Institute on Alcohol Abuse and Alcoholism agrees with this estimate, but the Rutgers Center for Alcohol Studies subscribes to a figure about 50% lower. Although many authorities estimate that alcoholics constitute about 7% of the U.S. population, most agree that the actual proportion remains unknown (Horton and Leslie 1974:539; McNall 1975:204; USNIMH n.d.:10).

About 50% of those who are alcoholics are between the ages of 25 and 54, the incidence of alcoholism dropping off sharply both before and after these ages (NcNall 1975:205; USNIMH 1967:20). The age distribution of alcoholics has been altered somewhat in recent years as there has been a marked increase in alcoholism among people in their twenties and thirties (Amelar *et al.* 1977:205; Mayer-Gross *et al.* 1969:390). Studies have shown that alcoholics typically have their first drinking experience at about age 16 and are alcoholic within 9–15 years thereafter (Clinard 1968:420; Suinn 1970:284). Women may begin this process later than men, but they develop more rapidly into alcoholics (Linbeck 1972:568; Rosen *et al.* 1972:313).

Traditionally, men were thought to have higher rates of alcoholism than were women, even taking into consideration that a smaller though unknown proportion of female alcoholics are counted than are male alcoholics because women are better able to mask their drinking by confining most of it to the home (Schafer *et al.* 1975:32). During the 1950s, for example, the ratio of male to female alcoholics was considered to be 5 or 6 to 1. The estimated ratio during the 1960s, however dropped to 4 to 1 and even lower (USNIMH, n.d.:10). Today, some physicians who specialize in the treatment of alcoholism believe that there are already as many women as men who are alcoholic (Galton 1978:10; Linbeck 1972:568). However, workers often question whether this increase in female alcoholism is more apparent than real, suggesting it may primarily reflect increased visibility of female alcoholics (cf. Kinsey 1966:6). There is a growing willingness of women alcoholics, for instance, to seek treatment (USNIMH, n.d.:10), yet it is still true that far fewer women than men alcoholics actually get help (Galton, 1978:10).

It is not known how many pregnant women are alcoholic, but one clinical series suggests that it might be as high as 14%. Forfar and Nelson (1973:632) report that of 911 pregnant women, 12% abstained from alcohol during their pregnancy, 43% took it occasionally, 31% took it regularly, and 14% were heavy drinkers.

It is frequently claimed that the rate of alcoholism in the United States is mounting rapidly (Gould 1976:262; Lieber 1972:326). However, though this may be an accurate assessment, there is no conclusive evidence supporting it, due to methodological and data problems (USNIMH, n.d.:11).[3] The National Institute of Mental Health does show an increase in the admission rate of alcoholics to state mental hospitals and in the number of clinics and beds in general hospitals that treat alcoholics (USNIMH, n.d.:11). Other trends also point to an overall increase in alcoholism, including two already mentioned: the recent increase in alcoholism among people in their twenties and thirties and the increase among women. Studies also report that young people appear to be drinking more frequently, in greater quantities, and more often to the point of drunkenness than ever before, trends that may feed an upward movement in the alcoholism rate (Gould 1976:262).

Alcoholism rates vary by population, culture, race, religion, socioeconomic status, urban–rural location, and other variables (Clinard 1968:418; Horton and Leslie 1974:543; Lieber 1972:326; Mauss 1975:281; Mayer-Gross et al. 1969:390; and Rosen et al. 1972:314). For instance, in developing countries and among individuals living within a simple culture, it is generally agreed that alcoholism is rare (Mayer-Gross et al. 1969:390).

---

[3]Petersen (1975:253–254) believes that the best index of alcoholism, particularly in a demographic context, is the number of deaths from associated ailments. He utilizes a formula devised by Jellinek that was designed to estimate the prevalence of alcoholism from the total number of deaths from diagnosed cirrhosis of the liver. Based on Jellinek's formula, Petersen concludes that alcoholism prevalence did not increase from the mid-1940s to 1960 and that any increase in the total number of alcoholics reflects the change in population number and structure rather than in prevalence. However, the value of this formula is very much in doubt. Statisticians state that it is unreliable, and Jellinek himself recommended in 1959 that it no longer be used (USNIMH, n.d.:11). This is a good example of why it is important for demographers to get a better understanding of the medical literature before utilizing it, especially an up-to-date understanding.

However, there is evidence that alcoholism is a serious and increasing problem in the urban areas of Africa (cf. Eisenberg 1973:2187) and is also gradually spreading to parts of Asia (cf. Garner 1971:219). Alcoholism can almost always be found in highly developed and affluent societies, but the prevalence varies widely. Alcoholism is an especially serious problem in France, where it is estimated that 12% of the population are alcoholics (Schafer *et al.* 1975:3), and in Russia, where it is virtually a national disease (Morrow 1977:49). A recent report (*Time* 1978b:58) indicates that alcoholism is also reaching epidemic proportions in Japan, where 6% of the population are alcoholic or problem drinkers—a fourfold jump since World War II. The prevalence of alcoholism in Japan will probably continue to soar because an increasing number of men and women of all ages are becoming dependent on the drug. Japanese women are becoming alcoholic at a faster rate even than Japanese men. And fully 63% of the male population believe that their lives are not possible without a few drinks. The diffusion of the problem to the younger age groups is evidenced by the fact that 20% of high school students admit that they need alcohol several times a week to relieve the pressures of academic life.

Population Subfecundity

Alcoholism is seldom investigated or even mentioned as a cause of population subfecundity, though a few historical and anthropological references do exist. From 1720 to 1750, England was swept by a "gin epidemic," the result of a law that lifted the traditional restrictions on distilling, leading to the availability and excessive consumption of inexpensive and plentiful gin. Several authors conclude that the concomitant fertility decline that is thought to have occurred was due to spreading alcoholism and its deleterious effect on fecundity (cf. Warner and Rossett 1975:1396–1397). Alcoholism has also been mentioned by anthropologists as a possible causal factor in the depopulation of various South Pacific societies (cf. Scragg 1957:7), and occasionally a demographer makes an incidental remark that alcoholism might affect population fecundity and ultimately fertility (e.g., Ryder 1959:417; U.N. 1973:77). However, the relationship between alcoholism and fecundity is all but ignored in the demographic literature.

This disregard on the part of demographers is clearly imprudent in view of the evidence presented here. Though the potential for alcoholism to influence population fecundity remains uncertain, there are several reasons to suspect that its influence can be substantial.

First, alcoholism can be prevalent enough to be a population factor. This is true even on the national level, as in France, where as many as 12% of the adult population are alcoholics. And, under the right social conditions, there is no reason why this rate cannot be exceeded. Indeed, alcoholism may be very common in certain population subgroups, particularly those experiencing social disintegration, such as Indians,[4] Eskimos, blacks, and Chicanos in the United States. There is a rough estimate, for instance, that 10–25% of families of welfare recipients have drinking problems (Green 1974:715).

Second, alcoholics are likely to be subfecund because of the tendency for subfecund people to become alcoholics and because alcoholism and its associated illnesses lead to subfecundity. The proportion of alcoholics who are subfecund and the amount of subfecundity they experience are unknown. If these facts were known, a definitive judgement could be made about the overall influence of alcoholism on population fecundity. However, alcoholism is considered by most subfecundity specialists as a serious threat to male and female reproductive potential because, as described above, alcoholics tend to be less able coitally, more infertile, and less capable of bringing a pregnancy to a successful conclusion than is the general population (cf. Babson and Benson 1971:19; Behrman and Kistner 1968:6; Brown 1965:133; Kleegman and Kaufman 1966:10; Siegler 1944:27). Van Thiel and Lester (1974:252), for instance, consider alcoholism as almost certainly the most common cause of nonfunctional coital inability and conceptive failure in the United States. Moreover, the recent upsurge of medical research into matters related to the effect of alcoholism on fecundity (e.g., hypogonadism, fetal alcohol syndrome) has invariably produced findings that point to a more substantial impact of alcoholism on fecundity than was previously thought.

Another reason why alcoholism may be a population fecundity factor is that the onset of alcoholism and its related subfecundity may occur early in reproductive life. It is known that more than 50% of alcoholics in the United States are currently within their reproductive period and that alcoholism has experienced a marked increase among people in their twenties. The onset of subfecundity related to alcoholism may vary with the particular condition experienced, but certainly many adverse effects, especially those attributable simply to excessive consumption, have an early onset. This is evidenced by the fact that many of the subfecund alcoholics in studies cited here were young. Since the majority of alcoholics are reluctant to seek medical attention for their condition and its associated illnesses and typically delay treatment inordinately (McNall 1975:204; Wallgren and Barry 1970:724), their subfecundity likewise persists indefinitely and for large chunks of their remaining reproductive careers.

[4]One bit of folklore about American Indians is that they have an inherited intolerance to alcohol and are less able to drink than whites. Evidence is accumulating that challenges this belief. Bennion and Li (1976:9) tested both groups and found no racial difference in the rate at which alcohol disappeared from the bloodstream. The high rates of alcoholism are probably due to the intense social disorganization that Indians experience.

In sum, the potential for alcoholism to influence population fecundity is unknown. However, a study of 28 alcoholic women and 28 controls by Wilsnack (1973:79–80) provides an inkling of how significant a population fecundity factor alcoholism might be. She found that more than 25% of the married alcoholics were unable to have children, as contrasted with only 4% of the married controls. A striking differerence in the incidence of gynecological and obstetrical disorders was also found. Of the ever-married alcoholics, 78% reported such disorders, in comparison to only 35% of the controls. Difficulties in conceiving, permanent sterility, and repeated abortion were the most common problems cited among the alcoholics.

Thus, it is distinctly possible that alcoholism may be an important determinant of population fecundity. And, due to wide variations in prevalence, this effect would be variable from population to population, subgroup to subgroup, and so forth. Therefore, alcoholism could be one explanatory factor in fertility trends and differentials.

Other Intermediate Variables

In addition to its effects on fecundity, alcoholism can lower fertility through other intermediate variables, the most important of which are coital frequency and marital disruption.

COITAL FREQUENCY

Although a minority of female alcoholics are promiscuous due to increased vulnerability or need for money (Gebhard 1965:485; Oliven 1965:479), and although the coital frequency of an occasional anhedonic, depressed individual, or one with an inhibitory-type impotence may be increased by alcohol (cf. Oliven 1965:434), most of the meager research evidence available indicates that alcoholics have diminished interest in heterosexual relationships and have relatively low rates of sexual activity (cf. Beckman 1975:809; Gebhard 1965:485; Jellinek 1952:35; Johnson 1968:32; Kinsey 1966:10–11, 1968:1464; Lisansky 1957:591; Money 1967:285; Ostow 1965:351; Rosen et al. 1972:304; Sherfey 1955:23–24; and USDHEW 1973:102). These observations of reduced libido are in agreement with the findings discussed previously that testosterone levels (which maintain libido) are seriously reduced in alcoholic men.

When one partner in a sexual union is alcoholic, the chances are perhaps greater than 3 out of 4 that the sexual relationship will be disordered (Busch et al. 1973:179). An unusually low coital frequency is the most common disorder observed, and this occurs regardless of which partner is alcoholic.

The most often cited study of the sexual activity of alcoholics is that of Levine (1955), which reviewed the sexual histories of 63 male and 16 female alcoholics who had received treatment at a state-operated outpatient clinic. Levine found that the sex life of many of these individuals was markedly disturbed, deficient, and ineffectual. The majority had sexual intercourse infrequently. Only 19 (30%) of the 63 men said that intercourse occurred at least once every 3 months. However, 8 of these 19 were relatively indifferent to heterosexual relations, their coital frequency being attributed to the wife's demands. Of the remaining 44 (70%), 12 did not participate in intercourse at all, and 16 had intercourse less than once or twice a year. All 44 of the individuals engaging in little or no intercourse expressed relative indifference or complete lack of interest in coitus, verbalizing that sex was an unimportant urge. Five of the 16 women alcoholics were promiscuous, but each had an almost complete absence of orgasm. One of these 5 women was bisexual, with a homosexual preference. Of the 11 remaining women, 8 denied having heterosexual relations, and 3 were frigid, though they did have frequent sexual relations (Levine 1955:676–677).

Blane (1968) also notes that alcoholic women are generally hyposexual. He states:

> The general aspect of sexuality in female alcoholics is inhibition rather than expression. And when it is expressed, sexual activity is less pleasurable than it is symptomatic of profound distress and disturbance of feelings about oneself and one's sexual role. Investigations repeatedly reveal that sexual inhibition is a common factor in alcoholic women. They find sexual relations frightening, uncomfortable, and painful; sexual activity is minimal, sometimes nonexistent. Frigidity and unresponsiveness replace warmth and participation [pp.115–116].

And Orford and Edwards (1977:66) report that the coital frequency of their study's 100 married male alcoholics and their wives was lower than the average frequency reported by Kinsey and his associates (1948, 1953) for the general population. This differential is greater than a simple comparison of these two figures would indicate, as Kinsey's coital frequency data are low relative to contemporary reported frequencies. However, one study by Burton and Kaplin (1968:603) challenges the view that male alcoholics are hyposexual. They found that a small select group of 16 alcoholics and their wives had no difficulty relating at a mature heterosexual level.

In addition to the effect of alcoholism on the libido of the alcoholic, their coital frequency is often reduced by the behavior of their mate. James and Goldman (1971:379) note that withdrawal from the male alcoholic is one style of coping behavior often used by wives. This entails sleeping alone, locking the husband out of the bedroom, sexual abstinence, and so forth. Oliven (1974) portrays many wives of alcoholics during coitus as "resentful of

alcoholized sex, submitting passively and with her teeth clenched [p.403]."
Surely such women probably avoid intercourse as much as possible, and
their behavior could also reduce their alcoholic husband's libido as well.

MARITAL DISRUPTION

Alcoholism may also depress fertility through marital disruption, as
many studies and reviews have reported that alcoholics have abnormally
high rates of marital desertion, separation, and divorce (cf. Bailey et al.
1965:19; Clinard 1968:418; Kessel 1966:133; Kinsey 1966:82–86; Linbeck
1972:575; McNall 1975:205, 211; NCMDA 1973:196; Oliven 1965:220; Rathod
and Thomson 1971:47; Schafer et al. 1975:32; Scott 1958:599; Strauss and
Bacon 1951:239; USNIMH, n.d.:14; and Wallgren and Barry 1970:725). In one
study of 65 ever-married female alcoholics and 67 matched controls, Medhus
(1974:6) found that only 38.5% of the alcoholics were still married, as opposed to 82.1% of the controls. In another series, Rathod and Thomson
(1971:47) report that 15 of 30 male alcoholics were divorced or separated and
that 18 of 30 alcoholic women were in a similar situation. Orford and Edwards
(1977:66) also found high rates of separation and divorce among alcoholics.
Within the 3 years prior to being interviewed, 23 of 100 wives of alcoholics
initiated divorce or legal separation proceedings, and 29 others had tried
temporary separation on at least one occasion. The National Commission on
Marihuana and Drug Abuse (1973) states:

> The alcoholic marriage is generally unstable and disturbed. Chafetz et al. (1971)
> found marital instability in 41% of the families of alcoholics. Intense conflict
> appeared in 60% of alcoholic homes (27% of the homes of non-drinkers) in a
> study by McCord and McCord (1960). The Robins (1966) study revealed that 55%
> of previously married alcoholics had been divorced. Separations or divorces
> were found in 60% of the alcoholics' family units by Lemert (1960). In fact, the
> higher the degree of alcoholic involvement, the lower the likelihood of an intact
> marriage (U.S. Department of Transportation, 1970A). In a review of 22 studies
> conducted between 1944 and 1965, for example, Gillespie (1967) found that
> 18–55% (median 32%) of alcoholics are divorced or separated. Pittman and
> Gordon (1967) noted that among their sample of chronic drinkers, 19% were
> divorced and 32% were separated [p. 196].

It is noteworthy that in the United States alcoholism is grounds for divorce in
40 states (Horton and Leslie 1978:194). Analyses of divorce court testimony
have found that excessive alcohol   consumption is a frequent source of marital
dissatisfaction and complaint (Orford and Edwards 1977:27).

Since temporary separation can be an important cause of reduced fertility, it is significant that many studies linking alcoholism to marital disruption,
including some previously cited, found high rates of temporary separation,

not just divorce. Indeed, even in those marriages that do not break apart, the spouses of alcoholics, particularly wives, almost always try separations of varying lengths as a tactic to save the marriage (cf. James and Goldman 1971:379). Thus, there is a considerable amount of marital disruption among alcoholics, even among those who do not become divorced.

It is not difficult to appreciate why chronic alcoholism is incompatible with marriage and why it is frequently the cause of separation and divorce (Oliven 1965:279; Orford and Edwards 1977:26). As Straus (1976) notes:

> Alcoholism clearly contributes to family stress and instability . . . the wives, husbands, and children of alcoholics have relatively high rates of physical, emotional, and psychosomatic illness. Alcoholics usually demand a great deal of emotional support from others but provide little or no such support in return. Also, because of their preoccupation with alcohol, because of personality traits associated with alcoholism, or merely because of the impotence resulting from the sedative impact of alcohol, alcoholics are often unsatisfying sexual partners. Additional stress for families stems from the economic burdens often associated with the relatively high cost of alcohol and the loss of income resulting from alcohol pathology [pp.210–211].

In addition, alcoholism is a leading cause of spouse and child abuse (Horton and Leslie 1978:192, 193), problems that can also lead to separation and divorce.

As previously mentioned, causality or even the direction of causality is sometimes not easily discernible when investigating the relationship between alcoholism and a second factor, such as marital disruption. Thus, in some cases, marital disruption leads to the alcoholism, rather than vice versa (Linbeck 1972:570). And a third factor may cause both the marital disruption and the alcoholism. Masters and Johnson (1970:149–150), for instance, describe a case in which subfecundity, in the form of sexual dysfunction, caused a man to become alcoholic and also divorced.

FURTHER INTERMEDIATE VARIABLES

There is little information about the relationship between other intermediate variables and alcoholism. However, there are indications that, due to the growing recognition of the fetal alcohol syndrome, more and more physicians and family planning counselors are encouraging alcoholic women to avoid childbearing. Hanson et al. (1976:1458) note that alcoholic women should be encouraged to take effective contraceptive measures, and Jones et al. (1974:1078) suggest that induced abortion may be the best course for those who do become pregnant.

9

Cigarette Smoking

Cigarette smoking is a form of drug abuse. Thus, like other forms of drug abuse such as alcoholism and heroin addiction, it is a psychopathological disorder classifiable under the personality disorder heading.[1] Although the public does not consider tobacco smoke as a drug (Mauss 1975:238), experts do, for it meets all the necessary criteria (cf. Forfar and Nelson 1973:633; NCMDA 1973:9; Rosen *et al.* 1972:316; Royal College of Physicians (RCP) 1971:40). The active ingredient intobacco,nicotine, is classified as a stimulant because of its initial effects: raised blood pressure, increased heartbeat, gland stimulation, appetite suppression, and so forth (Perry and Perry 1976:364).

Cigarette smoke, like alcohol or heroin, is habit forming. Some authorities have suggested that heavy cigarette smokers are true addicts who display real, though mild, withdrawal effects if smoking is stopped (Rosen *et al.* 1972:318). These effects may include drowsiness, headaches, diarrhea, and constipation (Perry and Perry 1976:364). Indeed, recent research by Schacter and his associates (1977:3–40) indicates that the primary reason for smoking is probably addiction. An advanced report in *Time* (1977:Feb. 21) includes the following passage:

[1]Cigarette smoking has also been classified as a social disorder, a heading that includes many of the same problems found under personality disorders. This classification was used by Petersen (1975:253), a demographer.

"Don't ask me why I smoke," says the grim-looking man in the Winston cigarette ad. Columbia Psychologist Stanley Schacter, 54, agrees that is better not to ask. The Winston man—or any other heavy smoker—would probably say he smokes for pleasure, or because it calms his nerves, gives him something to do with his hands or solves his Freudian oral problems. "Almost any smoker can convince you and himself that he smokes for psychological reasons or that smoking does something positive for him—it's all very unlikely," says Schacter, a virtual chain smoker. "We smoke because we're physically addicted to nicotine. Period." [p. 48].

And although individuals, especially teenagers, may begin smoking due to a desire to appear sophisticated and mature, they often continue to smoke after that motive has lost its relevance, because they have become dependent on nicotine (Eckholm 1978:25).

Psychopathologists have devoted relatively little study to smoking, and some authorities see this as an example of the discipline's misplaced priorities. Mechanic (1970:10–11) notes that psychopathologists focus too much on disorders that pose little risk to the individual, such as low self-esteem, and recommends that they pay more attention to high-risk behavior, such as smoking. The effects on the human body of many of the substances found in cigarette smoke, such as coal tars, formaldehyde, arsenic, and cyanide (Perry and Perry 1976:364), are devastating.[2] The number of diseases associated with smoking are many (cf. Eckholm 1978:9–14; Hammond 1962:39–51; Mays 1973:520–523; and RCP, 1971:48–107), and the list grows longer as research continues (Horton and Leslie 1974:588). Of particular importance are coronary heart disease, lung disease, and cerebrovascular disease. The following passage by Mays (1973) provides statistics regarding the impact of smoking on morbidity and mortality in the United States:

> It has been estimated that there are 11,000,000 more cases of chronic illness annually in the United States adult population than there would be if all the population had the same chronic disease prevalence rate as nonsmokers. Simi-

[2]Dr. Benjamin Byrd, former president of the American Cancer Society, describes the physiological stresses and the large number of noxious chemicals encountered by smoking a single cigarette (cf. Eckholm 1978):

> Within seconds after a smoker inhales cigarette smoke, his blood pressure starts rising by 10 to 20 points, his heart rate increases by 25 beats per minute, his skin temperature drops 5 or 6 degrees—because nicotine constricts the small blood vessels in his skin—and even his eyesight is adversely affected. And when he exhales, up to 90 percent of that true tobacco taste stays in his tissues as submicroscopic particles of about 1,200 chemicals—among them acids, glycerol, aldehydes, ketones, aliphatic hydrocarbons, aromatic hydrocarbons, and phenols, most of which are in chimney smoke or automobile exhausts. . . . Sixty percent of the smoke is made up of a dozen noxious gases, including propane, butane, methane, formaldehyde, ammonia, and hydrogen cyanide. Perhaps the most dangerous of all is carbon monoxide, which replaces up to 15 percent of the oxygen in the smoker's blood [p. 10].

larly, it has been estimated that one-third of all male deaths between the ages 35–59 would not have occurred if cigarette smokers had the same death rate as nonsmokers. Furthermore, in 1965, 36 percent of all United States' deaths were from diseases which have a causal or highly probable relationship to tobacco use [p.520].

Thus, premature deaths and disabling illnesses due to cigarette smoking have now reached epidemic proportions in Western nations (RCP 1971:1) and will probably increase further still since the full effects of recent increases in the proportion of such populations who smoke have yet to be felt. The question this chapter raises is whether smoking's negative effect on fecundity is large enough to be demographically significant. The following sections explore this possibility, beginning with a discussion of the effects of smoking on coital ability.

Coital Inability

Many health scientists (e.g., Cooper 1972:549; Kaufman 1967:137; Masters and Johnson 1970:184; Ochsner 1971:89; Subak-Sharpe 1974:53), and even a few social scientists (e.g., Horton and Leslie 1974:590; Perry and Perry 1976:364), have expressed the belief that cigarette smoking may cause impotence. Although this belief has a long history, with references in the literature dating back to 1622 (cf. Larson *et al.* 1961), only a handful of scientific studies of this relationship have been undertaken. Unfortunately, these studies (cf. Larson *et al.* 1961; Larson and Silvette 1968, 1971; Ochsner 1971; Subak-Sharpe 1974) generally contain severe methodological deficiencies (cf. Sterling and Kobayashi 1975), and it is probably a fair assessment that no hard evidence yet exists supporting the hypothesis that smoking is a cause of impotence (Eysenck 1965:21; Sterling and Kobayashi 1975:201).

Thus, the hypothesis that smoking can cause impotence in humans arises more from clinical and personal impressions than from experimental studies or statistical series (Larson *et al.* 1961:642). The literature is full of case studies of men whose impotence is linked to smoking (cf. Ochsner 1971; Subak-Sharpe 1974). A causal connection is often made because the smoker regains potency almost immediately after smoking is terminated (cf. Hastings 1968:239; Johnston 1952:480; Ochsner 1971:89, 92). This causal relationship may or may not exist, for, as Kaufman (1967) notes:

In some individuals, nicotine decreases peripheral flow of blood to a marked degree. It is occasionally gratifying to find potency restored in nicotine-sensitive individuals after the cessation of smoking. A man who smokes two or three packs of cigarettes and also has precarious potency may just be reflecting a basic emotional tension in two separate symptoms; on the other hand, there may be a cause-and-effect relationship, and the potency may improve if the nicotine consumption is decreased [p.137].

Although Kaufman suggests that the impotence observed in some smokers could be due to a nicotine-induced reduction in peripheral blood flow, others, notably Briggs (1973), have focused on the drop in testosterone levels associated with smoking. In a comparison of two groups of healthy men, heavy smokers and a group of suitably matched lifelong nonsmokers, Briggs found that initial testosterone levels were higher among the nonsmokers. After a week's abstention from smoking, the nonsmokers still had higher hormone levels. However, the level of testosterone in the smokers increased significantly over the period, substantially decreasing the initial differential. Briggs hypothesizes that smokers experience decreased levels of testosterone synthesis due to elevated carbon monoxide levels in their blood. Though he does not relate these findings to reduced potency in smokers, it is recognized that testosterone is necessary for potency. But exactly what level is necessary for potency is still unknown (Sterling and Kobayashi 1975:209–210).

In sum, the effect of smoking on potency is controversial (Oliven 1974: 382). Those who are opposed to the hypothesis note that there is no hard evidence supporting it. Proponents rely on their clinical experience. Nevertheless, there is general agreement that impotence is a rare consequence of smoking (Cooper 1972:549; Masters and Johnson 1970:184)[3] assuming that there is any causal relationship at all. Thus, smoking probably has little, if any, effect on population fecundity via impotence. In addition, there are no indications in the literature that it impairs coital ability in any other way, either in men or in women.

Conceptive Failure

Tobacco smoking is considered by many writers (cf. Behrman and Kistner 1968:6; Kleegman and Kaufman 1966:10; Siegler 1944:16; Subak-Sharpe 1974:51) to be a possible cause of infertility in both men and women, though this view is contested (cf. Kaufman 1970: 29; Sterling and Kobayashi 1975:201).

In men, tobacco smoking has been linked to defects in sperm production and quality. Smoking has been cited as a cause of oligospermia, but hard data are lacking (Amelar 1966:19; Amelar et al. 1977:81; Behrman and Kistner 1968:5). Most information on the relationship between smoking and

---

[3]A notable exception is a Soviet physician who claims that smoking is one of the chief causes of impotence in the Soviet Union (cf. Larson and Silvette 1968:425).

oligospermia comes from clinical impressions, such as those of Mai *et al.* (1972:201), who observed that men with low sperm counts smoked twice as much as men with normal counts. And Shirren (cf. Subak-Sharpe 1974:51) suggests that men who smoke more than 20 cigarettes daily may suffer severe disturbances of sperm motility.

However, not all studies report a relationship between smoking and male infertility. Arora *et al.* (1961:365) found no difference in sperm count or motility between smokers and nonsmokers. And Tokuhata (1968a:353), in a study of 2016 couples, found no association between the husband's smoking history and a couple's infertility.

In sum, the link between smoking and male infertility has yet to be established. The consensus among medical workers, as stated by Paul Schneiderman, medical director of the U.S. National Clearinghouse for Smoking and Health, is decidedly noncommittal (cf. Subak-Sharpe 1974): "Not enough studies have been done yet, but the preliminary findings would indicate that in cases with no apparent cause of male infertility, smoking might be a factor [p.52]."

Studies indicate that smoking may be a cause of infertility in women (cf. Larson *et al.* 1961:643). In a study of 2016 women, for example, Tokuhata (1968a:357) found that 21% of the smokers as opposed to only 14% of the nonsmokers were infertile. Overall, smokers were half again as likely to be infertile as nonsmokers, and this differential held up under nine different demographic and socioeconomic controls. In addition, smokers had fewer lifetime pregnancies.

Larson *et al.* (1961:642) reviewed a study by Bernhard (1949) in which the clinical records of 458 smokers and 5000 nonsmokers who were similar in most other respects were compared. The following grid shows the percentage in each group that complained of various reproduction-related disorders:

	Smokers	*Nonsmokers*
Dysmenorrhea	25.5%	4.2%
Amenorrhea	3.5	.3
Oligomenorrhea	6.1	3.6
Polymenorrhea	17.5	5.7
Premature menopause	21.2	3.9
Premature aging	69.6	1.7

Bernhard (1962) conducted another study 13 years later with similar results (Larson and Silvette 1968:425). Hammond (1961:146) also reports that menstrual disorders are more frequent among smokers than nonsmokers between the ages of 30 and 49.

The high frequency of menstrual disorders among smoking women points to an impairment of ovarian functioning, a conclusion reached by Bernhard (1962). Mai *et al.* (1972:203), however, failed to establish any relationship between smoking and a common ovarian dysfunction, anovulation. One researcher (Tokuhata 1968a) suggests that it is the ovum itself that is negatively affected by smoking. Others suggest a far different tack. Briggs (1973:617), for instance, notes that an investigation of the effects of smoking on estrogen synthesis would be worthwhile.

Smokers probably have less time to conceive than nonsmokers, since the former tend to reach menopause sooner. This is evident from the Bernhard data shown in the preceding grid. A striking association between smoking and the onset of menopause has also recently been discovered by Jick and his associates (1977:1354). In a study of 3500 middle-aged women, they found that, at each age, women who were smokers were more likely to be past menopause than were those who had never smoked and that heavy smokers were more likely to be past menopause than were light smokers. They also report that, the more a woman smokes, the earlier her menopause is likely to occur. This relationship between smoking and menopause was similar in each of seven countries examined. The researchers suggest two possible mechanisms: (a) the effect of nicotine on the central nervous system possibly results in changes in the secretion of hormones involved in menopause; and (b) the effect of cigarette smoke on certain enzymes may influence the manner in which the body handles sex hormones.

In sum, the consensus in the literature is that smoking may cause infertility in both men and women, and physicians typically discourage smoking among infertile individuals (Brown 1965:132). However, as was true with respect to the relationship between smoking and coital inability, there are few scientific studies on the relationship between smoking and conceptive failure. Much of the consensus, therefore, is derived from clinical experiences and case reports describing, for example, an improvement in sperm count or sperm motility when smoking is stopped.

Pregnancy Loss

As many as 25% of pregnant women in the United States smoke cigarettes. With such a large fetal population at potential risk, it is not surprising that the relationship between smoking and pregnancy outcome has received considerable attention. A study by Tokuhata (1968a:356–357) of 2016 couples found that smoking wives had a pregnancy loss rate of 16% as compared to 11% for nonsmoking wives and that this differential held under nine different controls. This is one of the few studies that deals with pregnancy loss in its entirety. Most studies deal with a component of pregnancy loss, such as abortion or late fetal death, or with perinatal mortality, which includes pregnancy loss as well as postnatal mortality. Hence, discussion of the evidence linking smoking with pregnancy loss is divided here into three separate sections, one each for abortion, late fetal death, and perinatal mortality. As an aside, information on the relationship between smoking and neonatal mortality, infant mortality, and child development will also be briefly reviewed.

ABORTION

Abortion, as the term is used in this book, refers to pregnancy loss that occurs before the end of the twenty-eighth week of gestation.

Women who smoke during pregnancy may be more likely to abort than nonsmokers (Eckholm 1978:14; Mays 1973:522; RCP 1971:5; Tucker 1975:18).[4] A number of both retrospective and prospective studies (e.g., Hudson and Rucker 1945; O'Lane 1963; Palmgren and Wallander 1971; Underwood et al. 1965; Zabriskie 1963) have reported statistically significant associations between maternal smoking and spontaneous abortion. For instance, comparing nonsmokers with smokers, Zabriskie found that the latter had 43% more abortions; the same figure in the O'Lane study was 71%; in the Hudson and Rucker study it was 144% (Rush and Kass 1972:192–193).

In an important recent study (Kline et al. 1977:793), women who smoked during pregnancy were found to be nearly twice as liable as nonsmokers to lose their babies through spontaneous abortion. The study compared 574 women who had spontaneous abortions with 320 women who delivered babies. A significant feature of this study is that the two groups were matched according to age, income, ethnic group, education, and number of previous pregnancies. All told, 41% of the women who aborted were smokers, compared to only 28% of the women who had normal pregnancies.

Several studies (e.g., Palmgren and Wallander 1971; Underwood et al. 1965; Zabriskie 1963) have even found evidence supporting a strong dose–response relationship between the number of cigarettes smoked and the risk of spontaneous abortion (USPHS 1973:123). Palmgren and Wallander (1971), for instance, in a prospective study of abortion in a sample of 4312 pregnancies, found that smokers of 10 or fewer cigarettes per day had an abortion rate of 9.1%, which was not much higher than that of nonsmokers (7.8%). But the rate for smokers of more than 10 cigarettes per day was 14.5%, 59% higher than that of the light smokers and 86% higher than that of the nonsmokers.

However, a general criticism of many of the studies to date that report an

---

[4]For a review of the literature prior to 1961, see Larson et al. (1961); for the period 1961 to 1971, see Larson and Silvette (1968, 1971); for other reviews of the literature of the last two decades, consult USPHS (1971, 1972, 1973), RCP (1971), and Rush and Kass (1972).

association between smoking and spontaneous abortion is that other variables that may influence the incidence of abortion are not controlled. And there have been other studies that report little, if any, correlation between smoking and abortion (Larson and Silvette 1971:264; Longo 1970:333).

In sum, the studies to date do not provide enough information to permit a firm conclusion to be drawn concerning the relationship between smoking and abortion (USPHS 1972:83, 1973:124).

LATE FETAL DEATH

Late fetal death, or stillbirth, refers to pregnancy loss occurring after the twenty-eighth week of gestation. Several retrospective and prospective studies (e.g., Butler and Alberman 1969; Butler *et al.* 1972; Frazier *et al.* 1961; Kullander and Kallen 1971; Rumeau-Roquette *et al.* 1972; and Tokuhata 1968a) have found that smokers' infants have a higher stillbirth rate than do those of nonsmokers. Butler and Alberman (1969), for example, report stillbirth rates (per 1000 total births) of 27.6 for infants of smokers and 19.3 for those of nonsmokers. Similarly, these figures are 15.5 and 6.4, respectively, in the Frazier *et al.* (1961) study and 13.0 and 9.8, respectively, in the Kullander and Kallen (1971) report.

A study by Butler *et al.* (1972) further defined the risk by showing that rates of stillbirth varied according to when and how much the mother smoked. Stillbirth rates were 30% higher for women who smoked after the fourth month of pregnancy than for women who did not smoke at that time. And a dose—response relationship was apparent in their sample, the death rate being directly related to the number of cigarettes smoked (Butler *et al.* 1972:127).

There is evidence that cigarette smoking is most strongly associated with a higher stillbirth rate when the woman is from a lower social class or has a history of obstetrical problems (USPHS 1973:125). Several studies (e.g., Lubs 1973; Niswander and Gordon 1972; Rush and Kass 1972), for instance, have shown that the impact of smoking on stillbirth rates is much greater for black than for white women in the United States.

However, another group of retrospective and prospective studies (e.g., Comstock and Lundin 1967; Downing and Chapman 1966; Savel and Roth 1962; and Underwood *et al.* 1965, 1967) detected no real difference in the late fetal death rate among the infants of smokers and nonsmokers (Astrup *et al.* 1972:1221). Underwood *et al.* (1967), for example, report stillbirth rates (per 1000 total births) of 8.4 for infants of smokers and 8.7 for those of nonsmokers.

Despite the fact that some studies have failed to find that smokers' infants have higher rates of stillbirth, many researchers, probably the majority, are convinced that smoking does increase the incidence of stillbirth (cf. Babson and Benson 1971:19; Eckholm 1978:14; Mays 1973:522). Indeed, after a review of the pertinent literature, the U.S. Public Health Service (1972:83) concluded that there is strong evidence to support the view that smoking mothers have a significantly greater number of unsuccessful pregnancies due to stillbirth than do nonsmoking mothers. It has further been suggested that smoking is more strongly related to stillbirth when other problems related to pregnancy loss are present.

PERINATAL MORTALITY

Perinatal mortality includes late fetal deaths and infants deaths in the first 1–4 weeks of life. Only late fetal death is a component of subfecundity. However, many workers focus on perinatal mortality, and a review of this literature does provide some information about late fetal death.

A number of retrospective and prospective studies (e.g. Butler and Alberman 1969; Butler et al. 1972; Comstock and Lundin 1967; Comstock et al. 1971; Frazier et al. 1961; Kullander and Kallen 1971; Lowe 1959; Mulcahy and Knaggs 1968; Niswander and Gordon 1972; Ontario Department of Health (ODH) 1967a,b; and Rush and Kass 1972) have revealed a statistically significant relationship between cigarette smoking and increased perinatal mortality. Rush and Kass (1972:192–193), after reviewing a number of such studies, conclude that, taken as a whole, the positive association between smoking and perinatal mortality is impressive. Overall, smokers were found to have an excess perinatal loss of 34.4%, with a range among studies of 0–144%. One of the studies reviewed by Rush and Kass is the British Perinatal Mortality Survey (Butler and Alberman 1969). This study of more than 15,000 women found that smokers experienced 42.5% more perinatal mortality than did nonsmokers.

Several studies indicate that the relationship between smoking and perinatal mortality varies by race and/or socioeconomic status. For instance, in the Rush and Kass (1972) study of 3276 smoking women, black smokers had 86% more perinatal mortality than did black nonsmokers, whereas for whites the same differential was only 11%. Similarly, in the Butler and Alberman (1969) study previously discussed, there was in inverse relationship between social class and the amount of excess perinatal mortality that smokers in the various classes had over nonsmokers. Thus, as was the case for late fetal death, smoking has its greatest impact on perinatal mortality in cases in which conditions are already unfavorable for a successful pregnancy outcome.

However, other studies (e.g., Bailey 1970; Downing and Chapman 1966; O'Lane 1963; Peterson et al. 1965; Rantakallio 1969; Savel and Roth 1962;

and Underwood *et al.* 1967) have not found a significant positive relationship between cigarette smoking and perinatal mortality. Bailey (1970), for example, in a prospective investigation of 1300 pregnancies in New Zealand, found about the same perinatal death rates for infants born to smoking and nonsmoking mothers.

Nevertheless, the weight of evidence supports the observation that maternal smoking increases the risk of perinatal mortality (Meyer and Comstock 1972:7; USPHS 1972:83). Indeed, the U.S. Public Health Service (1973:134–135), after reviewing much of the literature, concludes that a strong, probably causal, association exists between maternal cigarette smoking and higher perinatal mortality rates.

NEONATAL MORTALITY, INFANT MORTALITY, AND CHILD DEVELOPMENT

The conclusion that smoking can lead to pregnancy loss is based not only on the kinds of smoking–pregnancy failure associations just discussed but also on the observation that smoking apparently has a negative impact on a child's earliest years and, perhaps, throughout his or her entire life.

The evidence linking cigarette smoking and neonatal mortality is impressive. Both the U.S. Public Health Service (1971, 1972, 1973) and Meyer and Comstock (1972) reviewed much of the work available, and their conclusion was the same, that is, that strong evidence exists that tobacco smoking increases neonatal mortality.

Meyer and Comstock (1972:9) present data from six studies in which the neonatal mortality rate of smokers' children ranged from 2 to 75% higher than that of nonsmokers' children. This figure for the six studies is as follows: Butler and Alberman (1969), 31.3%; Comstock *et al.* (1971), 40.0%; Frazier *et al.* (1961), 18.0%; Kullander and Kallen (1971), 74.5%; Underwood *et al.* (1967), 7.8%; and Yerushalmy (1971), 2.8% for whites and 25.8% for blacks. Comstock *et al.* (1971), in a study covering more than 12,000 births, found that the neonatal mortality rate, even when adjusted for environmental and socioeconomic factors, was one-third higher among infants born to smoking mothers than among those born to nonsmoking ones. Butler and associates (1972:127) report that smokers in their study had a neonatal mortality rate that was 26% higher than that of nonsmokers and note that the increase was positively related to cigarette consumption. Finally, heavy smoking has been found to nearly double neonatal mortality when other factors are present that imperil the newborn, such as poverty and poor maternal nutrition (Eckholm 1978:14).

It is not, however, accepted by everyone that smoking increases neonatal mortality. A widely cited study by Yerushalmy (1971), for instance, contends that smoking per se does nothing to increase neonatal mortality. But, again, racial variation is evident, with several studies finding that the association between smoking and neonatal mortality is far stronger in black women than in their white counterparts (cf. Lubs 1973; Yerushalmy 1971).

Infant mortality rates may also be higher in the offspring of smokers. Kullander and Kallen (1971) report that the risk of death in the first year of life was about 60% higher for the offspring of smoking women as compared to those of nonsmokers. Several studies also indicate that smoking during pregnancy compromises the child's future development. Butler and Goldstein (1973:573) report that physical and mental deficiencies due to smoking have been found in children at ages 7 and 11 and that these deficits increase with the number of cigarettes smoked after the fourth month of pregnancy.

MECHANISMS

Thus, the preponderance of evidence supports the hypothesis that smoking affects the developing fetus in ways prejudicial to successful pregnancy outcome (Babson and Benson 1971:18). The following mechanisms have been proposed to explain the negative effects on the fetus of maternal smoking (USPHS 1973:119–120):[5]

1. A direct toxic influence of constituents of cigarette smoke upon the fetus

2. Decreased placental perfusion

3. Decreased maternal appetite and diminished maternal weight gain with secondary effects upon the fetus

4. A direct effect upon the placenta

5. An oxytocic (stimulates contraction) effect on uterine activity

6. A disturbance of vitamin B-12 metabolism

7. A disturbance of vitamin C metabolism

The first two mechanisms are the most popular and usually speak to the effects on the fetus of elevated levels of carbon monoxide and nicotine-induced constriction of the placental blood vessels. It is believed that the fetus suffers from an oxygen debt under these conditions and, as a result, is retarded in its growth within the uterus. Indeed, the strongest link between smoking and any particular pregnancy outcome is that between smoking and intrauterine growth-retarded (IUGR) babies. These babies are born at, or

[5]For further suggestions and discussion of these and other mechanisms, see RCP (1971:95), Green (1974:715), and Tokuhata (1968a:353).

nearly at, full term. Thus, they are developmentally mature but have low birth weights.

Meyer and Comstock (1972:1) found that the birth weights of infants of smoking mothers were depressed by 150 to 300 grams. The U.S. Public Health Service (1973:103–122), after reviewing 42 studies on the relationship between smoking and birth weight, concluded that a causal relation existed between the two. Its most important observations were that:

1. Smokers have a two-fold greater risk of having a low-birth-weight infant than do nonsmokers.

2. A strong dose–response relationship exists between the number of cigarettes smoked and the incidence of low-birth-weight infants.

3. These associations cut across population and geographical boundaries.

4. Animal experiments support the hypothesis that elevated levels of carbon monoxide cause reduction in birth weight.

As low birth weight is associated with higher rates of perinatal mortality, IUGR is undoubtedly responsible for much of the stillbirth, late fetal death, and neonatal mortality observed in the offspring of smokers. (Increased infant mortality rates and developmental retardation during childhood may also be sequelae to stunted intrauterine growth.)

Some mortality may also be the result of certain obstetrical disorders that are found with greater frequency or severity in smoking mothers. Lubs (1973:66, 76) reports a strong correlation between the number of cigarettes smoked and the frequency of complications of pregnancy, particularly hemorrhage and anemia. And Kullander and Kallen (1971:82) found significantly more abruptio placentae in smoking mothers, a serious complication that carries a perinatal mortality risk of 50–80% (Babson and Benson 1971:58). Finally, despite the fact that smoking mothers tend to have lower blood pressure and are less liable to develop toxemia than nonsmoking mothers, the risk to the infant, if toxemia does occur, has been found to be so much higher in smoking women that the overall risk to their infants is increased (RCP 1971:96; USPHS 1973:142).

CRITICISMS

Despite what may appear to be overwhelming support for the hypothesis that cigarette smoking increases pregnancy loss, there are some researchers who believe that the evidence is not incontrovertible. They cite two reasons for their dissenting opinion: the failure of some studies to find a positive correlation between cigarette smoking and pregnancy loss and/or the failure of many studies that do show a positive correlation to properly control for other genetic, behavioral, and environmental factors that are found in association with the smoking habit and may themselves be the real causes of any pregnancy loss.

The failure of some studies to find a positive correlation between smoking and pregnancy loss may be due in part to differences in the definition of a "smoker." Yerushalmy (1971) defines smokers relatively broadly, that is, as those who smoke at least one cigarette a day during pregnancy. Butler *et al.* (1972) define smokers more strictly, including only those women who smoked regularly after the fourth month of pregnancy. Other studies define smokers in still different ways. Such definitional noncomparability is only one of numerous technical problems that could account for disparate findings.

A study may also fail to find a positive correlation between smoking and pregnancy loss if the study population is experiencing otherwise optimal birth circumstances. Under such circumstances, smoking may be a relatively unimportant factor, becoming a serious factor only when found in conjunction with other obstetrical risks. It has already been noted that among blacks, who suffer high rates of pregnancy loss as a group, rates of perinatal and neonatal mortality are greatly enhanced by smoking. Between white smokers and nonsmokers, the differentials are not nearly so great. From this perspective, smoking is the proverbial "straw that broke the camel's back," a negative influence that, when superimposed on other negative influences, produces a condition capable of causing pregnancy loss.

The failure of some studies that do find a positive correlation between smoking and pregnancy loss to properly control for other etiological factors has been the subject of criticism. Mothers who smoke during pregnancy, for example, tend to come from poorer social backgrounds, are older, and are of higher parity than nonsmokers (Butler *et al.* 1972:127). Therefore, the possibility is raised that smoking does not cause pregnancy loss but is only an index of a particular type of mother. Yerushalmy (1971:443), for instance, contends that smokers as a group are different from nonsmokers and that these differences, rather than smoking per se, account for observed differences in pregnancy outcome. In his study, he found differences in mode of life characteristics between smokers and nonsmokers. The former, for example, consumed more liquor and coffee, practiced less contraception and family planning, and generally impressed him as living at a less moderate pace than nonsmokers.

Despite these criticisms, the consensus is that smoking itself is the cause of pregnancy loss. As the editors of the *British Medical Journal* (1973) put it: "Many careful studies on pregnant women as well as animals suggest that it is smoking itself rather than the type of woman who smokes that is responsible for these effects [p.369]." This position is strengthened but not confirmed by experimental studies on animals, many of which have found smoking associated with low birth weight, abortion, stillbirth, and late fetal and neonatal death (cf. *British Medical Journal* 1973:369; Larson *et al.* 1961; Larson and Silvette 1968, 1971; Longo 1970:334; and USPHS 1971, 1972, 1973).

Incidently, there is no evidence linking male smoking to pregnancy loss. Tokuhata (1968a:357) did investigate this possibility but concluded that the male's history of smoking was not related to pregnancy loss.

Prevalence

Tobacco is the second most commonly used drug in the United States (Mauss 1975:240). The percentage of the 1970 U.S. population that smoked cigarettes is given in Table 9.1 by age and sex. Nearly half of all men and almost 40% of all women in the reproductive ages smoked cigarettes.

Cigarette smoking is a relatively recent phenomenon. Prior to World War I, the mode for tobacco consumption was mainly pipes, cigars, chewing tobacco, and snuff. The annual consumption of manufactured cigarettes in the United States per adult rose from 49 in 1900 to 611 in 1920 to 3888 by 1960 (cf. Hammond 1962; Mays 1973; Retherford 1972). And present consumption is substantially higher yet, despite recent campaigns against smoking. In the 5 years prior to 1975, per capita cigarette consumption increased almost 20% (*Interchange* 1977:2).

As Table 9.1 shows, fewer women than men smoke. However, the proportion of women who smoke has been rising steadily, both in the United States and in other Western countries (Mays 1973:520; RCP 1971:1). Between 1962 and 1972, for instance, the number of women smokers in the United

TABLE 9.1.
Percentage of Current Smokers of Cigarettes by Sex and Age, 1970

Age	Males	Females
18–24	47.0	31.1
25–34	46.8	40.3
35–44	48.6	39.0
45–54	43.1	36.0
55–64	37.4	24.3
65+	23.7	11.8

SOURCE: USPHS (1971:6)

States increased by 50%, while the number of men smokers increased only slightly. Women are fast approaching men in terms of the percent who smoke (Mays 1973:520). In fact, recent surveys of teenage Americans indicate that, although more boys than girls 10 years of age smoke, by the age of 17 the differential is reversed. The percent of teenage girls who smoke has risen from 22% in 1969 to 27% in 1975 (*Intercom* 1977b:6). It is Ochsner's (1971:82) contention that, if this trend continues, more women than men will be smoking within the next decade.

In light of the association previously discussed between smoking and pregnancy loss, it is ominous and highly significant that many women fail to heed medical advice stipulating that they refrain from smoking during pregnancy. The U.S. Public Health Service (1973:103) estimates that between 20 and 25% of all U.S. women smoke throughout their pregnancies. Other figures in the literature are even higher. For instance, in the National Collaborative Perinatal Project, 54% of the white women and 42% of the black women smoked during pregnancy (Hardy and Mellites 1972:1333). In the Baltimore area subgroup, these percentages were 77 and 54, respectively. Many British women also smoke during pregnancy. Forfar and Nelson (1973:634) found that 57% of 911 randomly selected mothers giving birth at a British hospital smoked during pregnancy, and 28% of these women smoked more than 10 cigarettes per day.

The United States is the premier cigarette-smoking country because many Americans smoke and because they smoke more cigarettes per day than do smokers in other countries. The nation with the second highest consumption of cigarettes is Japan, whose per capita consumption is only about 6% below that of the United States. An astonishing 75% of all Japanese men smoke, as compared with only 15% of Japanese women. Consumption is also high in Western European countries, ranging from about one-third to over two-thirds the U.S. rate. China, the world's leading tobacco-growing country, undoubtedly also has a high consumption rate. In Mexico, annual per capita cigarette consumption is over 700, whereas in developing African countries, such as Nigeria and Tanzania, it is still only a few hundred cigarettes. These national cigarette-consumption averages were assembled by Eckholm (1978:15, 18), who believes they provide little hint of the present and increasing smoking pandemic. In his words (1978):

> While the incidence of cigarette smoking may have peaked in some of the developed Western countries, the practice has entered a dramatic growth phase in most less developed countries. Cigarettes are catching on especially quickly in the cities of poor countries, the forges of modernization. A Pan American Health Organization survey in eight urban areas of Latin America reveals that 45 percent of the men in these cities smoke. . . . In contrast, 18 percent of the women in these major Latin American cities are smokers. . . . Cigarette smoking is not

yet as widespread in most of Africa and Asia as it is in Latin America—no doubt
in part because average personal incomes in Africa and Asia are generally much
lower than those in Latin America. . . . Smoking in poor countries is by no
means confined to affluent urban residents. Tobacco use of one sort or another
has long been entrenched in many rural regions [pp.18–20].

Thus, most developing countries are well on their way toward the high
cigarette-consumption rates of developed countries.

It is also worth noting that cigarette smokers are not the only ones who
inhale cigarette smoke. Many nonsmokers find themselves involuntarily breathing cigarette smoke, often on a regular basis. Nonsmokers inhale substantial
amounts of tars, nicotine, and carbon monoxide in a smoky room or car. One
study found that bartenders working an 8-hour shift in poorly ventilated
saloons inhale as many noxious fumes as they would by smoking 36 cigarettes
(Eckholm 1978:13). Thus some nonsmokers are subject to the same medical
risks as smokers, including any effects on fecundity.

Population Subfecundity

Although population students recognize that smoking has an impact on
morbidity and mortality of immense population dimensions (cf. Retherford
1972, 1974a,b), the possibility that smoking may also affect population fecundity and, ultimately, fertility is never mentioned. This chapter has tried to
demonstrate that this possibility is not farfetched.

Smoking does meet the two minimal requirements of a population subfecundity factor. It is a widespread phenomenon, and, according to many
authorities, it can depress individual fecundity.

Smoking's designation as a population subfecundity factor is due more
to its prevalence than to its ability to depress fecundity.[6] In the United States,
nearly half the population smokes. Moreover, since many smokers are married to nonsmokers, this means that substantially more than half of U.S.
couples contain at least one smoking member. Of further subfecundity significance is the finding that prevalence rates do not fall much among pregnant women, most of whom continue to smoke throughout pregnancy. Few
of the other subfecundity factors discussed in this book can match the
prevalence statistics of cigarette smoking.

[6]There is a popular notion that breathing city air is like smoking two packs of cigarettes a day. If
this were true, the deleterious effects of smoking on fecundity would apply to entire urban
populations. This popular notion, however, is a myth (cf. Adler 1973:86–106). For example, persons
smoking two packs of cigarettes daily for a year expose their lungs to about 19 times the amount of
benzpyrene (a possible carcinogen) than they would by breathing the polluted air of Los Angeles
for a year (Eckholm 1978:11).

The literature on the relationship between smoking and individual fecundity is conflicting, as this chapter has shown. However, many workers conclude that smoking can lead to coital inability, conceptive failure, and pregnancy loss. It is impossible, however, to determine how much of a deficit smoking can make in a couple's fecundity. The knowledge available to date on the smoking–subfecundity relationship is simply not sufficient to support that kind of estimate. It should be noted, however, that this review has not uncovered any evidence to suggest that smoking is one of the most important causes of individual subfecundity. It certainly does not have, for example, the impact of some of the other psychopathological factors, such as alcoholism.

Overall, therefore, the combination of very high prevalence together with a relatively small impact on individual fecundity renders smoking a marginally significant population subfecundity factor. As a subfecundity factor, smoking is probably more important among various subgroups that already have greater risks of reproductive failure: U.S. blacks, those of lower socioeconomic status, women who already have obstetrical problems, and so forth. Textbooks on subfecundity are filled with the idea that it commonly takes more than one subfecundity factor to prevent childbearing and that subfecund couples generally have several problems at once. Smoking, perhaps relatively unimportant per se, may be the pivotal factor causing subfecundity in many couples. And it is in just such cases that its influence would be overlooked.

It is worth noting that this chapter and most of the evidence it presents pertain to all cigarette smokers. Chances are that the fecundity of heavy smokers is more strongly affected by smoking than is that of smokers in general. The evidence of a dose–response effect between smoking and subfecundity found in a number of studies supports this idea. And heavy smokers represent a sizable population subgroup, since they are a substantial fraction of all smokers. In 1975, for instance, 39% of female smokers consumed a pack or more a day (*Intercom* 1977b:6).

The reader is again reminded that smoking, like many other subfecundity factors, may affect fertility through other variables besides subfecundity. There are reports in the literature (e.g., Ochsner 1971:89, 92; Subak-Sharpe 1974:53), for instance, suggesting that smoking diminishes sexual drive. However, others (e.g., Sterling and Kobayashi 1975:202) dispute this, and, even if such effects exist, they are probably not very significant. The widely publicized health risks of smoking and the increased antismoking militancy of nonsmokers may also affect fertility through marital variables. It is conceivable that some nonsmokers may exclude smokers as potential mates, thus limiting their choice and perhaps delaying their entrance into unions. In addition, conflicts over smoking could lead to separation and divorce in couples in which only one partner smokes. On the other hand, smoking can have at least one positive effect on fertility, this time via a contraceptive variable. Recent research has shown that the risk of birth-control-pill–associated blood clots and heart attacks is dramaticaly increased in women who smoke (Eckholm 1978:12). Women who smoke and use the pill are hence being strenuously urged to quit smoking or, barring this, to switch to other less effective means of contraception, a move that could increase the number of unwanted births and increase fertility in general.

10

Illicit Drug Abuse

A few population students have hinted that illicit drug abuse may have an impact on population fecundity. For instance, DeJong and Sell (1977:133) raise the possibility that subfecundity due to drug abuse may be partly responsible for the significant increase in marital childlessness in the United States since 1960. Thomlinson (1967:45) notes that narcotics have biological properties that tend to lower fecundity, and Hansluwka (1975:208) suggests that drugs may be responsible for a portion of spontaneous abortions. There is even a report in the population literature that drug abuse may have caused subfecundity in 25% of the Likonala, an African tribe (cf. Clark 1967:29). Nevertheless, with the exception of these and perhaps a few other references, the possibility that illicit drugs may affect population fecundity is ignored in the demographic literature. This chapter investigates whether illicit drug use, and, more particularly, illicit drug abuse, has a role in population subfecundity.

Illicit drugs are certain psychoactive substances that are either legally unobtainable or available only by prescription. A substantial portion of illicit drug use is drug abuse, and this is a form of psychopathology, that is, a personality disorder. The use of illicit drugs that are not prescriptible and the nonmedicinal use of those that are constitute drug abuse.

This chapter focuses on the following illicit drugs or drug groups, listed in order of their frequency of use in the United States: (a) barbiturates and tranquilizers; (b) stimulants; (c) marihuana; (d) hallucinogens; and (e) opiate narcotics. Barbiturates are depressants and are used primarily as sedatives and hypnotics. Well-known barbiturates include Veronal, Seconal, and Nembutal. Tranquilizers are divided into two groups. The first, major tranquilizers, includes drugs such as Thorazine and Serpasil. The second, minor tranquilizers, includes drugs such as Valium, Librium, Miltown, and Quaalude. Major tranquilizers are rarely abused (Goode 1973:15; Leavitt 1974:2), whereas minor tranquilizers are frequently used for nonmedicinal purposes. Frequently used stimulants are cocaine and the amphetamines Benzidrine and Methedrine. LSD, peyote, and marihuana are hallucinogens of note, the last-named being treated separately here because it has received relatively more attention in the literature than have the other drugs. Opiates such as opium, morphine, and codeine and synthetic opiates such as heroin and methadone are included in the opiate narcotics category and are referred to in this chapter simply as "narcotics."

Ideally, this chapter would provide a report on each illicit drug's potential to depress fecundity, but this is impractical given the scope of this book and the fact that little or nothing is known about the fecundity-impairing ability of many drugs. This is why this chapter focuses on drug groups rather than on individual drugs, although marihuana is an exception.

Research Problems

It is difficult, for several reasons, to evaluate the effect of illicit drugs on individual fecundity. Most important is the gross lack of research into virtually every aspect of drug effects. In few other important medicosocial areas is there such a scarcity of verifiable information (*Lancet* 1973:527). "The literature on drug side effects is mainly a bunch of unconnected fragments at the basic science level [p.v]," note Shader and Di Mascio (1970). "Even in the clinical domain, data on the incidence of side effects and on factors contributing to the emergence of many side effects are less firm that one might like [p.v]."

Another reason why it is difficult to determine the effect of illicit drugs on fecundity is that subfecundity in a drug user may be caused by a pharmacological action of the drug or may be due to a common factor, such as psychic stress, which leads simultaneously to both subfecundity and drug use, or due to associated factors and living conditions that often accompany drug use, such as venereal disease, or due to a combination of the above. A fifth possibility is that subfecundity may be the precipitating cause of drug use.

Greaves (1972:363–364) discusses the possibility that some third factor may lead simultaneously to drug use and to subfecundity. He remarks, for instance, that emotional disturbance may be at the root of both disturbed sexuality and illicit drug use and cites a study (Bell and Trethowan 1961) in which amphetamine use was seen to augment an already disturbed sexual pattern rather than to cause a primary sexual disturbance. Similarly, the typical valium abuser is an emotionally upset woman (Franklin 1978:1), in whom psychic stress may simultaneously account for both valium use and any subfecundity.

The fact that drug abusers may be subfecund due to other factors simply associated with the drug-using life style is frequently recited in the subfecundity literature (cf. Goode 1973:14; Leavitt 1974:170; Murphree 1971:332; NCMDA 1973:194–195; Poland et al. 1972:955; and Tucker 1975:5). Illicit drug abusers often live in overcrowded and unsanitary conditions and do not maintain proper nutrition and health habits. Thus, with respect to habitual amphetamine users, for instance, researchers are still trying to decide whether the pathological side effects exhibited are a function of the action of the amphetamine itself or simply a consequence of the hectic, sleepless, starvation regimen pursued (Goode 1973:14). Drug abusers are also known to be susceptible to a variety of communicable diseases (NCMDA 1973:195), some of which, like tuberculosis, cause subfecundity. Physicians have also noticed a high incidence of venereal disease among drug addicts, especially among those who use heroin (cf. Neuberg 1970:1118; Stoffer 1968:779, 782; and Tucker 1975:5). It is also relevant that, in nearly all reported series of drug-dependent pregnant women, antenatal care is virtually absent (Neuberg 1972:867). Given the health problems these women face, this lack of care undoubtedly results in increased subfecundity in the form of pregnancy loss and even subsequent infertility. Thus, these and other associated factors make it difficult to determine the fecundity-impairing effect of the drugs alone. Indeed, Neuberg (1970) suggests that, for research concerning certain groups of drug users, it is almost impossible to find suitable controls. With respect to heroin users, he states that "there is no non-narcotic control group for comparison which has an equivalent lack of antenatal care, and a similar degree of physical deterioration, malnutrition, and ill health [p. 1119]."

To complicate matters even further, it is distinctly possible that among some drug abusers subfecundity may be the cause rather than the effect of drug abuse (Sterling and Kobayaski 1975:208). Some authors observe that impotence or sexual difficulty often precedes heroin addiction (Talkington 1971:27), and it has been suggested that persons not sure of their identity or doubtful of their masculinity and sexual ability may take drugs in order to have the feelings and sensations of orgasm without having to bother with the anxieties of sexual intercourse or of warm interpersonal relationships (cf. Talkington 1971:27).

It is also difficult to evaluate the effect of drug abuse on fecundity because the subfecundity literature is so conflicting. On the one hand are the "pathologizers," as Goode (1975:41) labels them, who produce findings that link illicit drug use to damage to an organ or to a function of the body, including those of the reproductive system. These findings are often challenged by the "nonpathologizers," who conduct similar studies but reach the opposite conclusion, that is, that drugs do not cause such damage. Goode (1975:41) notes that, at least with respect to marihuana,[1] the trend of support has recently swung away from the viewpoint of the "pathologizer" toward that of the "nonpathologizer." Though marihuana is only one of many illicit drugs, it is probably safe to say that the effects of illicit drugs on the body have been generally exaggerated (cf. Brecher 1975:145; Denisoff and Wahrman 1975:351).

In the following review of the relationship between illicit drug abuse and the component parts of subfecundity, the reader should keep the aforementioned problems in mind.

Coital Inability

Illicit drugs have a reputation for increasing sexual appetite or capacity in both men and women (Oliven 1974:443). In fact, drug abusers are not infrequently characterized as oversexed and even sexual menaces (Denisoff and Wahrman 1975:352; Witters and Jones-Witters 1975:251), but this reputation is basically false, and the characterization mythical. Some illicit drugs in small amounts may promote sexual activity by lowering inhibitions, but large amounts of the same drugs can decrease sexuality (Gebhard 1965:485). Indeed, many illicit-drug users frequently participate in little or no sexual activity.

In men, this lack of sexual activity can be the result of drug-induced primary and secondary impotence (Amelar et al. 1977:205; Cooper 1972:549; Masters and Johnson 1970:143, 184; Shader 1970b:63; Stewart 1975:42; and Stoffer 1968:782). As Oliven (1974) attests, "Men addicted to narcotic, stimulant, psychedelic and certain other drugs are subject to major disturbances of sexual potency [p.443]." This may be particularly true of adolescent and young drug users (Talkington 1971:27). Evidence that the impotence can be

---

[1]For an excellent review of research that alleges a negative effect of marihuana on health, including subfecundity, see Brecher (1975:143–145). This article also presents the conflicting evidence that is generally more satisfying (1975:145–149).

caused by the drugs themselves is provided by the fact that it is frequently reversible by the termination of drug use.

BARBITURATES AND TRANQUILIZERS

Many barbiturates and tranquilizers can produce impotence as a side effect (Hastings 1960:430; Johnson 1968:33; Kaufman 1967:137; Masters and Johnson 1970:184; Oliven 1974:445; Talkington 1971:27). This, incidently, is the most important reason why psychiatric patients avoid taking their prescribed medication (Marshall, 1971:656). Examples of tranquilizers whose excessive use may produce impotence include Thorazine, Compazine, Mellaril, Phenergan, and Sparine (Cross 1973:2). Potency is usually immediately restored after cessation of use of such impotence-causing tranquilizers (Dubin and Amelar 1972:580).

STIMULANTS

The effect of amphetamines on coital ability is apparently dose related (Cross 1973:2). Small amounts usually have little if any effect. Larger doses may enhance orgasmic feeling, and this may be one of the major reasons for their use (Leavitt 1974:316). Some authors believe that amphetamine users are relatively active sexually, even promiscuous (Greaves 1972:363). Even larger doses, however, may depress coital ability and result in impotence (cf. Cooper 1972:549; Masters and Johnson 1970:184; Oliven, 1974:444). As Cross (1973) notes:

> High doses such as one gram intravenously in 24 hours usually produce withdrawal and loss of interest in sex as well as everything else. Men who use the drug in this amount frequently go through two states. First, they are able to maintain erections for long periods without ejaculation. Later the second state causes a loss of erectile ability. Usually the results are reversed back to normal after a period of abstinence from drug use [p.2].

Cocaine, another stimulant, increases sexual appetite in most users, especially females, and male potency may be temporarily heightened. However, long-term male users may develop priapism, a malady often followed by impotence (Oliven 1974:445).

MARIHUANA

The relationship between marihuana use and coital ability is unclear. Arguing against a negative influence is the fact that surveys of users consistently find that increased sexual enjoyment is a frequent reason given for beginning and continuing to use the drug (cf. Leavitt 1974:317). However, some heavy users report progressive loss of sexual interest (Oliven 1974:444), and a few studies (e.g., Harmon and Aliapoulios 1972) indicate that heavy use of marihuana may adversely affect sexual function (cf. Amelar *et al.* 1977:81).

Kolodny and his associates have raised the possibility that marihuana may lead to impotence in some users. In one of their studies (1974), they investigated blood testosterone levels of 20 frequent marihuana users and 20 nonusers. Though within the normal range, the testosterone levels in the marihuana users were lower than those in the nonusers. Moreover, the testosterone level was inversely related to the amount of marihuana used. Two of the 20 marihuana users complained of impotence, which might be related to the low testosterone levels. One of these men regained potency after stopping use of the drug. In general, abstention from marihuana usually produced marked increases in testosterone (Kolodny *et al.* 1974:872).

In another study (cf. *Time* 1975c:54), Kolodny and his associates confined 20 male volunteers to a metabolic research ward where they were forbidden to smoke cigarettes, drink coffee or alcohol, or use marihuana for 11 days before their testosterone levels were measured. After this period, each participant was permitted a daily average of 5 marihuana cigarettes containing a known quantity of its active ingredient, and the consumption of these cigarettes was monitored closely throughout the 3-month test. After 4 weeks, the men's production of luteinizing hormone, one of the substances that causes the testes to produce testosterone, significantly dropped. The researchers reported decreases in the men's testosterone levels after the fifth week, and, by the end of the eighth week, production of follicle-stimulating hormone, which is involved in sperm production, was also dramatically down. Within 9 weeks, testosterone levels decreased on the average by one-third and, in some cases, to within the range in which impotence could occur. The conclusion, therefore, was that long-term marihuana smoking can interfere with the production of reproductive hormones, suppressing the supply of the male sex hormone testosterone enough to produce impotence. The researchers expressed doubt, however, that casual marihuana use would seriously affect sexual performance. The study also reported that the testosterone level and the ability to perform sexually of all subjects returned to normal 2 weeks after giving up the drug.

However, other researchers discount suggestions that marihuana reduces the amount of testosterone circulating in the blood (Gould 1976:261). In one study, Mendelson and his associates (1974) selected 27 young male users who had consumed at least 2 marihuana cigarettes daily for the past year and who had been using the drug for at least several years. For 2 weeks prior to the start of the experiment and during the first 6 days, no marihuana was allowed. Testosterone levels were measured daily and were found to be in the upper range of normal adult levels the first 6 days. During the next 21 days marihuana was smoked under observation in order to ensure its consumption. Some of the subjects smoked large quantities. The researchers found that the testosterone levels of the men did not fall and concluded that "high-dosage marihuana intake was not associated with suppression of testosterone levels [p. 1051]."

Thus, although the possibility that marihuana may lead to impotence has received carefully controlled study, this work has yielded conflicting results, and further research is required.

HALLUCINOGENS

LSD is considered to be an enhancer of sexual pleasures. There is little, if any, evidence that it causes or contributes to coital inability. In fact, some psychiatrists believe that LSD can be an effective agent in the cure of impotence, as well as of homosexuality (cf. Leavitt 1974:317; Oliven 1974:444). Not much is known about the relationship between peyote and coital ability. Fernberger reported that peyote greatly reduced the ability of his study subjects to become erotically aroused, but Kluver, who has extensively studied the drug, believes that peyote has no effect on sexual performance or desire (cf. Leavitt 1974:318).

In general, hallucinogens are thought to have a positive effect on sexual enjoyment (cf. Witters and Jones-Witters 1975:101, 104–106).

NARCOTICS

Many authors note that narcotics, especially heroin and morphine, can lead to impotence (e.g., Cross 1973:2; Johnson 1968:33; Talkington 1971:27). Some even contend that impotence is common or regularly found in narcotics addicts (e.g., Hastings 1960:430; Mayer-Gross et al. 1969:162; Stewart 1975:42). Oliven (1974:445–446) observes that more severe addicts frequently become totally impotent, but, as dilution increases, such side effects become milder. In one study (Chein et al. 1964:166), nearly half of 100 heroin users were found to be impotent. Indeed, Fraser (1972:868) observes that impotence has been blamed for the high incidence of subfecundity among heroin users.

Ironically, one of the main objections to methadone, a substitute drug used in the treatment of heroin addiction, is that it too causes sexual disturbances, including impotence (Cassidy 1972:112; Lennard et al. 1972:882). Methadone-maintenance participants often experience impotence for several months (Oliven 1974:382).

Conceptive Failure

Although it is apparent from the medical literature that illicit drugs are viewed as possible causes of infertility in both men and women, there is little information about the nature of such effects. As is so often the case with psychopathological disorders, an association with subfecundity is noted, without rigorous testing to prove causality or to determine the mechanisms involved.

Illicit drugs may cause infertility in the male by interfering with sperm transmission or by affecting the quantity or quality of sperm available for fertilization (Stewart 1975:42). In women, illicit drugs can lead to conceptive failure as a result of menstrual abnormalities and anovulation. Relatively more is known about drug-induced infertility in women than in men.

At the Lexington Clinical Research Center, many physicians have noted the high incidence of menstrual abnormalities and infertility among various kinds of drug-addicted women (Stoffer 1968:779). In a study of 115 such women, Stoffer (1968:780) found that, whereas 16% were infertile before using drugs, 63% became so while they used drugs. Similarly, though 10% had menstrual abnormalities before drug taking, 80% had them during drug taking, and 43% continued to have them after they stopped taking the drugs. Moreover, a number of women who had regular periods while using illicit drugs were nonetheless infertile at this time (Stoffer 1968:782). In another study (Fraser 1972:867), 7 of 15 drug-addicted women gave a history of either oligomenorrhea or amenorrhea. Similarly, after reviewing data from a prospective study of 136 women with a variety of drug habits, Poland et al. (1972:956) noted that irregular menstrual cycles and amenorrhea were not unusual.

BARBITURATES AND TRANQUILIZERS

Barbiturates and tranquilizers may cause infertility in males. Ejaculatory disorders, for instance, are a side effect of some common major and minor tranquilizers (cf. Johnson 1968:33, 64; Leavitt 1974:314; Shader 1970b:63; Stewart 1975:42). Major tranquilizers were cited as the cause of ejaculatory incompetence in 27% of 30 men presenting at an infertility clinic (Girgis et al. 1968:581). A popular minor tranquilizer, Librium, has also been reported to be a cause of ejaculation problems (Shader 1970b:63). In addition, some workers have noted decreased sperm quantity and quality in those using tranquilizers. Shader (1970b:63) has cited oligospermia as a possible result of tranquilizer use, and Oliver (1965:192) has observed that these drugs may alter sperm structure and function.

Barbiturates and tranquilizers may also produce infertility in women.

There is evidence, for instance, that tranquilizers can interfere with ovulation (cf. Defeo and Reynolds 1956, cited in Gaulden et al. 1964:156; Whitelaw 1960:176; Witters and Jones-Witters 1975:203). Menstrual irregularities, particularly amenorrhea, may also be a consequence of barbiturate and tranquilizer use (cf. Shader et al. 1970:10–15; Witters and Jones-Witters 1975:189, 203). In a random sample of Swedish women aged 15–35, Fries (1974:473, 477) found that women with secondary amenorrhea used tranquilizers and hypnotics twice as often as did the controls. In the Stoffer (1968:780) study, of the two tranquilizer-addicted women, one became amenorrheic and the second became polymenorrheic. But none of the four barbiturate-addicted women had any menstrual irregularities. However, 7 of the 8 women who used both heroin and barbiturates reported menstrual abnormalities coincident with drug use, whereas only 1 had a predrug history of such disorders. The study of Gaulden et al. (1964:158) tends to confirm this observation that combined heroin–barbiturate use is particularly disruptive to the menstrual cycle. In their study, 5 of 6 (83.3%) users of heroin and barbiturates had menstrual abnormalities, whereas only 25 of 35 (71.4%) users of heroin alone showed such disorders. These researchers feel that barbiturates enhance the interfering effect of heroin on the menstrual cycle.

STIMULANTS

In men, the use of amphetamines can result in difficulties in achieving orgasm and in ejaculatory incompetence (Witters and Jones-Witters 1975:161). Long-term heavy use of these drugs is particularly apt to have this consequence (Oliven 1974:444).

Though Poland and his associates (1972:956) observe that amenorrhea and irregular menstrual cycles are not uncommon in women who use amphetamines steadily, Stoffer (1968:78) found that women using amphetamines had no higher rate of menstrual abnormalities during use than before. And those who used amphetamines together with narcotics were observed to have a lower rate of menstrual abnormalities than those who used narcotics alone. Gaulden and his associates (1964:158) suggest that amphetamines may reduce the negative effect of heroin on the menstrual cycle, reporting that in their study oligomenorrhea and amenorrhea occurred in only 29.4% of the 17 heroin and stimulant users, in comparison to a 71.4% rate for the 35 users of heroin alone.

MARIHUANA

The evidence linking marihuana use to male infertility rests primarily on the observation of Kolodny et al. (1974:872) that 6 of 17 (35%) heavy marihuana users had oligospermia. They hypothesized that a dysfunction of the hypothalamic—pituitary—gonadal axis underlies the abnormally low sperm counts. However, as mentioned earlier, the relationship between marihuana use and abnormal male reproductive physiology is still largely unresolved.

Though recent animal studies have indicated that the active substance in marihuana (THC), in doses comparable to what a human would be exposed to by smoking only 2 marihuana cigarettes, inhibits the action of a hormone (luteinizing hormone) necessary for conception (cf. *Philadelphia Bulletin* 1977:June 11, 1), there is apparently little evidence linking marijuana use to infertility in women. In fact, Gaulden and his associates (1964:158) suggest that marihuana use may reduce the negative impact of heroin on the menstrual cycle.

HALLUCINOGENS

Little is known about the impact of hallucinogens on conceptive ability. In one study (Jacobson and Berlin 1972:1371) of pregnant LSD users, 12 women expressed a desire for a repeat pregnancy, but only 4 were able to conceive within 18 to 30 months. The authors submit that it was too soon to conclude definitely that their fecundity was compromised by the drug, although the data strengthen the belief that LSD may cause infertility.

NARCOTICS

Of all the illicit drug groups, narcotics probably have the most deleterious impact on the ability to conceive. In men, narcotics can have a downgrading effect on sperm structure and function, and ejaculation is often retarded or not achieved, and in women the menstrual functions tend to suspend themselves (Oliven 1965:192, 384, 1974:446).

Heroin use may inhibit the ability of men to bring about conception. Addicts may have delayed or absent ejaculation (Murphree 1971:332). And there is evidence that the ejaculate volume, seminal vesicular and prostatic secretions, serum testosterone levels, and sperm motility of heroin users are all lower than normal (cf. Cicero *et al.* 1975:882).

Amenorrhea and anovulation are well-recognized and frequent features of heroin addiction (cf. Fraser 1972:867; Murphree 1971:332; Neuberg 1970:1117; Oliven 1974:446; Pelosi *et al.* 1974:966—969; Wallach *et al.* 1969:1226; Weir 1972:869; and Witters and Jones-Witters 1975:251). Menstruation usually stops after 1—4 months of heroin use and usually returns shortly after withdrawal from the drug (Neuberg 1970:1117). Gaulden and his associates (1964) investigated the effect of heroin use on the menstrual cycle of 74 women. Their findings are summarized in the following passage:

> It can be readily seen that before the period of drug addiction, almost all of the women had normal cycles, while during heroin usage 64.9 percent had abnormal cycles. Cessation of the addictive period led to a return to normalcy in most subjects. In all cases but one the menstrual abnormality produced by heroin addiction was the prolongation of the cycle length or complete elimination of the menstrual periods [p.157].

The authors further conclude that heroin, in sufficiently large doses, will suppress ovulation in women, though they note that other factors, such as malnutrition and environmental stress, cannot be adequately assessed.

In a similar study, Stoffer (1968:779) found that whereas only 6% of 81 eventual heroin users had abnormal menses prior to drug use, 90% had abnormal menses during their addiction. Sixty-three percent of these were amenorrheic, and 10% were oligomenorrheic. In addition, 6 of 8 (75%) users of narcotics other than heroin had abnormal periods during drug use, as opposed to only 2 (25%) prior to the habit.

The relationship between frigidity and infertility is unknown, though some workers believe that the two may be related, perhaps causally (see Chapter 3). In this event, it is worth noting that, according to Mayer-Gross and associates (1969:162), frigidity is regularly found in heroin addicts.

Methadone, a substitute drug used in the treatment of heroin addiction, is also linked to infertility in both men and women (Witters and Jones-Witters 1975:256). A proportion of men using this drug become inorgasmic (Oliven 1974:446). And Cicero et al. (1975) report that the function of the secondary sex organs of 29 methadone users were found to be markedly impaired. In their words:

> The ejaculate volume and seminal vesicular and prostatic secretions were reduced by over 50 percent in methadone clients, as compared to 16 heroin addicts and 43 narcotic-free controls. Serum testosterone levels were also approximately 43 percent lower in methadone clients than in controls or heroin users. Although the sperm count of methadone clients was more than twice the control levels, reflecting a lack of sperm dilution by secondary-sex-organ secretions, the sperm motility of these subjects was markedly lower than normal [p. 882].

In women, the evidence linking methadone and amenorrhea is conflicting. On the one hand, Cassidy (1972:113) found that 3 of 4 methadone users developed amenorrhea subsequent to administration of methadone; the fourth had only been taking the drug for less than a month. However, Wallach et al. (1969:1227–1228) report that 82 of 83 former heroin addicts began to

menstruate regularly 1–2 months after the beginning of methadone maintenance. This strikingly uniform return to regular menstruation may be attributed, suggest the authors, either to a pharmacological effect of the
methadone itself or possibly to the concurrent return to the more orderly
existence that the drug permits. But the effect could also be due to the
absence of the pharmacological effect of heroin.

Pregnancy Loss

Recent studies both retrospective and prospective have shown that pregnant women consume many drugs, 80% of which are not prescribed by a
physician (Eriksson et al. 1973:199). One prospective study of 240 women
revealed that during the first trimester of pregnancy women were exposed to
an average of 3.1 drugs, many of which were readily avoidable (Zellweger
1974:345). Tucker (1975:3) reports that 92% of women take at least one drug
during their pregnancy, and about 4% take 10 or more. Moreover, pregnant
women dependent on illicit drugs are no longer a rarity (Neuberg 1972:867).
In one clinical series (Hill 1973:655) of 156 middle- to high-socioeconomic-
class women, 5% were using narcotics and 24% were taking barbiturates and
tranquilizers. In another series of 911 randomly selected mothers, 28% were
taking barbiturates and 4% were taking tranquilizers (Forfar and Nelson
1973:633). In 1972 at the New York Metropolitan Hospital, 1 in every 27
deliveries was to a narcotic-addicted woman (Zelson 1973:1393). The fact
that drugs are administered to or taken for nonmedicinal purposes by almost
all pregnant women may be relevant to population fecundity, since drugs can
have an adverse effect on the fetus and can even increase the rate of
pregnancy loss (Eriksson et al. 1973:199).

However, it is difficult to assess the specific nature of the relationship
between various drugs and pregnancy loss because little is known concerning the exact action of drugs on the embryo or fetus (Scott 1974:123) and
addiction to illicit drugs is associated with other variables, such as poor
prenatal care, that could adversely influence pregnancy outcome (cf. Fraser
1972:868; Neuberg 1970:1118; and Tucker 1975:5).

Research problems abound in the effort to elucidate the mechanisms by
which illicit drugs may effect pregnancy loss. Reliable studies about the
effects of most drugs on the human fetus are scarce (Forfar and Nelson
1973:639), and what is known often cannot be applied to all pregnancies
(Tucker 1975:3). Animal studies are often irrelevant because of species differences, and it is difficult to isolate the effects of drugs on humans. It is
noteworthy that the two best known fetotoxic drugs, thalidomide and diethyl-
stilbestrol, were identified primarily because they caused problems that

were otherwise rare. Even at that, thalidomide (a sedative) had been in extensive use for 4 years before detection. Thus, obstetrical texts are limited to lamely cautioning physicians against the use of most drugs during pregnancy (Hellman 1973:625).

Evaluating the impact of illicit drugs on pregnancy loss suffers not only from the lack of data and the research problems just mentioned but also from the difficulty of extracting subfecundity due to the drug itself from subfecundity due to problems associated with the life style of a drug addict. Such problems, which were touched upon earlier in this chapter, include habitation in overcrowded, unsanitary places, poor nutrition that predisposes to diseases such as TB, an increased incidence of venereal disease, and the almost complete absence of prenatal care. In Stern's (1966:257) series of 66 pregnant addicts, for example, there was an average of less than one prenatal-visit per woman. Addicts resist prenatal hospital admission unless they are ill, and they frequently present themselves to a physician for the first time when in labor (Neuberg 1972:867).

Despite these difficulties, physicians, impressed by the high rates of pregnancy loss apparent among drug addicts (cf. Stoffer 1968:779), do consider illicit drugs, including barbiturates, tranquilizers, hallucinogens, narcotics, and so on, as actual or potential teratogenic and/or fetotoxic agents (Babson and Benson 1971:36–37). Pregnancy loss in the form of abortion, stillbirth, and perinatal mortality has been recorded (cf. Poland *et al.* 1972:957–958). And, although it is not a component of pregnancy loss, it is pertinent that the offspring of users of some illicit drugs also have higher rates of neonatal and infant mortality (cf. Stoffer 1968:781).[2] Finally, prematurity, low birth-weight, and obstetric complications, which may contribute to pre- and postnatal mortality, have been linked to illicit drug use (cf. Poland *et al.* 1972:957–958).

Some data on the rates of unfavorable pregnancy outcome are presented by Niswander and Gordon (1972) and Stoffer (1968). Reporting on a

[2]Infants of mothers addicted to narcotics, for instance, can suffer withdrawal syndrome at birth, and, if this condition is not recognized and treated, these babies can go on to convulsions, coma, and death (Asch 1965:468; *British Medical Journal* 1972a:63; Desmond *et al.* 1961:432–433; *Medical Letter* 1972:95; Tucker 1975:9). Neonatal addiction occurs in at least 50% of the infants of mothers who regularly use narcotics (Babson and Benson, 1971:38). The proportion of addicted infants who die depends on whether or not they are recognized as addicted and on the effectiveness of the treatment administered (Priestley 1972:870). In 1956, Goodfriend and associates (1956:35) found a neonatal mortality rate of 93% in symptomatic, untreated infants of addicted mothers. At the other extreme, Zelson *et al.* (1971:178) report a mortality rate of 3.6%, essentially the same as that of infants whose mothers were not addicts. Most other studies report rates somewhere in between those of these two studies (see Desmond *et al.* 1961:432; Leavitt 1974:170; Neuberg 1970:1118). Interestingly, the offspring of narcotic-using men also have higher mortality (*Science News* 1975:116). In addition to narcotics, some barbiturates and tranquilizers can cause a severe withdrawal syndrome more hazardous than narcotic withdrawal (*British Medical Journal* 1972a:64).

large prospective study (The Collaborative Perinatal Project), Niswander and Gordon (1972:263–265) found that the rates (per 1000 births) of stillbirth and low birth-weight were 58.8 and 187.5 for white drug-addicted women; the same rates for normal women were 21.1 and 70.4. And the study by Stoffer (1968:781), one of the most complete accounts of prenancy outcome in drug-addicted women, reports that only 43% of such pregnancies produced surviving progeny. Of the pregnancies, 30% spontaneously aborted, and 18% were terminated by criminal abortion. Of the babies born alive, 58% were drug addicted, and one-third of these subsequently died. Thus, only 33 infants survived out of a total of 77 pregnancies.

The role of each drug group on pregnancy outcome will now be examined.

BARBITURATES AND TRANQUILIZERS

Barbiturates and tranquilizers are commonly used during pregnancy. In one series (Forfar and Nelson 1973:633), over 30% of the women used them during pregnancy. Thus, if these drugs cause pregnancy loss, a substantial amount of population subfecundity would result.

There is evidence that there may be a risk of teratogenicity, albeit a low one, if barbiturates are taken during pregnancy (Babson and Benson 1971:37; Crombie et al. 1970:178; Forfar and Nelson 1973:640; Mathews 1973:800). Large doses of barbiturates may also depress the fetus late in gestation or at the time of delivery, such that respiration is not adequately established (Forfar and Nelson 1973:641), and late fetal death or stillbirth may result. Moreover, the abrupt termination of barbiturates can cause a severe withdrawal syndrome in the mother that is more hazardous to the fetus than is narcotic withdrawal (cf. British Medical Journal 1972a:64; Neuberg 1970:1120).

The literature on the relationship between the minor tranquilizers and the fetus is similar. There is evidence that these drugs may be teratogenic (cf. Babson and Benson 1971:37). A recent study by Milkovich and van den Berg (1974:1268) reports that two widely used mild tranquilizers, Librium and Miltown, may cause serious birth defects if taken early in pregnancy. However, Hartz et al. (1975:726), in a similar study, found no link between these drugs and birth defects. The minor tranquilizers can produce physical dependence and give rise to withdrawal symptoms (Asch 1965:467), and these symptoms can be very hazardous to the fetus (British Medical Journal 1972a:64).

Though the major tranquilizers may be fetotoxic (cf. Babson and Benson 1971:37), no withdrawal symptoms occur to complicate pregnancy or delivery (Asch 1965:467).

STIMULANTS

Although some authors believe that stimulants have no adverse effects on the fetus (Neuberg 1970:1119), there is growing evidence that amphetamines may be teratogenic (cf. Forfar and Nelson 1973:640; Schenkel and Vorherr 1974:28). Recently, five physicians recommended that the U.S. Government ban the use of amphetamines, partially on the grounds that they may produce birth defects (*Philadelphia Bulletin* 1974:Nov. 10, 1). There are no withdrawal symptoms, however, to complicate pregnancy or delivery (Asch 1965:467). This also holds for cocaine.

MARIHUANA

Marihuana is the single most widely used illicit drug in the United States, especially among young people and those in their prime reproductive years (Neuberg 1970:1120). Therefore, if marihuana use causes pregnancy loss, it would be a significant determinant of population subfecundity. Though experiments on animals provide evidence that marihuana in high doses causes fetal loss (Leavitt 1974:172), there is no convincing evidence that marihuana causes pregnancy loss in humans. As with other illicit drugs, studies on the use of marihuana during pregnancy and its effects on the fetus are still inconclusive (Tucker 1975:14). It is fairly certain, however, that there are no physical withdrawal symptoms associated with this drug that complicate pregnancy or delivery (Asch 1965:467–468). However, some authors (e.g., Stenchever *et al.* 1974:110) feel that marihuana is associated with chromosome breakage and must be considered as a possible cause of the excessive pregnancy loss and reproductive dysfunctions reported among drug users (cf. Amelar *et al.* 1977:81).

The 8-year study by Stenchever and his associates (1974) concluded that persons using the drug on any regular basis have three times more chromosome damage than do nonusers. In addition, there was little difference in damage incidence between light and heavy users of the substance. It is also significant that the individuals studied in this series were college students who, unlike the subjects of many other drug-related studies, had good general health and nutrition. Another study (Gilmour *et al.* 1971) found a similar increase in chromosome breakage among heavy users of marihuana. However, no increase in chromosome aberrations were found for light users. Two studies of Persaud and Ellington (1967, 1968; cf. Neuberg 1970:1120) showed that marihuana resin is teratogenic in rats and causes fetal resorption in mice. Despite species differences, they feel that marihuana may possibly be harmful to the human fetus. Indeed, some researchers (e.g., Stenchever *et al.* 1974:110) are speculating that the fetal abnormalities and abortions observed in LSD users might have actually been caused by marihuana, since virtually all LSD users also smoke marihuana. It is noteworthy that all of the 140 couples in an oft-cited LSD study (Jacobson and Berlin 1972) also used marihuana.

Findings from a recent animal experiment (cf. *Philadelphia Bulletin* 1977:Aug. 26, 42) also suggest that marihuana may increase the risk of birth defects and fetal death in humans. Staab and Lynch report data linking the drug with a high incidence of kidney malformation, stunted growth, and death in the offspring of mice exposed to marihuana during pregnancy. What makes this study significant in terms of humans is that the marihuana was administered in relatively low doses through a smoke environment, which simulates the type of human exposure, rather than through an injection of resin into test animals.

However, though the possibility does exist, there is no conclusive evidence that chromosome breakage due to marihuana results in fetal abnormalities or subsequent pregnancy loss (Tucker 1975:14). Moreover, the evidence concerning the ability of the drug to break chromosomes is itself conflicting (cf. Brecher 1975:148−149). Nichols and his associates (1974:413), for instance, carried out a well-controlled study on this relationship and detected no chromosome damage. Also, several test tube studies (Neu *et al.* 1969; Pace *et al.* 1971; Stenchever and Allen 1972) failed to turn up a significant increase in chromosome breakage after exposure of cells to marihuana and some of its active ingredients. Stenchever *et al.* (1974:106) caution, however, that marihuana is a composite of a number of agents, and its effect on chromosomes is still to be defined.

HALLUCINOGENS

According to Tucker (1975:14), LSD has been shown to increase the rate of spontaneous abortion. And Neuberg (1970:1120) suggests that the time at which LSD is taken may affect this ability to cause abortions, since abortions apparently occur more frequently among those who take the drug either before or during early pregnancy. In one study (Jacobson and Berlin 1972:1367) of LSD-consuming women who enrolled in a study during the first trimester of pregnancy, 43% spontaneously aborted, a twofold increase in the commonly accepted figure of 15−20%. In another study, McGlothen and associates (1970:1483) report that 37% of pregnancies in LSD-consuming women were spontaneously aborted. Since the women in this sample had all taken LSD outside of medical supervision, it is possible that the LSD may have contained impurities and other drugs. Spontaneous abortions occurred significantly more frequently among couples where the woman, rather than the man, was the sole user of the drug. The authors also found that the frequency of abortion was within normal bounds for individuals exposed only to infrequent, low doses of medically administered LSD.

LSD is also frequently mentioned as a possible teratogen (e.g., Schenkel and Vorherr 1974:28; Babson and Benson 1971:36), there being some evidence that it may produce malformations in the fetus if taken early in pregnancy (cf. Assemany et al. 1970:1290; Eller and Morton 1970:395; *Medical Letter* 1972:95; and Neuberg 1972:867). However, others (cf. Eriksson et al. 1973:222; Smithells 1976:29), after reviewing the available evidence, conclude that there is little evidence that LSD is teratogenic in humans. Likewise, the most frequent explanation for observed abnormalities, the ability of LSD to damage chromosomes, is also disputed. Although the role of LSD in chromosome damage is frequently cited (cf. Babson and Benson 1971:36; Eriksson et al. 1973:222; Neuberg 1970:1120, 1972:867; Titus 1972:701; and Tucker 1975:14), the most recent studies have cast doubt on this hypothesis (cf. Brecher 1975:144; Goode 1975:42; Stenchever et al. 1974:106).

Although Witters and Jones-Witters (1975:114) note that chemical relatives of LSD have been associated with spontaneous abortion, they (1975:123) insist that more controlled studies must be carried out on the genetic effects of LSD and other hallucinogens and on their effects during pregnancy.

NARCOTICS

Narcotic addiction represents a serious threat to pregnancy (Babson and Benson 1971:36), since women who use illicit drugs report higher rates of abortion, of late fetal death, and of stillbirth (Leavitt 1974:170; Murphree 1971:332; Tucker 1975:8). Spontaneous abortion occurred in 30% of the pregnancies in Stoffer's (1968) study of drug-addicted women. Since the vast majority (89%) of study women were narcotic addicts, most of whom (86%) used heroin, this 30% figure likely approximates the spontaneous abortion rate of heroin addicts.

Stillbirth rates of narcotic-addicted women are approximately four times greater than those of the general obstetric population (Blinick et al. 1973:478; Rementeria and Nunag 1973:1155; Stern 1966:257; Wallach et al. 1969:1228). Five of 66 pregnancies (7.6%) reported by Stern terminated as stillbirths, as did 1 of 13 (7.7%) in the Wallach et al. study, 5 of 72 (6.9%) in the Blinick study, and 3 of 47 (6.4%) in the Rementaria and Nunag study. There are several studies, however, that report stillbirth rates similar to those of the general population for narcotic users. Blinick and associates (1969:999) and Statzer and Wardell (1972:275) found rates of 1.0 and 2.0%, respectively. Rementaria and Nunag (1973:1154) believe that one reason for such low rates is that most of the women in these series were on methadone maintenance and maintain that the withdrawal prior to childbirth was less severe than in heroin addicts. However, of the four series cited that report a 7% rate, two (Blinick et al. 1973 and Wallach et al. 1969) were also studies of methadone users.

Other authors have focused on the broader category of perinatal mortality. Babson and Benson (1971:38) report a 15–20% perinatal mortality rate in narcotic-addicted women.

Pregnancy loss associated with narcotic addiction may be attributable to a pharmacological action of the drug itself or to the adverse conditions that characterize the life style of addicts. Forfar and Nelson (1973:641) report that narcotics may depress the fetus. The establishment of fetal respiration, for example, may be depressed, thus compromising pregnancy outcome. Another known pharmacological effect of narcotics is physical dependence, which gives rise to severe withdrawal symptoms. This withdrawal may be deleterious to fetal survival (Asch 1965:467–468). It has been hypothesized that maternal withdrawal may cause increased fetal movement and sometimes death (Sutherland and Light 1965:793) and that the oxygen supply to the fetus may be lowered in severe withdrawal to the point that death occurs (Rementaria and Nunag 1973:1155).

The exact causes—pharmacological or life style—of the adverse circumstances intermediate to drug use and pregnancy loss, such as obstetric complications and low birth-weight, are also yet undetermined. But such adverse circumstances undoubtedly do occur with greater frequency in drug-addicted women. A high incidence of obstetric complications is observed in narcotic addicts (cf. Tucker 1975:8). In the Stern (1966:257) series, 41% of the 66 pregnancies were accompanied by at least one obstetric complication. Prematurity and intrauterine growth retardation are also frequently seen in the offspring of narcotics users (cf. Blinick et al. 1973:478; Fraser, 1972:868), some authors (e.g., Babson and Benson 1971:38; Neuberg 1970:1117; and Priestly 1972:870) reporting an incidence of approximately 50%. In one study (Zelson et al. 1973:1219) at the New York Metropolitan Hospital, 10% of the offspring of all women, but 44% of those of the heroin group and 48% of those of the methadone group, were low-birth-weight infants. It was considered noteworthy that the rate for methadone users was about the same as for that for heroin users, despite the supposedly more stable living conditions of the former.

Interestingly, animal studies indicate that male use of narcotics may also lead to higher fetal and infant mortality rates among their offspring. For instance, Smith and Joffe (1975:202–203) found that survival to 3 weeks occurred in only 26% of offspring sired by methadone-treated rats and 66% of those sired by morphine-treated rats. In contrast, the survival rate was between 90 and 95% for offspring of a control population. The researchers also report that the infant mortality rate is directly related to the size of the methadone dosage administered to the male parent and that the chances of infant mortality were greatest when insemination took place within 24 hours of treatment. Thus they (1975) conclude: "Our preliminary results suggest that it is necessary to investigate not only the drugs which were administered to the mother before and during pregnancy, but also those drugs used by the father [p. 203]." It is possible, then, that paternal drug use in humans causes congenital defects that contribute to infant mortality and that some of the more lethal defects are a cause of fetal loss as well.

Prevalence

Illicit drug abuse is widespread in the United States. The exact dimensions of the problem are unknown, however, due to the illicit nature of the drugs involved (Zelson 1973:1393). Data on the extent of illicit drug abuse are generally extrapolations from arrest data or are based on responses to sample surveys whose accuracy depends in part on individuals admitting illegal or deviant behavior. Moreover, much prescribed use is in fact nonmedicinal use or drug abuse, though the proportion is almost impossible to determine. Much of the data presented in the following is from a study done by the National Commission on Marihuana and Drug Abuse (1973). This study cautions the reader that it underestimates the prevalence of drug abuse, especially use of hallucinogens and narcotics, for the reasons just mentioned and, in particular, because the household surveys utilized do not pick up many "street" users. Thus, the reader should keep in mind that the following discussion of drug abuse prevalence probably errs on the low side.

BARBITURATES AND TRANQUILIZERS

As with illicit drugs in general, the extent of barbiturate and tranquilizer use in the United States is practically impossible to assess. In 1973, 10 billion doses of barbiturates, or 50 doses per capita, were produced legally, and the production of tranquilizers was even higher (Mauss 1975:248). For instance, about 4 billion Valium and Librium pills alone are dispensed annually to the U.S. public, enough to supply 20 per capita (Lawson 1976:28). The U.S. Commission on Marihuana and Drug Abuse (1973:51) found that 20% of American adults had used prescription barbiturates sometime in their lives and that 11% were recent users. The same percentages for prescription tranquilizer use were 24 and 17, respectively. Four percent of American adults admitted to nonmedicinal use of barbiturates, and 6% to nonmedicinal use of tranquilizers (NCMDA 1973:63). It has been estimated that as many as

1 million individuals in the United States are chronic users of these drugs (Goode 1973:16). In terms of gross abuse, Shulgin (1971:19) suggests that barbiturate and tranquilizer use may well constitute the most serious illicit drug problem in the United States.

STIMULANTS

Amphetamines are the most frequently used form of prescription stimulant. In 1971, 60 amphetamine doses per capita were manufactured in the United States, and half ended up on the illegal drug market. Amphetamine use is particularly widespread among college students, about one-third of whom report use of these drugs (McNall 1975:217). The National Commission on Marihuana and Drug Abuse (1973:51) found that 13% of the adult population had used amphetamines and that 8% were recent users. Five percent of the adult population admitted to nonmedicinal use of amphetamines (NCMDA 1973:63). The Commission also found substantial evidence that middle-class adults, particularly women, were chronic amphetamine users. When asked why they used these drugs, 43% of these adults stated that they "helped them accomplish something [Mauss 1975:248]."

The National Commission on Marihuana and Drug Abuse (1973:69) estimates that cocaine, another stimulant, has been tried at least once by 5 million Americans. However, more recent figures from the National Institute on Drug Abuse place this estimate at 8 million Americans, suggesting a continuing upward trend (cf. *Time* 1977b:50). However, because cocaine is so expensive under present circumstances, few can afford to use it often, thus minimizing its potential impact on population fecundity.

MARIHUANA

The use of marihuana in the United States is widespread and increasing. In 1973 the National Commission on Marihuana and Drug Abuse (1973:63) estimated that 26 million (16%) American adults have tried marihuana, and about half that number may be classified as regular users. More recent figures from the National Institute on Drug Abuse (cf. *Time* 1977b:50) show that as many as 36 million adults (22%) have used the drug. Marihuana is probably the single most widely used illicit drug among young people (Neuberg 1970:1120); about 50–60% of all college students have at least tried the drug, a proportion that is also increasing over time (cf. Horton and Leslie 1974:554; *Time* 1977b:50).

HALLUCINOGENS

About 5% of American adults have tried LSD or a similar hallucinogen at least once (NCMDA 1973:68). An estimated 16% of college students and 8% of high school students in 1970 and 1971 used LSD (Schafer et al. 1975:25), and 16% of college students and 14% of high school seniors used at least one hallucinogen in 1973 (NCMDA 1973:82–83).

NARCOTICS

The number of narcotic addicts in the United States has varied from a high of 600,000 during the early to middle 1970s (Horton and Leslie 1978:546) to a present estimate of 450,000 (Franklin 1978:6). The recent decline is apparently due to improved law enforcement, which has decreased supplies and has increased prices. Half to three-fifths of U.S. addicts live in New York (NCMDA 1973:173). Approximately 1.3% of American adults, 6% of college students, and 5% of high school seniors have used heroin at least once (NCMDA 1973:69, 82–83). In addition, there are about 70,000 opiate-dependent persons enrolled in methadone maintenance programs (NCMDA 1973:319).

Population Subfecundity

There are six reasons suggesting that illicit drug abuse may be a significant determinant of population subfecundity. First, illicit drugs have been linked to all three forms of reproductive dysfunction—coital inability, conceptive failure, and pregnancy loss. Second, the abuse of illicit drugs is prevalent in some populations, including that of the United States. Despite the aforementioned problems that routinely lead to underestimation of prevalence, available figures indicate that illicit drug abuse is characteristic of a substantial fraction of the U.S. population, in particular, its reproductive population.

Third, illicit drug abusers tend to be consumers of more than one such drug (and many use alcohol and tobacco in addition) (cf. Horton and Leslie 1978:551; NCMDA 1973:51, 70–71; Witters and Jones-Witters 1975:143, 160). Asch (1965:469) reports, for instance, that 25% of heroin addicts and many amphetamine users and alcoholics also abuse barbiturates and tranquilizers. Similarly, McNall (1975:214) relates that 49% of habitual marihuana users use LSD, 43% use amphetamines, and perhaps 20% use cocaine. Thus, many drug abusers subject themselves to a variety of drugs that can cause subfecundity.

Fourth, illicit drug abusers tend to be young, and many are in their prime reproductive years. For instance, the typical Valium abuser is a woman in her twenties. Narcotic abuse also has an early onset. The age at first opiate use of 2213 addicts admitted to two U.S. Public Health Service Hospitals in 1965 by sex are as follows: for males, 50% were under age 20, 75% under age 25, and 85% under age 30; for females, 33% were under age 20, 67% under age 25, and 75% under age 30 (Clinard 1968:314). Similar figures are given by the U.S. National Institute of Mental Health (1967:20). And Zelson (1973:1393) notes that 85% of heroin- and methadone-addicted women are in their childbearing years.

Fifth, the use of illicit drugs often persists for a substantial fraction of the usual reproductive period. In one study of 5553 men who had been regular users of narcotics, it was found that 34% had been addicted for 5 years, 40% for 6–9 years, 16% for 10–14 years, and about 10% for 15–50+ years. Three-quarters of these men terminated their addiction before the age of 36 (Clinard 1968:314–315), indicating that in most of these addicts long periods of drug use were coincident with their prime reproductive years.

And, finally, despite warnings from concerned physicians, many women consume drugs, including illicit drugs, during pregnancy.

In sum, illicit drug abuse meets the two minimal requirements of a population subfecundity factor: That is, it is prevalent, and it impairs individual fecundity. Moreover, illicit drug abusers tend to be consumers of more than one of these subfecundity-producing substances, are generally in the midst of their reproductive careers, use the substances for many years, and ingest large amounts even during pregnancy. However, it was indicated that it is presently impossible to determine how much of a deficit illicit drug abuse can make in a couple's fecundity, because of the limited data available and other research problems. Of all the research gaps, perhaps the most crucial is the lack of knowledge concerning the importance of illicit drugs as a cause of early, unrecognized pregnancy loss. Thus, the word "inconclusive" probably best describes the collective research upon which this chapter is based.

However, keeping in mind the deficiencies in present knowledge, it is, nevertheless, possible to draw some preliminary conclusions. To assist in this task, Table 10.1 was constructed to present this author's judgment concerning the ability of each of the drug groups to produce subfecundity. Also shown are estimates of the proportion of the U.S. population aged 15–44 who recently used the drugs for any reason and the proportion who are recognized as chronic abusers. In addition, an appraisal concerning the potential for the particular illicit drug abuse to influence population fecundity is offered.

TABLE 10.1

Ability of Illicit Drugs to Cause Coital Inability, Conceptive Failure, Pregnancy Loss, and Individual and Population Subfecundity; Also, Percentage of U.S. Population Ages 15–44 Who Are Recent Users and Chronic Abusers, 1973.

Illicit drugs	Coital inability	Conceptive failure	Pregnancy loss	Individual subfecundity	Recent use (%)	Chronic abuse (%)	Population subfecundity
Barbiturates and tranquilizers	yes	yes	yes	yes	25	2	improbable
Stimulants	yes	possible	possible	possible	10	3	improbable
Marihuana	possible	possible	possible	possible	10	10	improbable
Hallucinogens (LSD)	no	possible	possible		1	1	improbable
Narcotics	yes	yes	yes	yes	1	.7	improbable
All illicit drugs	yes	yes	yes	yes	30–40	10–15	yes

It is apparent from this table that the abuse of some drug groups has more of an impact on individual and population fecundity than does that of others. In particular, abuse of the most prevalent drug group, barbiturates and tranquilizers, and the least prevalent, narcotics, seems to have the most potential for fecundity impairment. All told, illicit drug abuse is judged to have only a small impact on population fecundity, but, nevertheless, an impact. The reader is again cautioned not to ignore or to consider trivial subfecundity factors of modest proportions, for, in so doing, the potential importance of the collective effect of many such factors on population fecundity would be overlooked. It is also worth noting that, although the vast majority of barbiturate, tranquilizer, and stimulant use is prescribed by physicians, a substantial portion of this use is de facto abuse merely masquerading as medicinal. Thus, the real impact of illicit drug abuse on fecundity is undoubtedly substantially higher than that based upon abuse figures alone.

It should also not escape the reader's attention that all illicit drug use, whether medicinal use or abuse, has an impact on population fecundity. More than half the adult population of the United States has used illicit drugs (cf. Witters and Jones-Witters 1975:5), and the data in Table 10.1 show that as many as 40% of the reproductive population are recent users of these drugs. The impact of this level of drug use on population fecundity is indeterminable given the present state of knowledge, but it might well be substantial.

Furthermore, this chapter has confined itself only to drugs that are classified as illicit. The reader should bear in mind that there are other sedatives, tranquilizers, and stimulants known as "proprietary" or "over-the-counter" drugs that are not considered illicit drugs but, nonetheless, have similar effects, especially in large doses. The National Commission on Marihuana and Drug Abuse (1973:51, 63) found that, among U.S. adults, 36% had used proprietary drugs, 21% had used them recently, and 7% admitted to excessive, nonmedicinal use. Thus, the effects of the use and abuse of proprietary drugs on fecundity must also be considered when a broader view of drug abuse is taken.

There is every reason to believe that the effect of illicit drug use and abuse on population fecundity varies over time, thus giving rise to fecundity differentials and, possibly, contributing to fertility differentials. In the United States, for instance, though no accurate figures exist, it has been estimated that as much as 2–4% of the population was addicted to narcotics in the late nineteenth century (Cohen and Goldsmith 1971:29; Schafer et al. 1975:22). During the first half of the twentieth century, the use of illicit drugs probably declined. However, in the last two decades, drug consumption has skyrocketed (Lancet 1973:527; Petersen 1975:255–257). In particular, the number of young women using drugs is increasing (Mauss 1975:246; Neuberg

1970:1117). Amphetamine production, as an example, rose from 20 tablets per capita in 1959 to 60 in 1971 (Mauss 1975:246; McNall 1975:217). However, there is recent evidence that this trend may be abating (Gould 1976:262; Schafer *et al.* 1975:18). There are also age, sex, racial, urban–rural, and other drug use differentials (which themselves vary over time; cf. Clinard 1968:311–313; Mauss 1975:245; Petersen 1975:255–257; and Rosen *et al.* 1972:318).

Narcotic use, for instance, is primarily an urban phenomenon, being concentrated in America's largest cities and their slums, and it is most often a feature of disadvantaged minority groups. In the following passage, Richardson and Frank (1977) show just how important narcotic addiction can be in one such city:

> The Newark [N.J.] Addiction Planning and Coordinating Agency estimates that city's hard core heroin addict population at around 20,000, or about 5 percent of the city's total population of 380,000. A 5 percent addiction rate is serious enough, but only when this figure is put into its proper perspective can we begin to understand its real impact.
>
> Most addicts are males, ranging between the ages of 15 to 35. It is estimated that of Newark's 20,000 hard-core addicts, about 17,000 are young men. According to the 1970 U.S. Census figures, Newark has a total population of 53,000 young males between the ages of 15 and 34. If 17,000 of these 53,000 young men are heroin addicts, it means that *one-third of all young men in Newark are heroin addicts* [p. 310].

Moreover Richardson and Frank consider Newark to be a typical eastern industrial city in terms of urban problems. Thus, although narcotic addiction may not be prevalent enough to significantly affect the fecundity of the entire U.S. population, it can have a substantial impact on that of sizable urban and other local populations.

Illicit drug use also varies from population to population. It is prevalent in most Western nations, though the situation in Europe is currently nothing like that in the United States (Clinard 1968:310). Certain drugs are readily available in developing countries. Opiates, for instance, are widely used among some Asiatic populations, and in South America cocaine is commonly obtained from chewing coca leaves (Rosen *et al.* 1972:322). Marihuana grows freely in many climates and is consumed in both developed and developing nations. In 1950, the U.N. noted that it was used principally in Asia and Africa, but this is no longer the case, since its consumption in Western nations and elsewhere has increased enormously since then (Grinspoon 1972:199; Witters and Jones-Witters 1975:137–139). In Jamaica 60–70% of the rural working-class population consumes some form of marihuana (Goode 1975:41). Amphetamine abuse is probably greater in Sweden than in any other country, and Japan also had high rates of amphetamine abuse in the recent past (Witters and Jones-Witters 1975:153).

The use of narcotics seems to be spreading. The International Narcotics Board recently expressed concern about the growing use of heroin in many countries where the narcotic had not been a problem in the past (Gould 1976:262).

Other Intermediate Variables

In addition to its effects on fecundity, illicit drug use can lower fertility through other intermediate variables, the most important of which are coital frequency, voluntary abortion, and union exposure.

Some female drug users, particularly narcotic addicts, have high rates of coital frequency because they are prostitutes. Women who become dependent on narcotics commonly have no means other than prostitution to support their habits (Horton and Leslie 1978:557). In the Stoffer (1968:780) study, for example, 67% of the heroin users had practiced prostitution. Also, casual use of drugs such as marihuana and cocaine sometimes leads to promiscuous behavior, especially among the young in developed countries. However, heavy drug users of both sexes generally exhibit depressed libido and low rates of sexual activity (cf. Ford and Beach 1951:238; Fraser 1972:868; Grinspoon 1972:204; Kaufman 1967:137; Money 1967:285; Murphree 1971:332; Oliven 1974:443–447; Ostow 1965:340; Pearlman and Kobashi 1972:300; Schafer et al. 1975:22; Shader 1970b:63; Stevens 1970:32; Stoffer 1968:782; Thomlinson 1976:173; Weir 1972:869; and Witters and Jones-Witters 1975:190, 203, 251, 256).

Illicit drug use may also increase the frequency of voluntary abortion. Indeed, some physicians suggest that very serious consideration should be given to termination when a patient has taken illicit drugs, such as LSD, in early pregnancy (Neuberg 1972:867). In one series (Jacobson and Berlin 1972:1367) of LSD-using women, 53 of 148 (36%) pregnancies were therapeutically aborted. Two other studies discussed in this chapter give the proportion of pregnancies that are voluntarily aborted among narcotic users. In one (Stoffer 1968:781), 14 of 77 pregnancies (18%) were voluntarily aborted, and, in the other (Blinick et al. 1973:478), 15 of 87 (17%) terminated in this fashion.

Illicit drug use may also be an obstacle to the establishment of unions, particularly for narcotics users. They tend to remain disproportionately single, especially males (Mauss 1975:245). Narcotic addicts are generally a dubious marital risk, and some states prohibit their marriage (Oliven 1965:220). Drug use can also be a cause of marital discord and disruption (Mauss 1975:245; Oliven 1965:279). Furthermore, a concealed premarital drug habit may be grounds for annulment (Oliven 1965:220). Addicts are also frequently separated from their mates. Approximately 10–15% of U.S. narcotic addicts are in prison, and others are in hospitals (Schafer *et al.* 1975:18). Finally, unions are not infrequently interrupted by death. Indeed, middle-aged or elderly addicts are uncommon. As Horton and Leslie (1974) put it, "With rare exceptions, those who are not 'clean' by middle age are dead [pp. 590–591]."

Finally, illicit drugs may decrease the effectiveness of contraception. Certainly, the chances of contraceptive error are increased while under the influence of drugs. And it has recently been discovered that certain drugs, such as tranquilizers, may inhibit the effectiveness of oral contraceptives by speeding up the enzymes that break down the contraceptives (Witters and Jones-Witters 1975:86).

11

Conclusion

The goal of this study has been to determine whether psychopathology can depress population fecundity and, if so, to what extent. The conclusion is that psychopathology can definitely affect population fecundity, although the magnitude of the effect remains unknown for many reasons. Indeed, common to every form of psychopathology discussed in this book is the observation that much remains to be learned before its quantitative impact on population fecundity can be assessed. A significant implication of this situation should not escape the reader's attention, to wit, that currently no one, not psychiatrists, psychologists, sociologists, demographers, or any other scientists, can accurately estimate the importance of psychopathology as a cause of population subfecundity. Thus, any statements in the population literature purporting to do this, including those that deny that psychopathology is influential, must be recognized for what they are, that is, speculations uninformed by empirical research.

Though it is presently not possible to determine the exact potential of psychopathology to affect population fecundity, it is clear that the effect is not negligible. This is because psychopathology easily fulfills the two necessary and sufficient requisites of a determinant of population subfecundity. First, it can have a considerable impact on individual fecundity, and, second, it can affect a substantial proportion of a population's potentially fecund members.

Evidence for an impact of psychopathology on individual fecundity is reviewed first, followed by a discussion of the prevalence of psychopathology among the reproductive members of an actual population. The population of the United States during the early 1970s is used in this example.

Effect on Individual Fecundity

Table 11.1 summarizes this author's appraisals of the ability of psychopathology and its various forms to cause individual subfecundity. It uses the words "definite," "likely," "possible," "improbable," and "none" as points on a descending scale that describe the likelihood of a causal relationship between psychopathological disorders and subfecundity. Here the word possible, admittedly imprecise, denotes only those relationships that fall between improbable and likely.

Five important facets of the relationship between psychopathology and subfecundity deserve attention. Two are illustrated in Table 11.1, namely: (a) the importance of psychopathology-induced subfecundity in both the male and the female; and (b) the ability of psychopathology to cause reproductive failure anywhere from coitus to childbirth. Other important facets are (c) the tendency for one form of subfecundity-producing psychopathology to lead to others (in the affected individual and in the mate); (d) the tendency for many of these disorders to occur early in life and to persist for much of the reproductive period; and (e) the importance of the indirect effects of psychopathology on fecundity. Each of these will be discussed in turn.

First, demographers and even clinicians specializing in subfecundity have generally ignored the possibility of male subfecundity. This has certainly been true as regards psychopathology-induced subfecundity. But Table 11.1 indicates that psychopathology exerts an influence on male as well as on female fecundity. In fact, it is not even possible to state with any assurance that psychopathology causes more subfecundity among women than among men.

Second, it is also evident from Table 11.1 that psychopathology can exert a negative influence on each of the principal components of subfecundity; it is a major cause of coital inability, conceptive failure, and pregnancy loss. In fact, psychopathology is the most important cause of coital inability, probably accounting for about 75–90% of cases (cf. Golden and Golden 1967:54; Johnson 1968:94). Psychopathology is also the primary cause of sexual disorders, such as premature ejaculation, that are involved in conceptive failure. Indeed, groups suffering from psychopathology almost always have a higher prevalence of sexual difficulties than do normal controls (Coppen

TABLE 11.1.
Ability of Psychopathological Disorders to Cause Coital Inability, Conceptive Failure, Pregnancy Loss, and Individual Subfecundity

Form of psychopathology	Sex (1)	Coital inability (2)	Conceptive failure (3)	Pregnancy loss (4)	Individual subfecundity (5)
Psychic stress (includes neuroses, psychophysiological disorders, and everyday stress)	male	definite	definite	none	definite
	female	definite	definite	definite	definite
Psychoses — All	male	definite	possible	none	definite
	female	possible	definite	unknown	definite
Schizophrenia	male	definite	definite	none	definite
	female	possible	possible	unknown	definite
Manic-depressive	male	definite	definite	none	definite
	female	possible	definite	unknown	definite
Sexual deviations — All	male	definite	likely	none	definite
	female	definite	improbable	none	definite
Homosexuality	male	definite	likely	none	definite
	female	definite	unknown	none	definite
Others	male	definite	likely	none	definite
	female	possible	improbable	none	possible
Alcoholism	male	definite	definite	possible	definite
	female	unknown	definite	likely	definite
Cigarette smoking	male	possible	possible	none	possible
	female	none	possible	likely	likely
Illicit drug abuse — All	male	definite	definite	improbable	definite
	female	none	definite	definite	definite
Barbiturates and tranquilizers	male	definite	definite	unknown	definite
	female	none	definite	likely	definite
Stimulants	male	definite	possible	unknown	definite
	female	none	possible	unknown	improbable
Marihuana	male	unknown	unknown	unknown	unknown
	female	none	none	possible	improbable
Hallucinogens	male	none	possible	improbable	improbable
	female	none	possible	possible	possible
Narcotics	male	definite	likely	definite	definite
	female	definite	definite	possible	definite
Psychopathology (total)	male	definite	definite	possible	definite
	female	definite	definite	definite	definite

1965:166). Aside from sexual disorders, psychopathology has a whole arsenal of other mechanisms to bring about conceptive failure, probably the most important being the frequently seen anovulatory amenorrhea. In addition, psychopathology, especially psychic stress, may be one of the main causes of pregnancy loss. And sizable fractions of alcoholic, smoking, and drug-addicted women continue their habits throughout pregnancy, seriously jeopardizing the health of their unborn child.

Third, the ability of psychopathology to decrease fecundity is enhanced by the tendency for one form of subfecundity-producing psychopathology to cause others. Often underlying narcotic habituation, for instance, is psychic stress; homosexuality may lead to alcoholism; and so forth. The fecundity of the partner may also be challenged when psychopathology exists in the mate. This is particularly relevant to the psychosexual disorders; impotence leads to vaginismus, premature ejaculation to female inorgasmy, and so forth. Indeed, if the union remains intact, it is probable that psychopathology in one partner generally alters the fecundity of both members of the union to some extent (cf. Abse 1966:133).

Fourth, the ability of psychopathology to affect fecundity is also enhanced by the fact that many forms tend to appear early in life and to persist for much of the reproductive period. This prolongation of both the disorder and any subsequent subfecundity is frequently abetted by the tendency for psychopathology to go untreated or to be treated ineffectively.

Fifth, it is also important to note that the effect of psychopathology on fecundity may be indirect. That is, psychopathology may be causally associated with other subfecundity factors, such as disease and malnutrition, that are the direct cause of the subfecundity. For example, psychic stress can increase the incidence, duration, and severity of tuberculosis, an important cause of subfecundity. Also, homosexuality is often associated with venereal diseases that can limit or abolish reproductive potential. And illicit drug abuse frequently leads to another subfecundity cause, malnutrition. It is important to evaluate these indirect effects when assessing the impact of psychopathology on fecundity.

Thus, psychopathology ably fulfills the first requirement of a determinant of population subfecundity, that is, it is an important cause of individual subfecundity.

Prevalence

Psychopathology can also be prevalent among the members of a population during their reproductive ages, the second requisite of a population subfecundity factor. To illustrate this point, the prevalence of psychopathology in the reproductive population of the United States during the early 1970s is examined in this section. Prevalence estimates are presented in Column 3 of Table 11.2, where the letter "S" means substantial and expresses a prevalence level that is unknown but thought to exceed 2%.

Although the current prevalence of psychopathology in the United States is unknown, it is certain that the frequency is far greater than is given in any official statistical report. Large-scale studies of psychopathology have been carried out in many areas, and virtually all yield evidence of widespread psychological impairment (Horton and Leslie 1974:528; Kramer *et al.* 1972:1). The findings of two of these studies, one dealing with an urban and the other with a rural (albeit Canadian) population, are reviewed by Clinard (1968) in the following passage:

> One of the most intensive metropolitan surveys ever made in the field of mental health involved a cross-section of a heterogeneous midtown Manhattan residential population of 110,000 persons. From interviews with 1660 residents the conclusion was reached that only 18.5 percent were free enough of emotional symptoms to be considered "well." A total of 58.1 percent were found to have mild to moderate symptoms, such as tensions, nervousness, and other indications of emotional disturbances, although not to the extent of impairing life functioning. Marked, severe, and incapacitating symptoms were found in 23.4 percent of cases.
>
> An intensive survey of Sterling County, Nova Scotia, using techniques similar to the Midtown Manhattan Study, found that two thirds of the residents exhibited symptoms of mental disorder, most of them neurotic, but only a small proportion were urgently in need of care [pp. 469–470].

Though these and similar studies have been criticized by some for their methodology and, in particular, for too-inclusive definitions of what constitutes psychopathology, most experts agree with Horton and Leslie (1978:527) that, *by any standard, the amount of psychopathology in the U.S. population is very large.*

Not only is the prevalence of psychopathology in general unknown, but, with the exception of cigarette smoking, so are the frequencies of the types discussed in this study. Thus, the estimates contained in Column 3 of Table 11.2 for the reproductive population are really just guesses. For some of these disorders, a prevalence range is given, whereas for others a single value is presented, one that either is generally recognized as the best or is the only one that could be found.

Despite this imprecision, it is clear from Table 11.2 that psychopathology is widespread in the U.S. reproductive population. One factor alone, psychic stress, is a common phenomenon and probably touches virtually everyone in the population through its component, everyday stress. Rather than submitting that the whole population is subject to psychic stress and thus, to psychopathology, an effort is made in Table 11.2 to estimate the proportion

TABLE 11.2.
The Ability of Psychopathological Disorders to Cause Individual and Population Subfecundity in the United States in the 1970s

Form of psychopathology	Sex (1)	Individual subfecundity (2)	Prevalence: Estimated percentage of population aged 15–44 (3)	U.S. population subfecundity (4)
Psychic stress				
Coital inability				
Impotence	male	definite	2	definite
Vaginismus	female	definite	0–1	improbable
Dyspareunia	male	definite	0–1	none
	female	definite	1–2	improbable
Conceptive failure				
Spermatogenic disorders	male	definite	S	likely
Premature ejaculation	male	definite	2	improbable
Ejaculatory incompetence	male	definite	0–1	none
Anovulation/amenorrhea	female	definite	S	definite
Frigidity	female	unknown	7–12	unknown
Inorgasmy	female	unknown	10–20	unknown
Pregnancy loss				
	male	none	0	none
All	female	definite	S	definite
	male	definite	S	definite
	female	definite	S	definite
Psychoses				
All	male	definite	1–2	improbable
	female	definite		possible
Schizophrenia	male	definite	.7–1.5	improbable
	female	definite		possible
Manic-depressive	male	definite	.1–.5	none
	female	definite		none

Sexual deviations				
All	male	definite	S	likely
	female	definite	S	improbable
Homosexuality	male	definite	4	likely
	female	definite	1.5	improbable
Others	male	definite	S	likely
	female	possible	S	improbable
Alcoholism	male	definite	7	definite
	female	definite	3–5	definite
Cigarette smoking	male	possible	50	possible
	female	likely	40	likely
Illicit drug abuse				
All	male	definite	10–15	definite
	female	definite		definite
-Barbiturates and tranquilizers	male	definite	2	improbable
	female	definite		improbable
Stimulants	male	definite	3	improbable
	female	improbable		improbable
Marihuana	male	unknown	10	unknown
	female	improbable		improbable
Hallucinogens	male	improbable	1	none
	female	possible		improbable
Narcotics	male	definite	.7	improbable
	female	definite		improbable
Psychopathology (total)	male	definite	S	definite
	female	definite	S	definite

NOTE: The letter "S" means substantial and expresses a prevalence level that is unknown but is thought to exceed 2%.

of the population actually experiencing specific kinds of subfecundity due to psychic stress. For the other forms of psychopathology, namely, psychoses, sexual deviations, and drug abuse, total prevalence is given. However, the estimated proportions of these latter disorders that actually decrease fecundity are factored into the judgments (Column 4 of Table 11.2) concerning whether these disorders substantially decrease population fecundity in the United States.

It should be noted that the estimates in Column 3 of Table 11.2 are not additive, since the same individual may have more than one disorder. Nevertheless, when added together and allowing for two or more forms in many individuals, the fact remains inescapable that a sizable fraction of the U.S. reproductive population has their fecundity jeopardized by psychopathology. In the face of the many unknowns catalogued in this study, it is difficult to provide even an approximate estimate of this fraction. However, it is this author's judgment that an estimate of 15–20% would be an exceedingly conservative one.

Population Subfecundity

The ability of each of the various forms of psychopathology to decrease population fecundity, again using the U.S. population as an example, is appraised in Column 4 of Table 11.2. In brief, the conclusion is that, for both males and females, psychic stress, alcoholism, and illicit drug abuse each have a prevalence and an individual fecundity impact sufficient to decrease the fecundity of the U.S. population. Female cigarette-smoking and male sexual deviations, though not in the definite group, likely have the same power. Finally, the female psychoses and male cigarette-smoking are considered to be possible depressants of U.S. fecundity. Within the psychic stress stress category, two factors, impotence and psychogenic amenorrhea, are strong enough by themselves to have an impact on U.S. population fecundity. It is considered likely that psychic-stress-induced spermatogenic disorders also have this effect.

Psychic-stress-induced vaginismus, dyspareunia, premature ejaculation, and ejaculatory incompetence probably do not have the capacity to impair U.S. population fecundity individually. Neither do the male psychoses, lesbianism, or any one of the illicit drug groups. However, it must again be emphasized that the minor impact of such factors on population fecundity should not be ignored, because, in doing so, the potential importance of their collective effect on population fecundity would be overlooked. For example, none of the illicit drug groups is considered to have the power to alter U.S.

population fecundity. But, together, under the heading of "Illicit Drug Abuse," they are considered to have a definite impact.

Population Variability

The prevalence of psychopathology in general and in its specific forms varies widely between populations, between subgroups within a population, and over time. The amount of psychopathology-induced subfecundity will vary accordingly.

INTERPOPULATION VARIABILITY

There is general agreement that psychopathology is substantially more prevalent in developed than in developing societies (cf. Gyongyossy and Szaloczy 1972:590–591; Kroger 1962b:633, 1962f:103; Kroger and Freed 1951:282; Milojkovic et al. 1966:829; and Vero and Szany 1972:429). Indeed, some workers even suggest that in modern urban societies virtually everyone suffers from some form of psychopathology (Clinard 1968:447). The following statements are typical of those in the medical literature that propose a link between the psychological pressures of modern society and subfecundity:

> It [impotence] is thought to be more prevalent now than in past centuries because of the increasing complexity and stressfulness of our social and cultural organization [Braiman 1970:739].

> The tension and impact of modern living has contributed much to tubal spasm, irregular menses, anovulatory cycles, and amenorrhea [Whitelaw 1960:175].

> It may also be open to question whether the modern complexity of our present civilization with its attendant tension, lack of relaxation, mental anxiety, and excesses of tobacco and alcohol may not also be possible etiologic factors [of subfecundity] [Siegler 1944:16].

Since fertility surveys, even those with designs that tend to underestimate the prevalence of subfecundity, repeatedly find that 30–40% of the U.S. reproductive population is subfecund (cf. Introduction) despite excellent health care and relatively low rates of such subfecundity factors as disease and severe malnutrition, the hypothesis that psychopathology may account for a substantial portion of this subfecundity deserves serious consideration.

There is considerable disagreement concerning the prevalence of psychopathology in primitive and developing societies. Some believe it is common; others believe it is rare (cf. Hammer 1972:423). However, the consensus seems to be that, although the level of psychopathology is considerably lower than in developed societies, it is more common than was previously thought. Consequently, the amount of psychopathology-induced subfecundity is probably also greater than is generally accepted. The following statement by a World Health Organization committee (1975) is significant because it aligns itself with the view that psychological factors have a definite role to play in the fecundity of developing societies: "Congenital abnormalities of the female genital tract, endocrine factors, and psychological factors causing infertility and pregnancy wastage are not discussed here since, although they represent some of the main causes of infertility, there is no evidence that they have any increased significance in Africa south of the Sahara [p. 16]."

In addition, many developing populations are in the process of modernizing, and the rapid sociocultural change and disorganization accompanying this process has led to increased psychopathology. This is particularly true in urban areas, where the clash between traditional and modern cultures is sharpest. A recent example of this phenomenon is provided by the Eskimos, among whom the social dislocations caused by the intrusion of Western ways upon their simple hunting and fishing society have been followed by a severe outbreak of mental illness (Trumbull 1974:8). Thus, subfecundity due to psychopathology probably assumes far greater importance in transitional societies than in traditional ones. However, little research attention has been directed toward this hypothesis. Adadevoh (1974) comments in the following passage about this situation with respect to Africa:

> Although several psychological variables are of possible relevance as determinants of sub-fertility and infertility, these have received little study despite the rapid socio-cultural, political, and economic changes being experienced in most African countries. Impotence induced by fear, lack of emotional compatibility between partners, homosexuality, changing sexual partners and patterns due to widespread use of contraceptive devices, fatalism, marital adjustment problems and changing cultural values could play a role of influencing fertility [p. 14].

In Chapter 1 it was noted that, although early workers believed that psychopathology accounted for a substantial portion of the depopulation of many primitive societies undergoing transition, later workers rejected this hypothesis. Based on the research assembled here, there is no strong evidence against the proposition that psychopathology could have contributed materially to depopulation in these societies, in part by depressing fecundity. Lorimer (1954:248) has concluded that acute social disorganization can, under certain circumstances, lead to the spread of subfecundity and to behavioral modes prejudicial to fertility, such as infrequent coitus and marital disruption, and that these effects can persist even to the point of population extinction. In such populations, psychopathology is undoubtedly a key intermediate variable between the acute social disorganization and both subfecundity and behavior that depresses fertility.

INTRAPOPULATION VARIABILITY

The prevalence of psychopathology also varies substantially between subgroups within a population. In the United States, for example, there are social class, occupational, and racial differences in the amount and type of psychopathology experienced, and psychopathology-induced subfecundity would be expected to vary accordingly. The reader may recall the study in Chapter 3 that proposed that the higher infertility rate among recent rural-to-urban migrants as compared to nonmigrants was due to stress-induced oligospermia. And it is interesting to note that the Hutterites, who have the highest fecundity of any group in the United States, also have very low rates of psychopathology. According to Eaton and Weil (1955):

> We judge that the Hutterite lifetime risk of all types of mental disorders is as low as or lower than that of any contemporary Euro-American group within the Judaeo-Christian complex of cultures for which comparable data were available [p. 210].

> [The Hutterites have] a relatively low level of social stress, in the sense that [their] way of life lacks many of the unresolved tensions and contradictions of the contemporary American melting pot cultural system [p. 209].

> The most clear-cut quantitative finding was the virtual absence of severe personality disorders, obsessive-compulsive neuroses, psychopathology, and psychoses associated with syphilis, alcoholism and drug addiction [p. 215].

> No Hutterite has been involved in a sex crime which came to the attention of the authorities. We know of no act of overt homosexuality [p. 143].

TEMPORAL VARIABILITY

The prevalence of psychopathology (and resulting subfecundity) was also found to vary over time. It was noted, for instance, that among U.S. women the rates of alcoholism, smoking, and illicit drug abuse have all increased considerably over the last several decades. And particular attention was paid to the possibility that the prevalence of sexual disorders, such as impotence and frigidity, is particularly responsive to social change.

An interesting research question is whether psychopathology, especially psychic stress and all forms of drug abuse, may increase during economic recessions and depressions. Bellak (1952) suggests that this may be true, especially for pregnant women. In his words:

> The pregnant woman is in a remarkably helpless state, and emotional insecurity
> can be mobilized in the face of economic insecurity. The stress and strain of
> pregnancy is particularly unrewarding if the gestation is to culminate with added
> responsibility for which the family is unprepared. This is especially true in the
> case of multiparas, where another pregnancy can represent an added burden in
> an intolerable life situation [p. 210].

If psychopathology does become more prevalent during periods of economic
stress, subsequent increases in subfecundity might partially cause, directly
and/or indirectly, the lower fertility characteristic of such periods by improv-
ing the chances that birth control will be effective. Brenner (cf. *Intercom*
1975), arguing that few areas of life are not intimately affected by the state of
the economy, points to the impact of recession on neonatal and infant
mortality as follows:

> Infant mortality is influenced by certain risk factors (high blood pressure, higher
> levels of cholesterol, increased smoking and use of alcohol) accompanying
> "major social stress," and the relationship between economic downturns
> and infant mortality is most striking in babies that die within a day after birth. In
> these cases, the mother suffered from the stresses of economic recession. Her
> blood pressure went up, she smoked and drank more, and, as a result, she gave
> birth to a baby that could not survive [p. 7].

Perhaps the same factors may increase pregnancy loss, especially during the
vulnerable period of early gestation, and other forms of reproductive dysfunction as well.

Other Intermediate Variables

This study has repeatedly pointed out that psychopathology can reduce
fertility through intermediate variables other than subfecundity. These
variables—especially the proportion marrying, marital disruption, birth control, and coital frequency—are important intermediaries between psychopathology and fertility, perhaps even more important than subfecundity
itself.

Slater and associates (1971:S64, S67) provide a good example of the
negative influence of psychopathology on mate exposure and, by implication, fertility. As a measure of the relative periods of risk of legitimate mater-
nity and paternity, they compared the number of years between the ages of
20 and 44 inclusive (25 years) that the general population of Britain and
various groups with a psychopathological disorder spent in the married
state. (The married state was defined to include periods of separation and to
exclude time spent after the death of a spouse or a divorce.) Their results,

TABLE 11.3
*Mean Number of Years Spent in the Married State
(Not Single, Widowed, or Divorced) during the 25
Years from Age 20 to 44 Inclusive*

Population	Males	Females
General population (British, 1961)	17.8	20.1
Schizophrenia	7.5	12.1
Manic-depression	13.9	17.6
Obsessional neurosis	13.0	18.7
Neurosis	15.7	18.4
Personality disorder	12.1	15.1

SOURCE: Slater *et al.* 1971:S65, S67.

which are presented in Table 11.3, reveal substantially lower rates of mate exposure among the disordered groups.

Such findings are typical. Indeed, persons suffering from psychopathology almost invariably display values for intermediate variables that, in comparison to those for normal individuals, are prejudicial to fertility.

Summary

Aside from a few remarks suggesting that psychopathology may have caused subfecundity in primitive societies undergoing rapid social transition and may currently be a factor in reducing fecundity in modern societies, the effect of psychopathology on fecundity has been ignored in the population literature. This study is a long overdue effort to examine this relationship systematically. The information presented here establishes psychopathology as a substantial cause of population subfecundity. However, an accurate assessment of the quantitative impact of psychopathology on population fecundity is currently impossible because of research problems, especially lack of data. Thus, this study is only a preliminary effort in the quest for a definitive, quantitative evaluation of the relationship between psychopathology and population fecundity.

Appendix A

Bogue's Appraisal of the Relationship between Subfecundity and Fertility

The Introduction describes the shallow niche occupied by subfecundity factors within population fertility thinking and assesses the scope and limitations of the treatment these factors generally receive. That discussion can be augmented by a detailed review of one such treatment by Donald Bogue (1969). Bogue's passage, presented as follows,[1] was selected because it is clear and unequivocal.

A surprisingly large proportion of the female adult population is childless, even at the end of the childbearing period. Part of it is due to spinsterhood, but much of it is due to involuntary or voluntary sterility. Table A1.1 reports data, tabulated by age, for a few nations of the world for which recent valid statistics are available. The highest degree of childlessness reliably reported for women of completed fertility is in the United States and Hungary—18 percent for ages 45 to 49 years. Even in nations where almost 100 percent of the population marries and where fertility rates are high and fertility control is very weak, about one woman in fifteen (6 to 8 percent) reaches menopause without bearing a child. Examples are Fiji, Samoa, Puerto Rico, Malaya, and Guinea. Childlessness is very high of course, before age 20, but there are very great variations among the populations in childlessness at these earlier ages—due to differences in age at marriage. Despite its very high fertility, more than 90 percent of the women 15 to 19 years of age in Western Samoa are childless, whereas only 44 percent of United States ever-married girls in their late teens are childless. There is a

[1]Reprinted by permission of John Wiley and Sons, Inc.

TABLE A1.1.

*Proportion of Women Aged 40 or Over Who Have
Borne No Children, Selected Nations of the World*

Nation	Age group	Percentage childless
Africa		
Central African Republic	45–49	18.7
Congo (Brazzaville)	45–49	15.5
Gabon	45–49	32.1
Guinea	45–49	5.7
Kenya	45–49	5.4
Niger	45–49	7.2
Senegal	45–49	5.6
South Africa	45–49	6.0
Sudan	50+	9.6
Togo	45–49	—
Zanzibar	46+	23.7
North America		
Baham	45–54	20.8
Barbados	45–64	24.6
Bermuda	45–49	26.8
British Honduras	45–49	19.7
Canada	45–49	13.1
Jamaica	45–54	19.8
Mexico	40–49	21.8
Nicaragua	45–54	12.7
Panama	50+	11.7
Puerto Rico	45–49	11.5
Trinidad and Tobago	45–64	22.0
United States	45–49	18.1
Virgin Islands	45–54	2.1
South America		
British Guinea	45–64	16.8
Chile	45–49	24.7
Peru	45–49	11.8
Asia		
Brunei	45–49	6.8
Cyprus	45–49	10.2
Israel	45–49	9.2
Japan	45–49	8.1
Jordan	45–49	5.3
Korea	45–49	3.7
Kuwait	50+	16.0
Macau	45–49	11.6
Malaya	45–49	8.2
Sabah	45–49	9.0
Sarawak	45–49	9.7
Ryukyu Islands	45–49	5.9

Europe

Czechoslovakia	45–49	15.4
Hungary	45–49	18.7
Ireland	45–49	12.5
Monaco	45–49	36.2
Netherlands	45–49	14.2
Norway	45–49	12.0
Portugal	45–49	12.0
Switzerland	45–49	19.7
United Kingdom	45–49	12.6

Oceania

American Samoa	45–49	12.6
British Solomons	45–49	11.3
Fiji Islands	45–49	8.8

SOURCE: United Nations Demographic Yearbook, 1965, Table 9. Reproduced from Bogue 1969:725.

marked tendency for nations with lower fertility rates to have a high percentage of childlessness at ages 35 and above and for nations with high fertility to have low proportions of childlessness. However, this relationship is only very approximate and needs to be interpreted. The low level of living that prevails in many nations does not appear to affect the fecundity of couples. It might have been supposed that inadequate diet, frequent illness, and poor general health may predispose couples toward involuntary sterility. Where health conditions are poor and the bearing of children is itself a risk to the mother's life, it might easily have been expected that a disproportionately large percentage of sterile women would survive to reach age 40 and would therefore comprise a larger proportion of all women aged 40. If this were ever true, it appears to be true no longer, because, as has already been observed, the proportion of childlessness among most high-fertility populations is quite low. Voluntary lifelong sterility is not a necessary ingredient in obtaining a state of demographic equilibrium.

If we study the adjustment of Japan, which has one of the world's lowest fertility rates, we find a low rate of childlessness in comparison with most nations of the world. In other words, Japan has managed to complete its demographic transition while maintaining a level of childlessness that is very nearly the same as that of the high-fertility nations. Where it exists, childlessness obviously helps to keep birthrates lower, but it is clearly not a necessary or important consideration among most populations in the modern world. Far more important is the ability of the population to avoid bearing more than 2 or 3 children per couple.

From the data in Table A1.1, together with the evidence of medical and biological research, we may conclude tentatively that not less than 5 percent of all couples around the world are physiologically unable to bear children and will remain sterile throughout their lives as a result. Unless hitherto undiscovered methods of promoting fertility are developed, it is valid to presume that one couple in 20 is sterile at the time of marriage or else will go throughout its marriage childless for physiological reasons. In addition, childlessness may be an incidental by-product of disruption of marriage by separation and divorce, late marriage, surgery, and psychological factors that make it impossible for a couple to have a child. Together these factors appear to be able to raise the proportion of childlessness among couples in particular populations by an additional 5 percent to a total of 10 percent. Sterility increases steadily with age and often occurs well before the normal time of menopause. It may be surprising to learn that Whelpton, Freedman, and Campbell found that in the United States 10 percent of all white couples with wife aged 18 to 39 years had been rendered surgically sterile. Of this 4 percent had had "remedial" surgery performed to remove a threat to life; removal of a cancerous growth or correction of a disorder of the reproductive system. Surgery in the remaining 6 percent had been performed for contraceptive reasons.

When childlessness rises above 10 percent in couples, we may infer that it is either primarily voluntary childlessness resulting from the use of contraceptives or else a result of very irregular exposure to childbearing [pp. 724–726].

The basis and merits of Bogue's argument are examined and organized into the following three comments.

Subfecundity Factors and Population Fertility

Bogue's initial argument is drawn from assembled fertility and childlessness data for a few nations of the world for which valid statistics are available. He reports a marked tendency for high fertility nations to have low childlessness and for low fertility nations to have high childlessness and thus posits an inverse relationship between fertility and childlessness.

Second, Bogue notes that virtually all high fertility nations experience low living standards. This proposition, coupled with his high-fertility–low-childlessness hypothesis, indicates that poverty and low childlessness coexist in many high fertility nations. From this, Bogue implicitly infers that a low standard of living does not increase childlessness.

Finally, Bogue uses national living standards as a proxy for the presence of subfecundity causes. That is, the lower the living standard, the higher the prevalence of such factors as disease, nutritional deficiencies, and poor health in general. Similarly, he uses childlessness as a proxy for subfecundity itself. By using these proxies, Bogue arrives at his final conclusion, which is that the subfecundity factors that are common in underdeveloped populations do not depress fecundity and therefore are not important fertility factors.

Thus, Bogue's argument hinges on an inverse relationship, a logical inference, and two proxy variables. Each of these components is now critically examined.

First, what about the inverse relationship between fertility and childlessness? Does it hold up under close examination? The answer is no. The scattergram shown in Figure A1.1 plots the childlessness data presented by Bogue in Table A1.1 against the crude birth rates for those populations.[2]

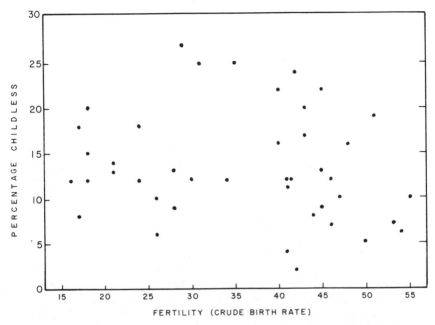

Figure A 1.1 *Scattergram of percentage of women aged 40 and over who have borne no children plotted against the crude birth rate for populations shown in Table A1.1.* SOURCE: *Percentage childless data from Bogue (1969:725); crude birth rates from Bogue (1969:664-669).* Several populations are not included because of missing data.

Judging from Bogue's own data, it is clear that there is neither a marked tendency for high fertility nations to have low childlessness nor a tendency for low fertility nations to have high childlessness. There is, in fact, much variation in the percentage childless among both high and low fertility populations and no perceivable overall pattern. In sum, the first part of Bogue's argument, the alleged inverse fertility–childlessness relationship, can be effectively challenged. What about the remainder?

The second part of his argument centers around the fact that virtually all high fertility nations have low living-standards. This is, of course, true. But, although all high fertility nations are poor, the reverse does not hold. Poor nations differ in many respects, including their fertility. Some poor nations have high fertility, but others have low fertility. In fact, as discussed in the opening section of the Introduction, a considerable number of less developed

[2]Although there are 51 populations in Table A1.1, only 42 are represented in Figure A1.1 because either the childlessness or the crude birth-rate for 9 populations was not given in the source material.

populations have been found to have unexpectedly low fertility. Indeed, it makes sense to argue a priori that many poor populations would be expected to experience low fertility, high subfecundity, and high childlessness on the basis of their relatively poor health care systems alone.

Moreover, some poor populations also have high rates of childlessness, as Tabbarah (1971) notes in the following passage:

> Statistics of childlessness among menopausal women reveal that relatively high percentages generally exist in backward areas: 12–18 percent in Kenya, Tanganyika, and Uganda, but these may be understated; 18 percent in Buhaya and 32 percent in Buganda, both in East Africa; 25 percent on the island of Zanzibar, excluding town, and 28 percent in the town; 25–35 percent among the Murut of Sabah in Malaya; and 42 percent among an Atoll population. It must be noted, however, that in a few backward areas the reported percentages are surprisingly low, i.e., under 10 percent [p. 267].

Thus, poor nations vary markedly with respect to fertility and childlessness. By focusing only on poor, high fertility populations, Bogue brushes aside this variation and, in the process, loses sight of the importance of the subfecundity factors that partially account for it.

In view of the above criticisms, the most Bogue can conclude concerning the relationship between low living standards and childlessness is expressed in the following syllogism:

> Some high fertility nations are low childlessness nations.
> All high fertility nations are poor nations.
> _____
> Therefore: Some poor nations are low childlessness nations.

Naturally, if only some poor nations have low childlessness and others experience high childlessness, not much can be deduced about the living-standard–childlessness relationship.

It is worth emphasizing that the logical problem underlying Bogue's argument lies in the fact that he is dealing with several universes that are not mutually exclusive or congruent, namely, the set of high fertility nations, the set of poor nations, and so forth. As a result, two critical set intersections, namely, the poor, low fertility nations and high fertility, high childlessness nations, fall outside of Bogue's analysis. And, unfortunately, it is in these very populations that subfecundity factors are undoubtedly most important.

Of course, Bogue is not primarily interested in living standards and childlessness per se. What he is trying to establish is that the usual subfecundity factors, such as disease, that are common in poor nations do not substantially affect their fecundity. The level of living is simply a proxy for subfecundity factors, and childlessness stands in for subfecundity itself. Even though the substantive aspects of Bogue's argument have already been challenged, it is still worth examining the grossly unrefined nature of these proxies, since similar ones are often encountered.

Because of the lack of primary research on the fundamental causes of subfecundity, population students are often forced to deal with such factors indirectly. What this means is that these factors are subsumed under broad, somewhat diffuse concepts, such as "level of living." Thus, when Bogue states that "the low level of living that prevails in many nations does not appear to affect the fecundity of couples [p. 724]," he is implying that the usual concomitants of a low living-standard, such factors as faulty diet and disease, probably do not affect fecundity either. But, unfortunately, though the level of living variable is expedient, it is hardly a suitable proxy for subfecundity factors. The level of living is a gross variable. At any given level, there is tremendous variation in the kinds of subfecundity factors present and in their eventual impact on population fertility.

In similar fashion, Bogue lets childlessness serve as a proxy for subfecundity, not an uncommon practice. But childlessness is a very poor proxy for subfecundity, for two reasons. First, subfecundity is only one possible cause of childlessness, there being other involuntary and also voluntary causes. Second, the effect of subfecundity on population fertility is not limited to producing childlessness, for it can cause other individuals to have fewer children than they would have had otherwise. So, even if it were possible to separate subfecundity from the other causes of childlessness, using childlessness to gauge the effects of subfecundity on fertility would omit the impact of subfecundity on the fertility of the nonchildless population. Thus, low childlessness and a high level of subfecundity in a population are not mutually exclusive. Indeed, considering their sociodemographic profiles, there are populations with lower-than-expected fertility, probably due in large part to subfecundity, which nevertheless have relatively low levels of childlessness. In fact, an inspection of Bogue's selected nations reveals at least five low childlessness populations[3] which are identified by Clark (1967:24) as having inexplicably low total fertilities. This situation could be accounted for by subfecundity factors that produce infecundity after childbearing has occurred or by factors, such as syphilis, that depress fecundity without completely eliminating the ability to bear children. Such factors cannot be accommodated by the childlessness proxy.

It is also worth noting that a high rate of involuntary childlessness does not necessarily go hand in hand with high population subfecundity. Brass (1968:365–367) presents data on two tribes in the Republic of Upper Volta, the Mossi and the Western. Though both have high crude birth rates (49.1

---

[3]These populations are Guinea, Kenya, Niger, Ryukyu Islands, and Senegal.

and 45.4), their childlessness rates are far apart. The Mossi have a low childlessness rate (4%), whereas the Western have a relatively high rate (12%). Thus, the Western tribe combines high fertility and high childlessness.

But, for the most part, high rates of involuntary childlessness are coincident with high rates of subfecundity at other parities. As Romaniuk (1968) observes: "Where many women are sterile in the sense of giving birth to no children, one would expect that many others might suffer fecundity impairment at parity one, two, or higher [p. 331]." This is because many of the factors that cause childlessness also cause subfecundity among women at other parities. But, as discussed earlier, the reverse is not necessarily true. Populations with high rates of subfecundity do not necessarily have high childlessness rates. Indeed, some of the most important population subfecundity factors are ones that cause secondary sterility due to infections following childbirth (or abortion).

Therefore, because high childlessness can coexist with relatively high and low subfecundity levels and because the same is true for low childlessness, childlessness is an inadequate and sometimes misleading proxy for subfecundity.

Thus, the "level of living" and "childlessness" proxies used for subfecundity causes and subfecundity, respectively, are grossly inadequate. But Bogue did not really have much choice. In the absence of fundamental research on subfecundity, populations students are often compelled to rely on such expedient, but imprecise, proxies. Basic information is needed before convincing arguments can be framed on either side of this question.

One also wonders whether groups of nations, or even single countries, as used by Bogue, represent the proper units by which to explore the relationship between subfecundity causes and population fertility. As a World Health Organization group (1975) suggests in the following passage, this relationship is more productively examined on a smaller scale: "It is not uncommon to find pockets of apparent infertility [subfecundity] even within areas that are characterized by high levels of fertility. In these circumstances, the ethnic or tribal group may be the best unit of study as the habitat, social conditions, and health problems are likely to be common to the whole unit [p. 9]." In Uganda, for instance, the frequency of subfecundity (and of its causes) varies widely from district to district (cf. *Uganda Atlas of Disease Distribution* 1968). Similarly, in the Congo, where the crude birth rate is about 45, the district birth rates range from 20 to 60, depending largely on the prevalence of subfecundity (Romaniuk 1968a:337). And Scragg (1957:63) found great variability (4–45%) between New Ireland population groups in the percentage infecund.

Finally, one might query what biases are introduced by only using data from "a few nations of the world for which recent valid statistics are available [p. 724]." Could it be that those nations with the poorest health and nutrition also have the fewest and least valid statistics and thus elude consideration?

The Classification of Subfecundity Causes

Bogue is surprised by the "large proportion of the female population that is childless, even at the end of the childbearing period." "Part of it is due," he states, "to spinsterhood, 4 but much of it is due to involuntary or voluntary sterility [p. 724]." Bogue divides the involuntary causes of childlessness into two groups, namely, the "physiological" causes and the "incidental by-product" causes, such as marital disruption. Voluntary childlessness is not subdivided. Thus, according to this scheme, childlessness (and subfecundity) may be due to either (a) physiological, (b) incidental by-product, or (c) voluntary causes.

The major difficulty with this classification is that the incidental by-product group contains imputed factors that belong in the other two groups. One result of this system, therefore, is that the importance of the physiological causes of childlessness is underestimated. For example, Bogue states that childlessness may be an incidental by-product of psychological factors that make it impossible for a couple to have a child. There is no doubt that psychological factors are important in almost every aspect of reproduction. But it is not clear what Bogue is referring to here as "incidental by-products." Psychological factors can cause childlessness physiologically through, for example, the psychosomatic mechanism or indirectly through such voluntary intermediate variables as birth control. Thus, psychological factors are not the sole province of any of Bogue's three groups.

In sum, the incidental by-product group contains factors that either are misassigned or fall within the limits of more than one category. One result is that the quantitative effect of the physiological group on fertility is understated, as is seen in the next comment.

An Estimate of Population Infecundity

Bogue believes that the level of lifelong infecundity is approximately the same for every population. In his view, "one couple in 20 is sterile at the time

---

4The term *spinster* categorizes women as "never-married" but reveals nothing about their sexual or fertility behavior. A spinster may, for example, enter a sexual union and bear illegitimate children. I think what is meant here by the term *spinster* is a woman who permanently refrains from sexual activity and is therefore childless. "Lifelong celibate" or "virgin" probably are better terms. Since the reasons for permanently refraining from sexual activity and, hence, childbearing, can be classified as either voluntary or involuntary, there is no need to devote a separate category to spinsterhood.

of marriage or else will go throughout its marriage childless for physiological reasons [p. 725]." Any additional childlessness among couples is considered either voluntary or due to the incidental by-product causes. Thus, according to Bogue, if 15% of the women in a population are childless, 5% have no children because of physiological reasons, and the remaining 10% are child-less voluntarily or due to incidental by-product causes.

First, Bogue's classification system and how it tends to underestimate the fertility-reducing strength of subfecundity causes have already been dealt with. This in itself would suggest that, ceteris paribus, this estimate of lifelong infecundity is too low.

Second, Bogue contends that the evidence of medical and biological research supports his position on the level of population infecundity. Unfortunately, he does not present this medical evidence, nor are there any relevant references in the chapter's extensive bibliography. On the contrary, after an extensive review of the medical literature, this author found no medical data to support the presumption that the level of infecundity is a universal constant. Indeed, it would be surprising if various populations, subject to different genetic makeups and environments, experience the same level of infecundity. Actually, empirical studies have suggested considerable variation in the proportion of populations that are infecund (cf. Bennett 1965:244; Brass 1968:427; Demeny 1968:493; Nag, 1962:110; Romaniuk 1968a:328; Scragg 1957:57; and van de Walle and Page 1969:6). The proportion of women over the age of 40 who are childless has been found to vary from as low as 2% for one cohort of ever-married Hutterites (Eaton and Mayer 1954:20) to as high as 50% for women in certain districts of the Congo (Romaniuk 1968a:328). Perhaps the following statement by a WHO group (1975) studying infecundity best places in perspective the fact that childlessness due to physiological causes varies widely:

> Involuntary infertility [infecundity] is a worldwide problem but its frequency varies from area to area. It seems that up to 5% of all couples are infertile [infecund] for complex reasons that are difficult to diagnose and for which present day treatment is therefore largely ineffective. Superimposed on this "hard core," additional factors may raise the prevalence of infertility [infecundity] to 30% or even higher in some communities [p. 5].

Discussion

Bogue's passage was examined not only because it conflicts with the perspective of this study but also because it is representative of a way of treating subfecundity or, in this case, subfecundity-induced childlessness, which is counterproductive to the development of fertility theory. This treatment makes the assumption that all populations experience the same amount of subfecundity or subfecundity-induced childlessness. Thus, Bogue suggests that about 5% of all populations are physiologically childless and that any additional childlessness is more or less voluntary. Similarly, Veevers (1972:269) uses the minimum rates of childlessness among women in high fertility, rural farm Quebec as an estimate of the maximum rates of physiological childlessness for other populations. Any amount of childlessness above these rates is considered to be due to nonphysiological causes. A similar formula, though opposite in conclusion, is advanced by Llewellyn-Jones (1974). He believes that it is voluntary childlessness that is low and relatively constant and that involuntary causes are variable and responsible for all the rest. He notes that "voluntary childlessness is relatively uncommon, and fewer than 5 percent of all married couples decide to have no children. It would seem from this that if a couple is childless the reason is an involuntary one in most cases [p. 126]." It is the point of this discussion that the preceding statements and approaches are not supported by empirical research and that the place of subfecundity in fertility theory cannot be determined until the causes of subfecundity are properly identified and their impact on individual and population fecundity is quantified.

References

Aal, H., A. El Atribi, A. Hafiz, and M. Aidaros. 1975. Azoospermia in bilharziasis and the presence of sperm antibodies. *Journal of Reproduction and Fertility*, **42**, 403.

Abelson, A., T. Baker, and P. Baker. 1974. Altitude, migration, and fertility in the Andes. *Social Biology*, **21**, 12.

Abramson, F. 1973. Spontaneous fetal death in man. *Social Biology*, **20**, 375.

Abse, D. 1966. Psychiatric aspects of human male infertility. *Fertility and Sterility*, **17**, 133.

Adadevoh, B. 1974. *Sub-fertility and infertility in Africa.* Ibadan, Nigeria:Caxton Press.

Adler, C. 1973. *Ecological fantasies.* New York:Dell.

Aitken, R. 1972. Methodology of research in psychosomatic medicine. *British Medical Journal*, **4**, 285.

Allen, E. 1935. Menstrual dysfunctions in disorders of the personality. *Endocrinology*, **19**, 255.

Amelar, R. 1966. *Infertility in men: Diagnosis and treatment.* Philadelphia:Davis.

Amelar, R., L. Dubin, and P. Walsh. 1977. *Male infertility.* Philadelphia:Saunders.

American Psychiatric Association. 1952. *Diagnostic and statistical manual of mental disorders.* Washington, D.C.:APA.

American Psychiatric Association. 1968. *Diagnostic and statistical manual of mental disorders,* 2nd ed. Washington, D.C.:APA.

Arieti, S. 1967. Sexual conflict in psychotic disorders. In C. Wahl (ed.), *Sexual problems,* pp. 228–237. New York:Free Press.

Arora, R., K. Saxena, and R. Choudhury. 1961. Sperm studies on Indian men. *Fertility and Sterility*, **12**, 365.

Arowolo, O. 1978. A demographic note on relative infertility in Nigeria. Forthcoming report derived from Segment 1 of the Changing African Family Project in Nigeria.

Asch, S. 1965. Psychiatric complications: Mental and emotional problems. In J. Rovinsky and A. Guttmacher (eds.), *Medical, surgical, and gynecologic complications of pregnancy,* pp. 461–472. Baltimore:Williams and Wilkins.

Assemany, S., R. Neu, and L. Gardner. 1970. Deformities in a child whose mother took LSD. *Lancet,* **1,** 1290.

Astrup, P., H. Olsen, D. Trolle, and K. Kjeldsen. 1972. Effect of moderate carbon monoxide exposure on fetal development. *Lancet,* **2,** 1220.

Babson, S., and R. Benson. 1971. *Management of high-risk pregnancy and intensive care of the neonate.* St. Louis:Mosby.

Badr, F., and R. Badr. 1975. Induction of dominant lethal mutation in male mice by ethyl alcohol. *Nature,* **253,** 134.

Bailey, M., P. Haberman, and H. Alksne. 1965. The epidemiology of alcoholism in an urban residential area. *Quarterly Journal of Studies on Alcohol,* **26,** 19.

Bailey, R. 1970. The effect of maternal smoking on the infant birth weight. *New Zealand Medical Journal,* **71,** 293.

Baker, A. 1967. *Psychiatric disorders in obstetrics.* Philadelphia:Davis.

Banks, A. 1962. Does adoption affect infertility? *International Journal of Fertility,* **7,** 23.

Banks, A., R. Rutherford, and W. Coburn. 1961. Fertility following adoption. *Fertility and Sterility,* **12,** 438.

Bardwick, J. 1971. *Psychology of women.* New York:Harper and Row.

Bardwick, J., and S. Behrman. 1967. Investigations into the effects of anxiety, sexual arousal, and menstrual cycle phase on uterine contractions. *Psychosomatic Medicine,* **29,** 468.

Barlow, D., G. Abel, E. Blanchard, and M. Mavissakalian. 1974. Plasma testosterone levels and male homosexuality: A failure to replicate. *Archives of Sexual Behavior,* **3,** 571.

Barrett-Connor, E. 1969. Infections and pregnancy: A review. *Southern Medical Journal,* **62,** 275.

Bass, M. 1978. Some issues concerning sexuality and mental retardation. Paper presented at the first annual conference of the Eastern Regional Chapter, Society for the Scientific Study of Sex, Atlantic City, April.

Beckman, L. 1975. Women alcoholics. *Journal of Studies on Alcohol,* **36,** 797.

Behrman, S., and R. Kistner. 1968. *Progress in infertility.* Boston:Little Brown.

Bell, D., and W. Trethowan. 1961. Amphetamine addiction and disturbed sexuality. *Archives of General Psychiatry,* **4,** 74.

Bellak, L. 1952. *Manic-depressive psychosis.* New York:Grune and Stratton.

Bellak, L. 1958. *Schizophrenia: A review of the syndrome.* New York:Grune and Stratton.

Bellak, L. 1969. Introduction, personal reflection and a brief review. In L. Bellak and L. Loeb (eds.), *The schizophrenic syndrome,* pp. 1–10. New York: Grune and Stratton.

Bellak, L., and L. Loeb (eds.). 1969. *The schizophrenic syndrome.* New York:Grune and Stratton.

Beller, A. 1977. *Fat and thin—A natural history of obesity.* New York:Farrar, Strauss, and Giroux.

Benedek, T., G. Ham, and R. Robinson. 1953. Some emotional factors in infertility. *Psychosomatic Medicine,* **15,** 485.

Bennett, F. 1965. The social, cultural, and emotional aspects of sterility in women in Buganda. *Fertility and Sterility,* **16,** 243.

Bennion, L., and T. Li. 1976. Alcohol metabolism in American Indians and whites. *New England Journal of Medicine,* **294,** 9.

Birk, L., G. Williams, M. Chasen, and L. Rose. 1973. Serum testosterone levels in homosexual men. *New England Journal of Medicine,* **289,** 1236.

Biskind, L. 1962. Emotional aspects of prenatal care. In W. Kroger (ed.), *Psychosomatic obstetrics, gynecology and endocrinology,* pp. 33–41. Springfield:Thomas.

Blacker, J. 1962. Population growth and differential fertility in Zanzibar Protectorate. *Population Studies,* **15,** 261.

Blackman, A. 1975. Baby boom not likely now. *Philadelphia Bulletin,* Nov. 2, WA, 1.

Blair, J. 1952. Question of histopathologic changes in testes. *Journal of Mental Science,* **98,** 464.

Blake, J. 1961. *Family structure in Jamaica.* Glencoe, New York:Free Press.

Blandau, R., B. Brackett, R. Brenner, J. Boling, S. Broderson, C. Hamner, and L. Mastroianni. 1977. The oviduct. In R. Greep and M. Koblinsky (eds.), *Frontiers in reproduction and fertility control,* pp. 132–145. Cambridge, Massachusetts:MIT Press.

Blane, H. 1968. *The personality of the alcoholic: Guises of dependency.* New York:Harper and Row.

Blau, M., B. Slaff, K. Easton, J. Welkowitz, J. Springarn, and J. Cohen. 1963. The psychogenic etiology of premature births. *Psychosomatic Medicine,* **25,** 201.

Bleuler, E. 1950. *Dementia praecox or the group of schizophrenias.* New York: International University Press.

Blinick, G. 1971. Fertility of narcotics addicts and effects of addiction on the offspring. *Social Biology,* **Supplement 18,** S34.

Blinick, G., E. Jerez, and R. Wallach. 1973. Methadone maintenance, pregnancy, and progeny. *Journal of the American Medical Association,* **225,** 477.

Blinick, G., R. Wallach, and E. Jerez. 1969. Pregnancy in narcotics addicts treated by medical withdrawal. *American Journal of Obstetrics and Gynecology,* **105,** 997.

Bliss, E. 1976. Participant in the colloquium, The biology of the schizophrenic process. *Advances in Behavioral Biology,* **19,** 50.

Block, R. 1972. Pregnancy in portal cirrhosis. *Journal of Reproductive Medicine,* **8,** 143.

Blum, L. 1959. Sterility and the magic power of the maternal figure. *Journal of Nervous & Mental Disease,* **128,** 401.

Bogue, D. 1969. *Principles of demography.* New York:Wiley.

Bondarevskii, Y. 1974. Alcoholism and venereal diseases (translation). *Zdravookhronenie rossiiskoi Federatsii,* **12,** 17.

Bos, C., and R. Cleghorn. 1956. Psychogenic sterility. *Fertility and Sterility,* **9,** 84.

Bourgeois-Pichat, J. 1967. Social and biological determinants of human fertility in nonindustrial societies. In *Population Problems, Proceedings of the American Philosophical Society,* November 11, 1966.

Bradshaw, B. 1969. Fertility differences in Peru: A reconsideration. *Population Studies,* **23,** 5.

Braiman, A. 1970. Psychosexual disorders of young adulthood. *Clinical Obstetrics and Gynecology,* **13,** 734.

Brass, W. 1968. The demography of French-speaking territories covered by special sample inquiries: Upper Volta, Dahomey, Guinea, North Cameroon, and other areas. In W. Brass *et al.* (eds.), *The demography of tropical Africa,* pp. 342–439. Princeton:Princeton University Press.

Brass, W., and A. Coale. 1968. Methods of analysis and estimation. In W. Brass *et al.* (eds.), *The demography of tropical Africa,* pp. 88–150. Princeton:Princeton University Press.

Brass, W., A Coale, P. Demeny, D. Heisel, F. Lorimer, A. Romaniuk, and E. van de Walle (eds.) 1968. *The demography of tropical Africa.* Princeton:Princeton University Press.

Brecher, E. 1975. Marijuana: The health questions. *Consumer Reports,* March, 143.

Briggs, M. 1973. Cigarette smoking and infertility in men. *Medical Journal of Australia,* **1**, 616.

Brill, N. 1969. General biological studies. In L. Bellak and L. Loeb (eds.), *The schizophrenic syndrome*, pp. 114–154. New York:Grune and Stratton.

British Journal of Venereal Disease. 1973. Homosexuality and venereal disease in the United Kingdom. **49**, 329.

British Medical Journal. 1955. Chronic alcoholism and fertility. **1**, 1170.

British Medical Journal. 1972. Neonatal behavior and maternal barbiturates. **4**, 63. (a)

British Medical Journal. 1972. ABO blood groups and abortion. **4**, 314. (b)

British Medical Journal. 1973. Smoking hazard to the fetus. **1**, 369.

Brodie, H., N. Gartrell, C. Doering, and T. Rhue. 1974. Plasma testosterone levels in heterosexual and homosexual men. *American Journal of Psychiatry*, **131**, 82.

Brown, J. 1965. Treatment of the infertile male. *Clinical Obstetrics and Gynecology,* **8**, 132.

Brown, J. 1972. Psychological and dietary aspects of secondary amenorrhea. In N. Morris (ed.), *Psychosomatic medicine in obstetrics and gynecology,* pp. 579–581. New York:Karger.

Brown, W., J. Donahue, N. Axnick, J. Blount, N. Ewen, and O. Jones. *Syphilis and other venereal diseases.* Cambridge, Massachusetts:Harvard University Press.

Burns, C. 1974. Alcoholism—The family disease. *New Zealand Medical Journal,* **79**, 748.

Burton, G., and H. Kaplin. 1968. Sexual behavior and adjustment of married alcoholics. *Quarterly Journal of Studies on Alcohol,* **29**, 603.

Busch, H., E. Kormendy, and W. Feuerlein. 1973. Partners of female alcoholics. *British Journal on Addiction,* **68**, 179.

Buss, A. 1966. *Psychopathology.* New York: Wiley.

Butler, N., and E. Alberman. 1969. *Perinatal problems.* Edinburgh:Livingstone.

Butler, N., and D. Bonham. 1963. *Perinatal mortality.* London:Livingstone.

Butler, N., and H. Goldstein. 1973. Smoking in pregnancy and subsequent child development. *British Medical Journal,* **4**, 573.

Butler, N., H. Goldstein, and E. Ross. 1972. Cigarette smoking in pregnancy: Its influence on birth weight and perinatal mortality. *British Medical Journal,* **2**, 127.

Caldwell, J. 1974. The study of fertility and fertility change in tropical Africa. *World Fertility Survey Occasional Papers,* **No. 7**. Voorburg, The Netherlands:International Statistical Institute.

Cameron, N. 1971. Abnormal psychology. *Encyclopaedia Britannica,* **18**, 745.

Campbell, A. 1976. Preface. In S. Newman and V. Thompson (eds.), *Population psychology:Research and educational issues,* p. iii. Washington, D.C.:U.S. Government Printing Office.

Carr-Saunders, A. 1922. *The population problem: A study in evolution.* Oxford:Clarendon Press.

Cassidy, W. 1972. Maintenance methadone treatment of drug dependency. *Canadian Psychiatric Association Journal,* **17**, 107.

Cassidy, W., N. Flanagan, M. Spellman, and M. Cohen. 1957. Clinical observations of manic-depressive disease. *Journal of the American Medical Association,* **164,** 1535.

Castelnuovo-Tedesco, P. 1967. The doctor's attitude and his management of patients with sexual problems. In C. Wahl (ed.), *Sexual problems,* pp. 238–246. New York:Free Press.

Centers, R., and G. Blumberg. 1954. Social and psychological factors in human procreation: A survey approach. *Journal of Social Psychology,* **40,** 245.

Chang, M., C. Austin, I. Bedford, B. Brackett, R. Hunter, and R. Yanagimachi. 1977. Capacitation of spermatozoa and fertilization in mammals. In R. Greep and M. Koblinsky (eds.), *Frontiers in reproduction and fertility control,* pp. 434–451. Cambridge, Massachusetts:MIT Press.

Chein, I., D. Gerard, R. Lee, and E. Rosenfeld. 1964. *Narcotics, delinquency, and social policy.* London:Tavistock.

Chertok, L. 1972. Psychosomatic aspects of childbirth. In N. Morris (ed.), *Psychosomatic medicine in obstetrics and gynecology,* pp. 7–12. New York:Karger.

Chez, R. 1967. The female patient's sexual history. In C. Wahl (ed.), *Sexual problems,* pp. 1–12. New York:Free Press.

Chisholm, I. 1972. Sexual problems in marriage. *Postgraduate Medical Journal,* **48,** 544.

Chodoff, P. 1976. The German concentration camp as a psychological stress. In R. Moos (ed.), *Human adaptation,* pp. 337–349. Lexington:Heath.

Cicero, T., R. Bell, W. Wiest, J. Allison, K. Polakoski, and E. Robins. 1975. Function of the male sex organs in heroin and methadone users. *New England Journal of Medicine,* **292,** 882.

Clark, C. 1969. *Population growth and land use.* London:Macmillan.

Clinard, M. 1968. *Sociology of deviant behavior.* New York:Holt.

Coale, A. 1966. Estimates of fertility and mortality in tropical Africa. *Population Index,* **32,** 173.

Coale, A. 1969. The decline of fertility in Europe from the French Revolution to World War II. In S. Behrman, L. Corsa, and R. Freedman (eds.), *Fertility and family planning: A world view,* pp. 3–24. Ann Arbor:University of Michigan Press.

Coale, A. 1973. The demographic transition. Vol. 1 of the IUSSP International Population Conference Meeting Papers, Liege.

Cohen, S., and J. Goldsmith. 1971. Epidemiology. In S. Epstein (ed.), *Drugs of abuse,* pp. 27–44. Cambridge, Massachusetts:MIT Press.

Cohler, B., D. Gallant, H. Grunebaum, J. Weiss, and E. Gamer. 1975. Pregnancy and birth complications among mentally ill and well mothers and their children. *Social Biology,* **22,** 269.

Comstock, G., and F. Lundin. 1967. Parental smoking and perinatal mortality. *American Journal of Obstetrics and Gynecology,* **98,** 708.

Comstock, G., F. Shah, M. Meyer, and H. Abbey. 1971. Low birth weight and neonatal mortality rate related to maternal smoking and socioeconomic status. *American Journal of Obstetrics and Gynecology,* **3,** 53.

Cooper, A. 1972. The causes and management of impotence. *Postgraduate Medical Journal,* **48,** 548.

Cooper, A. 1974. Aetiology of homosexuality. In J. Loraine (ed.), *Understanding homosexuality,* pp. 1–23. New York:Elsevier.

Copenhaver, W. 1964. Revisor of *Bailey's textbook of histology.* Baltimore:Williams and Wilkins.

Coppen, A. 1959. Psychosomatic aspects of pre-eclamptic toxemia. *Journal of Psychosomatic Research,* **2,** 241.

Coppen, A. 1965. The prevalence of menstrual disorders in psychiatric patients. *British Journal of Psychiatry,* **111,** 155.

Crombie, D., R. Pinsent, B. Slater, D. Fleming, and K. Cross. 1970. Teratogenic drugs—RCGP survey. *British Medical Journal,* **4,** 178.

Cross, R. 1973. Management of sexual dysfunction in family practice. Paper presented at the meetings of the Interstate Post-Graduate Medical Association, Chicago, November.

Cutright, P. 1971. *Illegitimacy in the United States: 1920–1968.* Final report to the U.S. Public Health Service.

Daly, M. 1970. The unwanted pregnancy. *Clinical Obstetrics and Gynecology,* **13,** 713.

Davis, K. 1966. Sociological aspects of genetic control. In *Genetics and the future of man: Proceedings of the Nobel Conference, 1965,* pp. 173–204. Amsterdam:North Holland Publishing Co.

Davis, K. 1976. Sexual behavior. In R. Merton and R. Nisbet (eds.), *Contemporary social problems,* pp. 218–261. New York:Harcourt Brace Jovanovich.

Davis, K., and J. Blake. 1956. Social structure and fertility: An analytic framework. *Economic Development and Cultural Change,* **4,** 211.

DeJong, G., and R. Sell. 1977. Changes in childlessness in the United States: A demographic path analysis. *Population Studies,* **31,** 129.

Demeny, P. 1968. The demography of the Sudan. In W. Brass *et al.* (eds.), *The demography of tropical Africa,* pp. 466–514. Princeton:Princeton University Press.

Denisoff, R., and R. Wahrman. 1975. *An introduction to sociology.* New York:Macmillan.

Desmond, M., R. Franklin, R. Blattner, and R. Hill. 1961. The relation of maternal disease to fetal and neonatal morbidity and mortality. *Pediatric Clinics of North America,* Symposium on the Newborn, **8,** 421.

Dimic, N., S. Pavlovic, S. Milojkovic, and S. Radosavijevic. 1972. The importance of psychosomatic factors as the origin of sterility in women. In N. Morris (ed.), *Psychosomatic medicine in obstetrics and gynecology,* pp. 475–477. New York:Karger.

Doerr, P. 1973. Plasma testosterone, estradiol and semen analysis in male homosexuals. *Archives of General Psychiatry,* **29,** 829.

Doerr, P., K. Pirke, G. Kockott, and F. Dittmar. 1976. Further studies on sex hormones in male homosexuals. *Archives of General Psychiatry,* **33,** 611.

Dohrenwend, B. P., and B. S. Dohrenwend. 1969. *Social status and psychological disorder: A causal inquiry.* New York:Wiley.

Dorland's Medical Dictionary. 1965. Philadelphia:Saunders.

Downing, G., and W. Chapman. 1966. Smoking and pregnancy: A statistical study of 5,659 patients. *California Medicine,* **104,** 187.

Dreher, K., and J. Fraser. 1967. Smoking habits of alcoholic out-patients, I. *International Journal of Addictions,* **2,** 259.

Dreher, K., and J. Fraser. 1968. Smoking habits of alcoholic out-patients, II. *International Journal of Addictions,* **3,** 65.

Dreikurs, R. 1962. Discussion of psychosomatic aspects of frigidity. In W. Kroger (ed.), *Psychosomatic obstetrics, gynecology and endocrinology,* pp. 415–417. Springfield:Thomas.

Dube, K., and N. Kumar. 1973. An epidemiological study of manic-depressive psychosis. *Acta Psychiatrica Scandinavica,* **49,** 691.

Dubin, L., and R. Amelar. 1971. Etiological factors in 1,294 consecutive cases of male infertility. *Fertility and Sterility,* **22,** 469.

Dubin, L., and R. Amelar. 1972. Sexual causes of male infertility. *Fertility and Sterility,* **23,** 579.

Dubos, R. 1978. Health and creative adaptation. *Human Nature,* **1,** 1, 74.

Dumond, D. 1975. The limitation of human population: A natural history. *Science,* **187,** 713.

Dunbar, F. 1962. Emotional factors in spontaneous abortion. In W. Kroger (ed.), *Psychosomatic obstetrics, gynecology, and endocrinology,* pp. 135–143. Springfield:Thomas.

Durand, J. 1967. Demographic transition. Report to Session II, IUSSP Sydney Conference.

Durand, J. 1972. The viewpoint of historical demography. In B. Spooner (ed.), *Population growth: Anthropological implications,* pp. 370–374. Cambridge, Massachusetts:MIT Press.

Duxon, M., and S. Dawkins. 1964. Non-consummation of marriage. *Medical Science and the Law,* **4,** 15.

Easterlin, R., R. Pollak, and M. Wachter. 1976. Toward a more general economic model of fertility determination: Endogenous preferences and natural fertility. U-NBER Conference on Economic and Demographic Change in Less Developed Countries, Philadelphia, September.

Eaton, J., and A. Mayer. 1954. *Man's capacity to reproduce: The demography of a unique population.* Glencoe, Illinois:Free Press.

Eaton, J., and R. Weil. 1955. *Culture and mental disorders.* Glencoe, Illinois:Free Press.

Eckholm, E. 1978. Cutting tobacco's toll. *World Watch Paper,* **18.**

Eisenberg, L. 1973. Syphilis in the Bantu of Soweto. *South African Medical Journal,* **47,** 2181.

Eller, J., and J. Morton. 1970. Bizarre deformities in offspring of user of lysergic acid diethylamide. *New England Journal of Medicine,* **283,** 395.

El-Mofty, A. 1962. Clinical aspects of bilharziasis. In G. Wolstenholme and M. O'Connor (eds.), *Bilharziasis,* pp. 174–197. Boston:Little Brown.

Elsdon-Dew, R. 1962. The pathognomy of bilharziasis. In G. Wolstenholme and M. O'Connor (eds.), *Bilharziasis,* pp. 207–214. Boston:Little Brown.

Eriksson, M., C. Catz, and S. Yaffe. 1973. Drugs and pregnancy. *Clinical Obstetrics and Gynecology,* **16,** 199.

Erlenmeyer-Kimling, L., S. Nichol, J. Rainer, and W. Deming. 1969. Changes in fertility rates of schizophrenic patients in New York State. *American Journal of Psychiatry,* **125,** 916.

Erlenmeyer-Kimling, L., J. Rainer, and F. Kallmann. 1966. Current reproductive trends in schizophrenia. In P. Hoch and J. Zubin (eds.), *Psychopathology of schizophrenia,* pp. 252–276. New York:Grune and Stratton.

Evans, R. 1972. Physical and biochemical characteristics of homosexual men. *Journal of Consulting and Clinical Psychology,* **39,** 140.

Eysenck, H. 1965. *Smoking, health, and personality.* New York:Basic Books.

Family Planning Perspectives, 1971. Abortion demand will increase. 3, 1, 59.

Farkas, G., and R. Rosen. 1976. Effect of alcohol on elicited male sexual response. *Journal of Studies on Alcohol,* **37,** 265.

Farley, R. 1970. *Growth of the black population.* Chicago:Markham. (a)

Farley, R. 1970. Fertility among urban blacks. *Milbank Memorial Fund Quarterly,* **43,** 183. (b)

Fawcett, J. 1970. *Psychology and population.* New York:Population Council.

Fawcett, J. (ed.). 1973. *Psychological perspectives on population.* New York:Basic Books.

Ferreira, A. 1965. Emotional factors in the prenatal environment. *Journal of Nervous & Mental Disease,* **141,** 108.

Flapan, M. 1976. Population psychology research focused on family formation and marital relationships. In S. Newman and V. Thompson (eds.), *Population psychology: Research and educational issues,* pp. 43–50. Washington, D.C.:U.S. Government Printing Office.

Fleck, S. 1970. Some psychiatric aspects of abortion. *Journal of Nervous & Mental Disease,* **151,** 42.

Foa, P. 1962. The mediation of psychic stimuli and the regulation of endocrine function. In W. Kroger (ed.), *Psychosomatic obstetrics, gynecology, and endocrinology,* pp. 550–559. Springfield:Thomas.

Ford, C., and F. Beach. 1951. *Patterns of sexual behavior.* New York:Harper.

Forfar, J., and M. Nelson. 1973. Epidemiology of drugs taken by pregnant women: Drugs that may affect the fetus adversely. *Clinical Pharmacology & Therapeutics,* **14,** 632.

Fox, V. 1966. Treatment of non-neurological complications of alcoholism. *Modern Treatment,* **3,** 502.

Franklin, S. 1978. Junkies shift habits. *Philadelphia Bulletin,* April 16, 1.

Fraser, A. 1972. Drug addiction in pregnancy—An obstetrician's experience. *Proceedings of the Royal Society of Medicine,* **65,** 867.

Frazier, T., G. Davis, H. Goldstein, and I. Goldberg. 1961. Cigarette smoking and prematurity: A prospective study. *American Journal of Obstetrics and Gynecology,* **81,** 988.

Freda, V. 1973. Hemolytic disease. *Clinical Obstetrics and Gynecology,* **16,** 72.

Freedman, R. 1963. *The sociology of human fertility.* Oxford:Basil Blackwell.

Freedman, R., P. Whelpton, and A. Campbell. 1959. *Family planning, sterility, and population growth.* Princeton:Princeton University Press.

Freund, K. 1974. Male homosexuality: An analysis of the pattern. In J. Loraine (ed.), *Understanding homosexuality,* pp. 25–81. New York:Elsevier.

Friederich, M. 1970. Foreword. *Clinical Obstetrics and Gynecology (Psychosexual Problems in Obstetrics and Gynecology),* **13,** 689. (a)

Friederich, M. 1970. Motivations for coitus. *Clinical Obstetrics and Gynecology (Psychosexual Problems in Obstetrics and Gynecology),* **13,** 691. (b)

Friedman, L. 1962. *Virgin wives.* London:Tavistock.

Fries, H., S. Nillius, and F. Pettersson. 1974. Epidemiology of secondary amenorrhea. *American Journal of Obstetrics and Gynecology,* **118,** 473.

Frisch, R. 1975. Demographic implications of the biological determinants of female fecundity. *Social Biology,* **22,** 17.

Fuller, J. 1974. *Fever: The hunt for a new killer virus.* New York:Ballantine.

Galton, L. 1978. Impotence: What medicine can do for it now. *Parade Magazine,* April 23, 20.

Galvao-Teles, A., D. Anderson, G. Burke, J. Marshall, C. Corbes, R. Brown, and M. Clark. 1973. Biologically active androgens and oestradiol in men with chronic liver disease. *Lancet,* **1,** 173.

Garner, T. 1971. Drugs and society. *British Journal of Addiction,* **66,** 219.

Gaulden, E., D. Littlefield, O. Putoff, and A. Seivert. 1964. Menstrual abnormalities associated with heroin addiction. *American Journal of Obstetrics and Gynecology,* **90,** 155.

Gebhard, P. 1965. Situational factors affecting human sexual behavior. In F. Beach (ed.), *Sex and behavior,* pp. 483–495. New York:Wiley.

Gebhard, P. 1972. Incidence of overt homosexuality in the United States and Western Europe. In J. Livingood (ed.), *National Institute of Mental Health Task Force on Homosexuality: Final reports and background papers,* pp. 22–29. Washington, D.C.:U.S. Government Printing Office.

Gelfand, M., C. Ross, D. Blair, W. Castle, and M. Weber. 1970. Schistosomiasis of the male pelvic organs: Severity of infection as determined by digestion of tissue and histologic methods in 300 cadavers. *American Journal of Tropical Medicine and Hygiene,* **19,** 779.

Gelfand, M., M. Ross, D. Blair, and M. Weber. 1971. Distribution and extent of schistosomiasis in female pelvic organs with special reference to the genital tract, as determined at autopsy. *American Journal of Tropical Medicine and Hygiene,* **20,** 846.

German, E. 1973. Medical problems in chronic alcoholic men. *Journal of Chronic Diseases,* **26,** 661.

Gilder, S. 1974. Alcohol, tobacco, and pregnancy. *Canadian Medical Association Journal,* **110,** 903.

Gilmour, D., A. Bloom, K. Lele, E. Robbins, and C. Maximilian. 1971. Chromosomal aberrations in users of psychoactive drugs. *Archives of General Psychiatry,* **24,** 268.

Ginsberg, G., W. Frosch, and T. Shapiro. 1972. The new impotence. *Archives of General Psychiatry,* **26,** 218.

Girgis, S., A. Etriby, H. El-Henfnawy, and S. Kahil. 1968. Aspermia: A survey of 49 cases. *Fertility and Sterility,* **19,** 580.

Gluckman, J., M. Kleinman, and A. May. 1974. Primary syphilis of the rectum. *New York State Journal of Medicine,* **74,** 2210.

Gluckman, L. 1966. Lesbianism—A clinical approach. *New Zealand Medical Journal,* **65,** 443.

Golden, J., and S. Golden. 1967. Varieties of sexual problems in obstetrical and gynecological practice. In C. Wahl (ed.), *Sexual problems,* pp. 53–70. New York:Free Press.

Gonick, P. 1976. Urologic problems and sexual dysfunction. In W. Oaks, G. Melchiode, and I. Ficher (eds.), *Sex and the life cycle,* pp. 191–197. New York:Grune and Stratton.

Goode, E. 1972. Drug use and sexual activity on a college campus. *American Journal of Psychiatry,* **128,** 92.

Goode, E. 1973. *The drug phenomenon: Social aspects of drug taking.* New York:Bobbs-Merrill.

Goode, E. 1975. Effects of cannabis in another culture. Book review of *Ganja in Jamaica* by V. Rubin and L. Comitas, The Hague, Mouton. *Science,* **189,** 41.

Goodfriend, M., I. Shey, and M. Klein. 1956. The effects of maternal narcotic addiction on the newborn. *American Journal of Obstetrics and Gynecology,* **71,** 29.

Gordon, G., K. Altman, A. Southern, E. Rubin, and C. Lieber. 1976. Effect of alcohol on sex hormone metabolism in normal men. *New England Journal of Medicine,* **295,** 793.

Gould, D. 1976. Drug abuse. *Encyclopaedia Britannica Yearbook,* 261.

Grabill, W., C. Kiser, and P. Whelpton. 1958. *The fertility of American women.* New York:Wiley.

Gray, R. 1977. Biological factors other than nutrition and lactation which may influence natural fertility. A review, paper presented at the IUSSP Seminar on Natural Fertility, Paris.

Greaves, G. 1972. Sexual disturbances among chronic amphetamine users. *Journal of Nervous & Mental Disease,* **155,** 363.

Green, H. 1974. Infants of alcoholic mothers. *American Journal of Obstetrics and Gynecology,* **118,** 713.

Green, P., and L. Rubin. 1959. Amenorrhea as a manifestation of chronic liver disease. *American Journal of Obstetrics and Gynecology,* **78,** 141.

Green, R. 1967. Sissies and tomboys: A guide to diagnosis and management. In C. Wahl (ed.), *Sexual problems,* pp. 89–114. New York:Free Press.

Greenfield, N., and A. Alexander. 1965. The ego and bodily responses. In N. Greenfield and W. Lewis (eds.), *Psychoanalysis and current biological thought,* pp. 201–214. Madison:University of Wisconsin Press.

Gregory, I. 1968. *Fundamentals of psychiatry.* Philadelphia:Saunders.

Grieve, J., T. Sommerville, G. Smith, and D. Piercy. 1972. To what extent is male infertility genetically determined? *Proceedings of the Royal Society of Medicine,* **65,** 20.

Grimm, E. 1967. Psychological and social factors in pregnancy, delivery, and outcome. In S. Richardson and A. Guttmacher (eds.), *Childbearing: Its social and psychological aspects,* pp. 1–52. Baltimore:Williams and Wilkins.

Grinspoon, L. 1972. Marihuana. In *Readings from Scientific American, Physiological Psychology,* pp. 199–208. San Francisco:W. H. Freeman.

Guilford, J. 1952. *General psychology.* New York:Van Nostrand.

Gyongyossy, A., and P. Szalozy. 1972. The ovulation-inhibiting effect of modern living. In N. Morris (ed.), *Psychosomatic medicine in obstetrics and gynecology,* pp. 589–592. New York:Karger.

Hagnell, O., and K. Tunving. 1972. Mental and physical complaints among alcoholics. *Quarterly Journal of Studies on Alcohol,* **33,** 77.

Hammer, M. 1972. Schizophrenia: Some questions of definition in cultural perspective. In A. Kaplin (ed.), *Genetic facts in schizophrenia,* pp. 423–450. Springfield:Thomas.

Hammond, E. 1962. The effects of smoking. *Scientific American,* **207,** 39.

Handlon, J. 1962. Hormonal activity and individual responses to stresses and easements in everyday living. In R. Roessler and N. Greenfield (eds.), *Physiological correlates of psychological disorders,* pp. 157–170. Madison:University of Wisconsin Press.

Hansluwka, H. 1975. Health, population, and socio-economic development. In L. Tabah (ed.), *Population growth and economic development in the Third World,* pp. 191–250. Belgium:Ordina.

Hanson, F., and J. Rock. 1950. The effect of adoption on fertility and other reproductive functions. *American Journal of Obstetrics and Gynecology,* **59,** 311.

Hanson, J., K. Jones, and D. Smith. 1976. Fetal alcohol syndrome: Experience with 41 patients. *Journal of the American Medical Association,* **235,** 1458.

Harding, R. 1970. A note on some vital statistics of a primitive peasant community in Sierra Leone. In T. Ford and G. DeJong (eds.), *Social demography,* pp. 638–642. Englewood Cliffs:Prentice-Hall.

Hardy, J., and E. Mellitis. 1973. Effect on child of maternal smoking during pregnancy. *Lancet,* **1,** 719.

Hare, E. 1967. The epidemiology of schizophrenia. *British Journal of Psychiatry,* **Special Publication 1,** 9.

Harmon, J., and M. Aliapoulios. 1972. Gynecomastia in marihuana users. *New England Journal of Medicine,* **287,** 936.

Harrison, R. 1977. The metabolism of mammalian spermatozoa. In R. Greep and M. Koblinsky (eds.), *Frontiers in reproduction and fertility control,* pp. 379–401. Cambridge, Massachusetts:MIT Press.

Harter, C. 1970. The fertility of sterile and subfecund women in New Orleans. *Social Biology,* **17,** 195.

Hartz, S., O. Heinonen, S. Shapiro, V. Siskind, and D. Slone. 1975. Antenatal exposure to meprobamate and chlordiazepoxide in relation to malformations, mental development, and childhood. *New England Journal of Medicine,* **292,** 726.

Hastings, D. 1960. Psychogenic impotence. *Postgraduate Medicine,* **27,** 429.

Hastings, D. 1968. Forms of impotence and contributing factors. *Journal of the American Medical Association,* **203,** 239.

Hawthorn, G. 1970. *The sociology of fertility.* London:Collier-MacMillan.

Heath, D. 1971. Psychiatry and abortion. *Canadian Psychiatric Association Journal,* **16,** 55.

Hedblom, J. 1973. Dimensions of lesbian sexual experience. *Archives of Sexual Behavior,* **2,** 329.

Heer, D. 1964. Fertility differences between Indian and Spanish-speaking parts of Andean countries. *Population Studies,* **18,** 71.

Heer, D. 1967. Fertility differences in Andean countries: A reply to W. H. James. *Population Studies,* **21,** 71.

Heiman, M. 1962. Toward a psychosomatic concept of infertility. In W. Kroger (ed.), *Psychosomatic obstetrics, gynecology, and endocrinology,* pp. 354–360. Springfield:Thomas.

Heiman, M. 1965. A psychoanalytic view of pregnancy. In J. Rovinsky and A. Guttmacher (eds.), *Medical, surgical, and gynecologic complications of pregnancy,* pp. 473–511. Baltimore:Williams and Wilkins.

Hellman, L. 1973. Keynote address of the Symposium on Drugs and the Unborn Child. *Clinical Pharmacology & Therapeutics,* **14,** 625.

Hemphill, R., and M. Reiss. 1948. Experimental investigations in the endocrinology of schizophrenia. *Proceedings of the Royal Society of Medicine,* **41,** 533.

Henin, R. 1968. Fertility differentials in the Sudan (with reference to the nomadic and settled populations). *Population Studies,* **22,** 147.

Henin, R. 1969. The patterns and causes of fertility differentials in the Sudan. *Population Studies,* **23,** 171.

Henry, L. 1965. French statistical research in natural fertility. In M. Sheps and J. Ridley (eds.), *Public health and population change,* pp. 333–350. Pittsburgh:University of Pittsburgh Press.

Hill, R. 1973. Drugs ingested by pregnant women. *Clinical Pharmacology & Therapeutics,* **14,** 654.

Hiraizumi, Y., C. Spradlin, R. Ito, and S. Anderson. 1973. Frequency of prenatal deaths and its relationship to ABO blood groups in man. *American Journal of Human Genetics,* **25,** 362.

Hirsch, H. 1972. Psycho-medical management of vaginism. In N. Morris (ed.), *Psychosomatic medicine in obstetrics and gynecology,* pp. 448–450. New York:Karger.

Hollingshead, A., and F. Redlich. 1958. *Social class and mental illness.* New York:Wiley.

Hollingsworth, T. 1977. Review of R. Lee (ed.), *Population patterns in the past,* New York:Academic Press. *Demography,* **14,** 548.

Hooker, E. 1972. Homosexuality. In J. Livingood (ed.), *National Institute of Mental Health Task Force on Homosexuality: Final reports and background papers,* pp. 11–21. Washington, D.C.:U.S. Government Printing Office.

Horton, P., and G. Leslie. 1974. *The sociology of social problems.* Englewood Cliffs:Prentice-Hall.

Horton, P., and G. Leslie. 1978. *The sociology of social problems.* Englewood Cliffs:Prentice-Hall.

Hudson, G., and M. Rucker. 1945. Spontaneous abortion. *Journal of the American Medical Association,* **129,** 542.

Humphrey, M. 1969. The adopted child as a fertility charm. *Journal of Reproduction and Fertility,* **20,** 354.

Humphrey, M. 1972. Childbirth following adoption: A myth revisited. In N. Morris (ed.), *Psychosomatic medicine in obstetrics and gynecology,* pp. 491–493. New York:Karger.

Hunt, E., N. Kidder, D. Schneider, and W. Stevens. 1949. The Micronesians of Yap and their depopulation. Report to the Pacific Science Board, from the Peabody Museum, Harvard University, Cambridge, Massachusetts.

Hunt, M. 1974. *Sexual behavior in the 1970s.* Chicago:Playboy Press.

Imielinski, K. 1969. Homosexuality in males, with particular reference to marriage. *Psychotherapy & Psychosomatics,* **17,** 126.

Interchange. 1977. American way of life: A way of death? *Population Reference Bureau,* **6,** 5, 1.

Intercom. 1975. Infant deaths. **3,** 1, 7.

Intercom. 1977. Studies link abnormalities to alcohol, coffee intake. **5,** 6, 3. (a)

Intercom. 1977. Study uncovers smoking, early menopause link. **5,** 7, 6. (b)

Israel, S. 1967. *Menstrual disorders and sterility.* New York:Harper and Row.

Isselbacher, K., and N. Greenberger. 1964. Metabolic effects of alcohol on the liver. *New England Journal of Medicine,* **270,** 351.

Jacobson, C., and C. Berlin. 1972. Possible reproductive detriment in LSD users. *Journal of the American Medical Association,* **222,** 1367.

Jacobsson, L., B. von Schoultz, and F. Solheim. 1976. Repeat aborters–first aborters, a social psychiatric comparison. *Social Psychiatry,* **11,** 75.

James, J., and M. Goldman. 1971. Behavior trends of wives of alcoholics. *Quarterly Journal of Studies on Alcohol,* **32,** 373.

James, W. 1966. The effect of altitude on fertility in Andean countries. *Population Studies,* **20,** 97.

James, W. 1969. The effect of maternal psychological stress on the fetus. *British Journal of Psychiatry,* **115,** 811.

Javert, C. 1962. Further follow-up on habitual abortion patients. *American Journal of Obstetrics and Gynecology,* **84,** 1149.

Jellinek, E. 1952. Expert Committee on Mental Health, Alcoholism Subcommittee, second report. *World Health Organization Technical Report Series,* **48,** (35).

Jick, H., J. Porter, and A. Morrison. 1977. Relation between smoking and age of natural menopause. *Lancet,* **1,** 1354.

Johnson, J. 1968. *Disorders of sexual potency in the male.* New York:Pergamon.

Johnston, L. 1952. Cure of tobacco smoking. *Lancet,* **2,** 480.

Jones, A. 1967. *Introduction to parasitology.* Reading, Massachusetts:Addison-Wesley.

Jones, K., and D. Smith. 1973. Recognition of the fetal alcohol syndrome in early infancy. *Lancet,* **2,** 999.

Jones, K., D. Smith, A. Streissguth, and N. Myrianthopoulos. 1974. Outcome in offspring of chronic alcoholic women. *Lancet,* **1,** 1076.

Jones, K., D. Smith, C. Ulleland, and A. Streissguth. 1973. Pattern of malformation in offspring of chronic alcoholic mothers. *Lancet,* **1,** 1267.

Jones, M. 1973. IQ and fertility in schizophrenia. *British Journal of Psychiatry,* **122,** 689.

Jordan, P., and G. Webbe. 1969. *Human schistosomiasis.* London:William Heinemann Medical Books.

Kallmann, F. 1938. *The genetics of schizophrenia.* New York:Augustin.

Karahasanoglu, A., P. Barglow, and G. Growe. 1972. Psychological aspects of infertility. *Journal of Reproductive Medicine,* **9,** 241.

Katz, S. 1972. Biological factors in population control. In B. Spooner (ed.), *Population growth: Anthropological implications,* pp. 351–369. Cambridge, Massachusetts: MIT Press.

Kaufman, J. 1967. Organic and psychological factors in the genesis of impotence and premature ejaculation. In C. Wahl (ed.), *Sexual problems,* pp. 133–148. New York:Free Press.

Kaufman, S. 1970. *New hope for the childless couple.* New York:Simon and Schuster.

Kellet, J. 1973. Evolutionary theory for the dichotomy of the functional psychoses. *Lancet,* **1,** 860.

Kendler, H. 1963. *Basic psychology.* New York:Appleton-Century-Crofts.

Kent, J., R. Scaramuzzi, W. Lauwers, and A. Parlow. 1973. Plasma testosterone, estradiol, and gonadotrophins in hepatic insufficiency. *Gastroenterology,* **64,** 111.

Kenyon, F. 1968. Studies in female homosexuality. *British Journal of Psychiatry,* **114,** 1337. (a)

Kenyon, F. 1968. Psychical and physical health of female homosexuals. *Journal of Neurology, Neurosurgery, & Psychiatry,* **31,** 487. (b)

Kenyon, F. 1970. Homosexuality in the female. *British Journal of Hospital Medicine,* **3,** 183.

Kenyon, F. 1972. Some characteristics of female patients referred with homosexual problems. In N. Morris (ed.), *Psychosomatic medicine in obstetrics and gynecology,* pp. 379–381. New York:Karger.

Kenyon, F. 1974. Female homosexuality—A review. In J. Loriane (ed.), *Understanding homosexuality,* pp. 83–120. New York:Elsevier.

Kessel, N. 1966. Alcoholism. In L. Platt and A. Parkes (eds.), *Social and genetic influences on life,* pp. 130–139. New York:Plenum.

Ketty, S. 1976. Participant in the colloquium on the biology of the schizophrenic process. *Advances in Behavioral Biology,* **19,** 37.

King, A. 1974. Homosexuality and venereal disease. In J. Loraine (ed.), *Understanding homosexuality,* pp. 186–204. New York:Elsevier.

Kinsey, A., W. Pomeroy, and C. Martin. 1948. *Sexual behavior in the human male.* Philadelphia:Saunders.

Kinsey, A., W. Pomeroy, C. Martin, and P. Gebhard. 1953. *Sexual behavior in the human female.* Philadelphia:Saunders.

Kinsey, B. 1966. *The female alcoholic.* Springfield:Thomas.

Kinsey, B. 1968. Psychological factors in alcoholic women from a state hospital sample. *American Journal of Psychiatry,* **124,** 1463.

Kiser, C. 1958. Fertility trends and differentials among nonwhites in the U.S. *Milbank Memorial Fund Quarterly,* **36,** 149.

Kiser, C. 1964. Psychological factors in infertility—A demographic appraisal. *Journal of the Indian Medical Profession,* **11,** 4927.

Kissane, J., and M. Smith. 1967. *Pathology of infancy and childhood.* St. Louis:C. V. Mosby.

Kistner, R. 1964. *Gynecology: Principles and practice.* Chicago:Yearbook Medical Publishers.

Kleegman, S., and S. Kaufman. 1966. *Infertility in women.* Philadelphia:Davis.

Kline, J., Z. Stein, M. Susser, and D. Warburton. 1977. Smoking: A risk factor for spontaneous abortion. *New England Journal of Medicine,* **297,** 793.

Knight, H. 1978. Impotence? The more you worry, the worse it gets: Conversation with Dr. Harold Lief. *Discover Magazine,* Feb. 26, 8.

Knowles, J. 1976. The struggle to stay healthy. *Time,* Bicentennial Essay, Aug. 9, 60.

Kole, J. 1975. Stress: The new sex killer. *Forum,* **4,** 8.

Kolodny, R., L. Jacobs, W. Masters, G. Toro, and W. Daughaday. 1972. Plasma gonadotrophins and prolactin in male homosexuals. *Lancet,* **2,** 18.

Kolodny, R., and W. Masters. 1973. Hormones and homosexuality. *Annals of Internal Medicine,* **79,** 897.

Kolodny, R., W. Masters, J. Hendryx, and G. Toro. 1971. Plasma testosterone and semen analysis in male homosexuals. *New England Journal of Medicine,* **285,** 1170.

Kolodny, R., W. Masters, R. Kolodner, and G. Toro. 1974. Depression of plasma testosterone levels after chronic intensive marihuana use. *New England Journal of Medicine,* **290,** 872.

Kramer, M., E. Pollack, R. Rednick, and B. Locke. 1972. *Mental disorders and suicide.* Cambridge, Massachusetts:Harvard University Press.

Kroger, W. 1962. New perspectives in obesity—An integrated approach. In W. Kroger (ed.), *Psychosomatic obstetrics, gynecology, and endocrinology,* pp. 531–548. Springfield:Thomas. (a)

Kroger, W. 1962. Fertility after adoption. In W. Kroger (ed.), *Psychosomatic obstetrics, gynecology, and endocrinology,* pp. 632–637. Springfield:Thomas. (b)

Kroger, W. 1962. Psychosomatic aspects of frigidity and impotence. In W. Kroger (ed.), *Psychosomatic obstetrics, gynecology, and endocrinology,* pp. 386–399. Springfield:Thomas. (c)

Kroger, W. 1962. Psychosomatic aspects of infertility. In W. Kroger (ed.), *Psychosomatic obstetrics, gynecology, and endocrinology,* pp. 339–342. Springfield:Thomas. (d)

Kroger, W. 1962. Psychosomatic aspects of functional uterine bleeding, amenorrhea, pseudocyesis, and dysmenorrhea. In W. Kroger (ed.), *Psychosomatic obstetrics, gynecology, and endocrinology,* pp. 255–261. Springfield:Thomas. (e)

Kroger, W. 1962. Psychophysiologic factors in toxemias of pregnancy. In W. Kroger (ed.), *Psychosomatic obstetrics, gynecology, and endocrinology,* p. 103. Springfield:Thomas. (f)

Kroger, W. 1962. Psychosomatic aspects of nausea and vomiting. In W. Kroger (ed.), *Psychosomatic obstetrics, gynecology, and endocrinology,* pp. 115–116. Springfield:Thomas. (g)

Kroger, W. 1962. Psychosomatic factors in spontaneous abortion. In W. Kroger (ed.), *Psychosomatic obstetrics, gynecology, and endocrinology,* pp. 133–134. Springfield:Thomas. (h)

Kroger, W. 1962. Evaluation of personality factors in the treatment of infertility. In W.

Kroger (ed.), *Psychosomatic obstetrics, gynecology, and endocrinology*, pp. 361–371. Springfield:Thomas. (i)

Kroger, W. 1962. Psychosomatic aspects of frigidity and postpartum frigidity. In W. Kroger (ed.), *Psychosomatic obstetrics, gynecology, and endocrinology*, pp. 383–385. Springfield:Thomas. (j)

Kroger, W. (ed.), 1962. *Psychosomatic obstetrics, gynecology and endocrinology*. Springfield:Thomas.

Kroger, W., and S. Freed. 1951. *Psychosomatic gynecology*, Philadelphia:Saunders.

Kuhr, M. 1973. Fetal risks in rubella vaccination. *Journal of the American Medical Association*, **226**, 1357.

Kullander, S., and B. Kallen. 1971. A prospective study of smoking and pregnancy. *Acta Obstetrica et Gynecologica Scandinavica*, **50**, 82.

Lancet. 1973. Maternal drug addiction and the neonate. **1**, 527.

Lane, E., and G. Albee. 1970. The birth weight of children born to schizophrenic women. *Journal of Psychology*, **74**, 157.

Larson, C., and G. Nyman. 1973. Differential fertility in schizophrenia. *Acta Psychiatrica Scandinavica*, **49**, 272.

Larson, P., M. Haag, and H. Silvette. 1961. *Tobacco: Experimental and clinical studies.* Baltimore:Williams and Wilkins.

Larson, P., and H. Silvette. 1968. *Tobacco: Experimental and clinical studies, Supplement I.* Baltimore:Williams and Wilkins.

Larson, P., and H. Silvette. 1971. *Tobacco: Experimental and clinical studies, Supplement II.* Baltimore:Williams and Wilkins.

Lawson, D. 1976. The natural tranquilizers. *Forum,* **5**, 8, 28.

Leavitt, F. 1974. *Drugs and behavior.* Philadelphia:Saunders.

Leevy, C., and W. tenHove. 1967. Pathogenesis and sequelae of liver disease in alcoholic man. In R. Maickel (ed.), *Biochemical factors in alcoholism,* pp. 151–166. London:Pergamon Press.

Lelbach, W. 1966. Leberschaden bei chronischem alkoholismus. *Acta Hepato–Splenologica,* **13**, 321.

Lemere, F., and J. Smith. 1973. Alcohol-induced sexual impotence. *American Journal of Psychiatry,* **130**, 212.

Lemoine, P., H. Haronsseau, J. Borteyeu, and J. Menuet. 1968. Les enfants de parents alcooliques; anomalies observees a propos de 127 cas. *Ouest Medical,* **25**, 476.

Lennard, H., L. Epstein, and M. Rosenthal. 1972. The methadone illusion. *Science,* **176**, 881.

Leridon, H. 1977. *Human fertility: The basic components.* Chicago:University of Chicago Press.

Lessa, W., and G. Myers. 1962. Population dynamics of an atoll community. *Population Studies,* **15**, 752.

Levin, R. 1975. The Redbook report on premarital and extramarital sex. *Redbook,* October, 38.

Levin, R., and A. Levin. 1975. Sexual pleasure: The surprising preferences of 100,000 women. *Redbook,* September, 51.

Levine, J. 1955. The sexual adjustment of alcoholics. *Quarterly Journal of Studies on Alcohol,* **16**, 675.

Lewis, A. 1958. Fertility and mental illness. *Eugenics Review,* **50**, 91.

Lewis, A. 1959. Families with manic-depressive psychosis. *Eugenics Quarterly,* **6**, 130.

Lewis, H., D. Roberts, and A. Edwards. 1972. Biological problems, and opportunities, of isolation among the islanders of Tristan da Cunha. In D. Glass and R. Revelle (eds.), *Population and social change.* pp. 383–417. London:Edward and Arnold.

Lidberg, L. 1972. Social and psychiatric aspects of impotence and premature ejaculation. *Archives of Sexual Behavior,* **2**, 135.

Lidz, T. 1973. *The origin and treatment of schizophrenic disorders.* New York:Basic Books.

Lieb, J. 1975. What causes anorexia. *Time,* Aug. 18, 8.

Lieber, C. 1972. Metabolism of ethanol and alcoholism: Racial and acquired factors. *Annals of Internal Medicine,* **76**, 326.

Lieber, C., and C. Davidson. 1962. Some metabolic effects of ethyl alcohol. *American Journal of Medical Sciences,* **33**, 319.

Linbeck, V. 1972. The woman alcoholic: A review of the literature. *International Journal of Addictions,* **7**, 567.

Linder, R. 1963. Homosexuality and the contemporary scene. In H. Ruitenbeek (ed.), *The problem of homosexuality in modern society,* pp. 100–110. New York:Dutton.

Lippincott Publishing Co. 1963. *Aspects of alcoholism, vol. 1.* Philadelphia:Lippincott.

Lippincott Publishing Co. 1966. *Aspects of alcoholism, vol. 2.* Philadelphia:Lippincott.

Lisansky, E. 1957. Alcoholism in women: Social and psychological concomitants. *Quarterly Journal of Studies on Alcohol,* **18**, 588.

Little, R., F. Schultz, and W. Mandell. 1976. Drinking during pregnancy. *Journal of Studies on Alcohol,* **37**, 375.

Livi-Bacci, M. 1977. *A history of Italian fertility.* Princeton:Princeton University Press.

Llewellyn-Jones, D. 1974. *Human reproduction and society.* New York:Pitman.

Lloyd, C., and R. Williams. 1948. Endocrine changes associated with Laennec's cirrhosis of the liver. *American Journal of Medicine,* **4**, 315.

London, D. 1972. Male infertility. *British Medical Journal,* **1**, 609.

Longo, L. 1970. Carbon monoxide in the pregnant mother and the fetus and its exchange across the placenta. *Annals of the New York Academy of Sciences,* **174**, 313.

Loraine, J., D. Adamopoulos, K. Kirkham, A. Ismail, and G. Dove. 1971. Patterns of hormone excretion in male and female homosexuals. *Nature,* **234**, 552.

Loraine, J., A. Ismail, D. Adamopoulos, and G. Dove. 1970. Endocrine function in male and female homosexuals. *British Medical Journal,* **4**, 406.

Lorimer, F. 1954. *Culture and human fertility.* Paris:UNESCO.

Lowe, C. 1959. Effect of mothers' smoking habits on birth weight of their children. *British Medical Journal,* **2**, 673.

Lubke, F. 1972. Psychological aspects of the problem of sterility. In N. Morris (ed.), *Psychosomatic medicine in obstetrics and gynecology,* pp. 482–487. New York:Karger.

Lubs, M. 1973. Racial differences in maternal smoking effects on the newborn infant. *American Journal of Obstetrics and Gynecology,* **115**, 66.

Lukianowicz, N. 1963. Sexual drive and its gratification in schizophrenia. *International Journal of Social Psychiatry,* **9**, 250.

Lynch, J. 1977. *The broken heart: The medical consequences of loneliness.* New York:Basic Books.

Macavei, I. 1971. Female anorgasmy in marriage as an indirect cause of infertility. Paper presented at the VII World Congress on Fertility and Sterility, Tokyo. Abstract in *Excerpta Medica,* **234**, 95.

Magee, B. 1966. *One in twenty: A study of homosexuality in men and women.* New York:Stein and Day.

Mai, F. 1969. Psychiatric and interpersonal factors in infertility. *Australian and New Zealand Journal of Psychiatry,* **3**, 31.

Mai, F. 1971. Conception after adoption: An open question. *Psychosomatic Medicine,* **33,** 509.

Mai, F., R. Munday, and E. Rump. 1972. Psychosomatic and behavioral mechanisms in psychogenic infertility. *British Journal of Psychiatry,* **120,** 199.

Mandy, T., and A. Mandy. 1962. The psychosomatic aspects of infertility. In W. Kroger (ed.), *Psychosomatic obstetrics, gynecology, and endocrinology,* pp. 343–353. Springfield:Thomas.

Mann, C. 1959. Habitual abortion. *American Journal of Obstetrics and Gynecology,* **77,** 706.

Mann, E., and E. Grimm. 1962. Habitual abortion. In W. Kroger (ed.), *Psychosomatic obstetrics, gynecology, and endocrinology,* pp. 153–159. Springfield:Thomas.

Margolese, M. 1970. A new endocrine correlate. *Hormones and Behavior,* **1,** 151.

Marshall, E. 1971. Why patients do not take their medication. *American Journal of Psychiatry,* **128,** 656.

Marshall, J., and T. Fraser. 1971. Amenorrhea in anorexia nervosa. *British Medical Journal,* **4,** 590.

Masnick, G., and S. Katz. 1976. Adaptive childbearing in a North Slope Eskimo community. In B. Kaplan (ed.), *Anthropological studies of human fertility,* pp. 37–58. Detroit:Wayne State Press.

Masnick, G., and J. McFalls. 1976. A new perspective on the twentieth-century American fertility swing. *Journal of Family History,* **1,** 217.

Masnick, G., and J. McFalls. Forthcoming. *The American fertility swing: Three generations of black natality.*

Masters, W., and V. Johnson. 1966. *Human sexual response.* Boston:Little Brown.

Masters, W., and V. Johnson. 1970. *Human sexual inadequacy.* Boston:Little Brown.

Masters, W., and V. Johnson, 1976. Personal communication. (a)

Masters, W., and V. Johnson. 1976. Personal communication. (b)

Mathews, D. 1973. Sedation in pregnancy. *British Medical Journal,* **1,** 800.

Maura, E. 1971. *Pregnancy and delivery complications in schizophrenic women.* Doctoral thesis, New School for Social Research, New York.

Maurer, R. 1975. Health care and the gay community. *Postgraduate Medicine,* **58,** 127.

Mauss, A. 1975. *Social problems as social movements.* Philadelphia:Lippincott.

Mayer-Gross, W., E. Slater, and M. Roth. 1969. *Clinical psychiatry.* London:Cassell.

Mays, E. 1973. Cigarette smoking: Its relationship to other diseases. *Journal of the National Medical Association,* **65,** 520.

McFalls, J. 1973. Impact of VD on the fertility of the U.S. black population, 1880–1950. *Social Biology,* **20,** 2.

McGlothlin, W., R. Sparkes, and D. Arnold. 1970. Effect of LSD on human pregnancy. *Journal of the American Medical Association,* **212,** 1483.

McKusick, V. 1964. *Human genetics.* Englewood Cliffs:Prentice-Hall.

McNall, S. 1975. *Social problems today.* Boston:Little Brown.

McNeil, T., and L. Kaij. 1973. Obstetric complications and physical size of offspring of schizophrenic-like and control mothers. *British Journal of Psychiatry,* **123,** 341.

McNeil, T., and L. Kaij. 1974. Reproduction among female mental patients: Obstetric complications and physical size of offspring. *Acta Psychiatrica Scandinavica,* **50,** 3.

McQuerter, G. 1978. Cancer: Clues in the mind. *Greater Wilmington Advertiser,* May 28, 1; reprinted from *Science News.*

Mechanic, D. 1969. *Mental health and social policy.* Englewood Cliffs:Prentice-Hall.

Mechanic, D. 1970. Problems and prospects in psychiatric epidemiology. In E. Hare and

J. Wing (eds.), *Psychiatric epidemiology,* pp. 3–22. London:Oxford University Press.

Medhus, A. 1974. Morbidity among female alcoholics. *Scandinavian Journal of Social Medicine,* **2,** 5.

Medhus, A. 1975. Venereal disease among female alcoholics. *Scandinavian Journal of Social Medicine,* **3,** 28.

Medical Letter on Drugs and Therapeutics. 1972. Drugs in pregnancy. **14,** 94.

Mednick, S. 1970. Breakdown in individuals at high risk for schizophrenia: Possible predispositional perinatal factors. *Mental Hygiene,* **54,** 50.

Mednick, S., E. Mura, F. Schulsinger, and B. Mednick. 1971. Perinatal conditions and infant development in children with schizophrenic parents. *Social Biology,* **Supplement 18,** S103.

Mednick, S., E. Mura, F. Schulsinger, and B. Mednick. 1973. Erratum and further analysis—Perinatal conditions and infant development in children with schizophrenic parents. *Social Biology,* **20,** 111.

Mednick, S., and F. Schulsinger. 1968. Some premorbid characteristics related to breakdown in children with schizophrenic mothers. In D. Rosenthal and S. Kety (eds.), *The transmission of schizophrenia,* pp. 267–292. New York:Pergamon.

Melchiode, G. 1976. Sexual dysfunction in the male. In W. Oaks, G. Melchiode, and I. Ficher (eds.), *Sex and the life cycle,* pp. 97–103. New York:Grune and Stratton.

Mendelson, J., J. Kuehnle, J. Ellingboe, and T. Babor. 1974. Plasma testosterone levels before, during, and after chronic marihuana smoking. *New England Journal of Medicine,* **291,** 1051.

Menniger, K. 1963. *The vital balance: The life process in mental health and illness.* New York:Viking.

Merari, A., A. Ginton, T. Heifez, and T. Lev-Ran. 1973. Effects of alcohol on mating behavior of the female rat. *Quarterly Journal of Studies on Alcohol,* **34,** 1095.

Meuwissen, J. 1967. Human infertility in Ghana. *Fertility and Sterility,* **18,** 223.

Meyer, M., and G. Comstock. 1972. Maternal cigarette smoking and perinatal mortality. *American Journal of Epidemiology,* **96,** 1.

Milkovich, L., and B. van den Berg. 1974. Effects of prenatal meprobamate and chlordiazepoxide hydrochloride on human embryonic and fetal development. *New England Journal of Medicine,* **291,** 1268.

Millar, D. 1972. Preconceptional pseudocyesis. In N. Morris (ed.), *Psychosomatic medicine in obstetrics and gynecology,* pp. 433–435. New York:Karger.

Milojkovic, A., S. Simic, and M. Dzumhur. 1966. Migration and place of work as a cause of male sterility. Proceedings of the Fifth World Congress on Fertility and Sterility, Stockholm, June, 828.

Molnar, J., and G. Papp. 1973. Alcohol as a possible enhancer of mucus in semen. *Andrologia (Berlin),* **5,** 105.

Money, J. 1967. Sexual problems of the chronically ill. In C. Wahl (ed.), *Sexual problems,* pp. 266–288. New York:Free Press.

Moran, P. 1972. Theoretical considerations of schizophrenia genetics. In A. Kaplan (ed.), *Genetic factors in schizophrenia,* pp. 295–309. Springfield:Thomas.

Morrow, L. 1977. The Russian Revolution turns 60. *Time,* Nov. 14, 46.

Mosley, W. 1977. The effects of nutrition on natural fertility. Paper presented at the IUSSP Seminar on Natural Fertility, Paris, March.

Mott, F. 1919. Normal and morbid conditions of the testes from youth to old age in 100 asylum and hospital cases. *British Medical Journal,* **2,** 737.

Mulcahy, R., and J. Knaggs. 1968. Effect of age, parity, and cigarette smoking on outcome of pregnancy. *American Journal of Obstetrics and Gynecology,* **101,** 844.

Murphree, H. 1971. *Drill's pharmacology in medicine.* New York:McGraw-Hill.

Nag, M. 1962. *Factors affecting human fertility in nonindustrial societies: A cross-cultural study.* New Haven:Yale University Publications in Anthropology.

Nag, M. 1972. Sex, culture and human fertility. *Current Anthropology,* **13,** 231.

National Commission on Marijuana and Drug Abuse. 1973. *Drug use in America: Problem in perspective.* Washington, D.C.:U.S. Government Printing Office.

National Institute on Alcohol Abuse and Alcoholism. 1978. *Alcohol and your unborn baby.* DHEW Publication No. (ADM) 78-521.

Neshkov, N. 1969. The state of spermatogenesis and sexual function in those who abuse alcohol (translation). Abstract in *Quarterly Journal of Studies on Alcohol,* 1970, **31,** 769.

Neu, R., H. Powes, S. King, and L. Gardner. 1969. Cannabis and chromosomes. *Lancet,* **1,** 675.

Neuberg, R. 1970. Drug dependence and pregnancy: A review of the problems and their management. *Journal of Obstetrics and Gynecology of the British Commonwealth,* **77,** 1117.

Neuberg, R. 1972. Drug addiction in pregnancy. A review of the problem. *Proceedings of the Royal Society of Medicine,* **65,** 867.

Newman, S., and V. Thompson. 1976. *Population psychology: Research and educational issues.* Washington, D.C.:U.S. Government Printing Office.

Newton, N. 1972. A woman's viewpoint on woman's problems. In N. Morris (ed.), *Psychosomatic medicine in obstetrics and gynecology,* pp. 13–19. New York:Karger.

Nichols, W., R. Miller, W. Heneen, C. Bradt, L. Hollister, and S. Kanter. 1974. Cytogenic studies on human subjects receiving marihuana and tetrahydrocannabinol. *Mutation Research,* **26,** 413.

Niswander, K., and M. Gordon. 1972. *The women and their pregnancies.* Philadelphia:Saunders.

Noyes, R., and E. Chapnick. 1964. Literature on psychology and infertility. *Fertility and Sterility,* **15,** 543.

Ochsner, A. 1971. Influence of smoking on sexuality and pregnancy. *Medical Aspects of Human Sexuality,* **5,** 81.

Odegard, O. 1960. Marriage rate and fertility in psychotic patients before hospital admission and after discharge. *International Journal of Social Psychiatry,* **6,** 25.

Ojo, O. 1968. The male factor in infertile marriages in Nigeria. *West African Medical Journal,* **17,** 210.

O'Lane, J. 1963. Some fetal effects of maternal cigarette smoking. *Obstetrics and Gynecology,* **22,** 181.

Oliven, J. 1965. *Sexual hygiene and pathology.* Philadelphia:Lippincott.

Oliven. J. 1974. *Clinical sexuality.* Philadelphia:Lippincott.

O'Loughlin, P. 1974. The islands of love: Trobriand Islands. *Philadelphia Bulletin,* Feb. 10, 1.

Omran, A. 1971. The epidemiologic transition. *Milbank Memorial Fund Quarterly,* **39,** 509.

Ontario Department of Health. 1967. *Second report of the Perinatal Mortality Study in ten teaching hospitals.* Toronto:ODH. (a)

Ontario Department of Health. 1967. *Supplement to the Second report of the Perinatal Mortality Study in ten university teaching hospitals.* Toronto:ODH. (b)

Orford, J., and G. Edwards. 1977. *Alcoholism.* Oxford:Oxford University Press.

Orr, D. 1941. Pregnancy following the decision to adopt. *Psychosomatic Medicine,* **3,** 441.

Ossofsky, H. 1972. Amenorrhea: Symptom of endogenous depression. *Medical Annals of the District of Columbia,* **41,** 744.

Ostow, M. 1965. Psychic energies in health and disease. In N. Greenfield and W. Lewis (eds.), *Psychoanalysis and current biological thought,* pp. 339–362. Madison: University of Wisconsin Press.

Pace, H., W. Davis, and C. Borgen. 1971. Teratogenesis and marihuana. *Annals of the New York Academy of Sciences,* **191,** 123.

Paffenbarger, R., and L. McCabe. 1966. The effect of obstetric and perinatal events on risk of mental illness in women of childbearing age. *American Journal of Public Health,* **56,** 400.

Paffenbarger, R., C. Steinmetz, B. Poller, and R. Hyde. 1961. The picture puzzle of the postpartum psychosis. *Psychiatry,* **13,** 161.

Palmer, R., E. Ouellette, L. Warner, and S. Leichtman. 1974. Congenital malformations in offspring of a chronic alcoholic mother. *Pediatrics,* **53,** 490.

Palmgren, B., and B. Wallander. 1971. Cigarette smoking and abortion: Consecutive prospective study of 4,312 pregnancies (translation). *Lakarrtidningen,* **68,** 2611.

Palti, Z. 1969. Psychogenic male infertility. *Psychosomatic Medicine,* **31,** 326.

Parkes, A. 1976. *Patterns of sexuality and reproduction.* New York:Oxford University Press.

Parks, G., S. Korth-Schutz, R. Penny, R. Hilding, K. Dumars, S. Frazier, and M. New. 1974. Variation in pituitary-gonadal function in adolescent male homosexuals and heterosexuals. *Journal of Clinical Endocrinology and Metabolism,* **39,** 796.

Pearlman, K., and L. Kobaski. 1972. Frequency of intercourse in men. *Journal of Urology,* **107,** 298.

Pelosi, M., J. Sama, H. Caterini, and H. Kaminetzky. 1974. Galactorrhea-amenorrhea syndrome associated with heroin addiction. *American Journal of Obstetrics and Gynecology,* **118,** 966.

Penrose, L. 1971. Congenital malformations in man and natural selection. In C. Bajema (ed.), *Natural selection in human populations,* pp. 111–118. New York:Wiley.

Perry, J., and E. Perry. 1976. *Face to face: The individual and social problems.* Boston:Education Associates.

Persaud, T., and A. Ellington. 1967. Cannabis in early pregnancy. *Lancet,* **2,** 1306.

Persaud, T., and A. Ellington. 1968. Teratogenic activity of cannabis resin. *Lancet,* **2,** 406.

Petersen, W. 1975. *Population.* New York:Macmillan.

Peterson, W., K. Morese, and D. Kaltreider. 1965. Smoking and prematurity: A preliminary report based on study of 7,740 Caucasians. *Obstetrics and Gynecology,* **26,** 775.

Philadelphia Bulletin. 1976. MDs urge U.S. to ban amphetamines. Nov. 11, 1.

Philadelphia Bulletin. 1977. Marihuana study. June 11, 1. (a)

Philadelphia Bulletin. 1977. Marihuana said to be linked to birth defects. Aug. 26, 42. (b)

Pillard, R., R. Rose, and M. Sherwood. 1974. Plasma testosterone levels in homosexual men. *Archives of Sexual Behavior,* **3,** 453.

Pincock, T. 1964. Alcoholism in tuberculous patients. *Canadian Medical Association Journal,* **91,** 851.

Pitt-Rivers, G. 1927. *The clash of culture and the contact of races.* London:Routledge.

Platt, J., I. Ficher, and M. Silver. 1973. Infertile couples: Personality traits and self-ideal concept discrepancies. *Fertility and Sterility,* **24,** 972.

Pohlman, E. 1970. Childlessness, intentional and unintentional. *Journal of Nervous & Mental Disease,* **151,** 2.

Poland, B., L. Wogan, and J. Calvin. 1972. Teenagers, illicit drugs, and pregnancy. *Canadian Medical Association Journal,* **107,** 955.

Pomeroy, W. 1969. *Task force on homosexuality: Background papers.* Washington, D.C.:U.S. Government Printing Office.

Potts, M., P. Diggory, and J. Peel. 1977. *Abortion.* New York:Cambridge University Press.

Presser, H. 1971. The timing of the first birth: Female roles and black fertility. *Milbank Memorial Fund Quarterly,* **44,** 329.

Price, J., E. Slater, and E. Hare. 1971. Marital status of first admissions to psychiatric beds in England and Wales in 1965 and 1966. *Social Biology,* **Supplement 18,** S74.

Priestley, B. 1972. Drug addiction in pregnancy. Drug addiction and the newborn. *Proceedings of the Royal Society of Medicine,* **65,** 870.

Prothero, R. 1972. Problems of public health among pastoralists: A case study from Africa. In N. McGlashan (ed.), *Medical geography,* pp. 105–118. London:Methuen.

Pumper-Mindlin, E. 1967. Nymphomania and satyriasis. In C. Wahl (ed.), *Sexual problems,* pp. 163–171. New York:Free Press.

Racz, I. 1970. Homosexuality among syphilitic patients. *British Journal of Venereal Disease,* **46,** 117.

Rantakallio, P. 1969. Groups at risk in low birth weight infants and perinatal mortality. *Acta Paediatrica Scandinavica,* **Supplement,** 193.

Rasidakis, N. 1972. Cancer and insanity. *Behavior Today,* **3,** 2.

Rathod, N., and I. Thomson. 1971. Women alcoholics: A clinical study. *Quarterly Journal of Studies on Alcohol,* **32,** 45.

Rawnsley, K. 1968. Epidemiology of affective disorders. *British Journal of Psychiatry,* **Special Publication 2,** 27.

Raymont, A., G. Arronet, and W. Arrata. 1969. Review of 500 cases of infertility. *International Journal of Fertility,* **14,** 141.

Razzell, P. 1977. *The conquest of smallpox: The impact of inoculation on smallpox mortality in eighteenth century Britain.* Sussex:Caliban.

Reed, S., C. Hartley, V. Anderson, V. Phillips, and N. Johnson. 1973. *The psychoses: Family studies.* Philadelphia:Saunders.

Rementeria, J., and N. Nunag. 1973. Narcotic withdrawal in pregnancy: Stillbirth incidence with a case report. *American Journal of Obstetrics and Gynecology,* **116,** 1152.

Renshaw, D. 1974. Homosexuality today. *Postgraduate Medicine,* **55,** 172.

Retherford, R. 1972. Tobacco smoking and the sex mortality differential. *Demography,* **9,** 203.

Retherford, R. 1974. Tobacco smoking and sex ratios in the United States. *Social Biology,* **21,** 28. (a)

Retherford, R. 1974. Cigarette smoking and widowhood in the United States. *Population Studies,* **27,** 193. (b)

Revue de Alcoolisme. 1975. Concerning the offspring of alcoholics. **21,** xvii.

Richardson, G., and I. Frank. 1977. *Junkie: The deadliest cover-up.* New York:Manor.

Richardson, S. 1967. Introduction. In S. Richardson and A. Guttmacher (eds.), *Childbearing: Its social and psychological aspects,* pp. vii–xvi. Baltimore:Williams and Wilkins.

Richardson, S., and A. Guttmacher (eds.). 1967. *Childbearing: Its social and psychological aspects.* Baltimore:Williams and Wilkins.

Rieder, R., D. Rosenthal, P. Wender, and H. Blumenthal. 1975. The offspring of schizophrenics: Fetal and neonatal deaths. *Archives of General Psychiatry,* **32,** 200.

Ritchey, M., and A. Leff. 1975. Venereal disease control among homosexuals. *Journal of the American Medical Association,* **232,** 509.

Roberts, G. 1957. *The population of Jamaica.* London:Cambridge University Press.

Roberts, S. 1927. *Population problems of the Pacific.* London:Routledge.

Rock, J., C. Tietze, and H. McLaughlin. 1965. Effect of adoption on fertility. *Fertility and Sterility,* **16,** 305.

Romaniuk, A. 1968. The demography of the Democratic Republic of the Congo. In W. Brass *et al.* (eds.), *The demography of tropical Africa,* pp. 241–341. Princeton:Princeton University Press. (a)

Romaniuk, A. 1968. Infertility in tropical Africa. In J. Caldwell and C. Okonjo (eds.), *The population of tropical Africa,* pp. 214–224. London:Longmans. (b)

Romm, M. 1967. Fetishism. In C. Wahl (ed.), *Sexual problems,* pp. 221–227. New York:Free Press.

Rommer, J. 1962. Some personality types and mechanisms in functional sterility and fertility. In W. Kroger (ed.), *Psychosomatic obstetrics, gynecology, and endocrinology,* pp. 372–378. Springfield:Thomas.

Rosen, E., R. Fox, and I. Gregory. 1972. *Abnormal psychology.* Philadelphia:Saunders.

Rosenbaum, M. 1976. Female sexuality, or why can't a woman be more like a woman. In W. Oakes, G. Melchiode, and I. Ficher (eds.), *Sex and the life cycle,* pp. 87–96. New York:Grune and Stratton.

Rossi, A. 1977. A biosocial perspective on parenting. *Daedalus,* **106,** 2, 1.

Royal College of Physicians of London. 1971. *Smoking and health now: A new report and summary on smoking and its effects on health.* London:Pitman.

Rubin, E., and C. Lieber. 1968. Alcohol-induced hepatic injury in nonalcoholic volunteers. *New England Journal of Medicine,* **278,** 869.

Rubin, E., C. Lieber, K. Altman, G. Gordon, and A. Southern. 1976. Prolonged ethanol consumption increases testosterone metabolism in the liver. *Science,* **191,** 563.

Rumeau-Rouquette, C., J. Goujard, M. Kaminski, and D. Schwartz. 1972. Perinatal mortality in relation to obstetric antecedents and tobacco usage (translation). Paper presented at the Third European Congress of Perinatal Medicine, Lausanne, April.

Rush, D., and E. Kass. 1972. Maternal smoking: A reassessment of the association with perinatal mortality. *American Journal of Epidemiology,* **96,** 183.

Russell, G. 1972. Psychological and physiological mechanisms contributing to amenorrhea in anorexia nervosa. In N. Morris (ed.), *Psychosomatic medicine in obstetrics and gynecology,* pp. 582–584. New York:Karger.

Russell, J. 1972. Psychosocial aspects of weight loss and amenorrhea in adolescent girls. In N. Morris (ed.), *Psychosomatic medicine in obstetrics and gynecology,* pp. 593–595. New York:Karger.

Rutherford, R. 1965. Emotional aspects of infertility. *Clinical Obstetrics and Gynecology,* **8,** 100.

Ryder, N. 1959. Fertility. In P. Hauser and O. Duncan (eds.), *The study of population,* pp. 400–436. Chicago:University of Chicago Press.

Sadikali, F. 1975. The association of syphilis with cirrhosis: The role of alcohol and serum hepatitis. *Postgraduate Medicine,* **51,** 69.

Saghir, M., and E. Robins. 1969. Homosexuality: Sexual behavior of the female homosexual. *Archives of General Psychiatry,* **20,** 192.

Saghir, M., E. Robins, and B. Walbran. 1969. Homosexuality: Sexual behavior of the male homosexual. *Archives of General Psychiatry,* **21,** 219.

Saghir, M., E. Robins, B. Walbran, and K. Gentry. 1970. Homosexuality, IV: Psychiatric disorders and disability in the female homosexual. *American Journal of Psychiatry,* **127,** 147.

Sameroff, A., and M. Zax. 1973. Perinatal characteristics of the offspring of schizophrenic women. *Journal of Nervous & Mental Disease,* **157,** 191.

Sanua, V. 1969. Socio-cultural aspects. In L. Bellak and L. Loeb (eds.), *The schizophrenic syndrome,* pp. 256–310. NewYork:Grune and Stratton.

Savel, L., and E. Roth. 1962. Effects of smoking in pregnancy: A continuing retrospective study. *Obstetrics and Gynecology,* **20,** 313.

Schacter, S., B. Silvestein, L. Kozlowski, and D. Perlick. 1977. Smoking and addiction. *Journal of Experimental Psychology,* **106,** 3.

Schafer, S., M. Knudten, and R. Knudten. 1975. *Social problems in a changing society.* Reston, Virginia:Reston Publishing Co.

Schellen, A., and G. Sassen. 1967. Fertility after adoption. *Bulletin de la Société Royal Belge de Gynecologie et d'Obstetrique,* **37,** 181.

Schenkel, B., and H. Vorherr. 1974. Non-prescription drugs during pregnancy: Potential teratogenic and toxic effects upon embryo and fetus. *Journal of Reproductive Medicine,* **12,** 27.

Schur, E. 1965. *Crimes without victims.* Englewood Cliffs:Prentice-Hall.

Science News. 1975. A man's drinking may harm his offspring. **107.** 116.

Sclare, A. 1970. The female alcoholic. *British Journal of Addiction,* **65,** 99.

Scott, A. 1974. Drugs and pregnancy. *Journal of the Irish Medical Association,* **67,** 123.

Scott, E. 1958. Psychosexuality of the alcoholic. *Psychological Reports,* **4,** 599.

Scragg, R. 1957. *Depopulation in New Ireland.* Administration of Papua and New Guinea.

Segal, B., V. Kushnarev, G. Urakov, and E. Misionzhnik. 1970. Alcoholism and disruption of the activity of deep cerebral structures. *Quarterly Journal of Studies on Alcohol,* **31,** 587.

Seixas, F. 1971. Treating alcoholics. *Medical Times,* **99,** 45.

Seward, G., P. Wagner, J. Heinrich, S. Bloch, and H. Myerhoff. 1965. The question of psychophysiologic infertility: Some negative answers. *Psychosomatic Medicine,* **27,** 533.

Shader, R. 1970. Ejaculation disorders. In R. Shader and A. DiMascio (eds.), *Psychotropic drug side effects,* pp. 72–76. Baltimore:Williams and Wilkins. (a)

Shader, R. 1970. Male sexual function. In R. Shader and A. DiMascio (eds.), *Psychotropic drug side effects,* pp. 63–71. Baltimore:Williams and Wilkins. (b)

Shader, R., and A. DiMascio (eds.). 1970. *Psychotropic drug side effects.* Baltimore:Williams and Wilkins.

Shader, R., J. Nahum, and A. DiMascio. 1970. Amenorrhea. In R. Shader and A. DiMascio (eds.), *Psychotropic drug side effects,* pp. 10–15. Baltimore:Williams and Wilkins.

Shaltuck, C., and W. Spellacy. 1965. Cirrhosis of liver in pregnancy. *Minnesota Medicine,* **48,** 171.

Shapiro, S., E. Schlesinger, and R. Nesbitt. 1968. *Infant, perinatal, maternal, and childhood mortality in the United States.* Cambridge, Massachusetts:Harvard University Press.

Shearer, L. 1975. Virgin wives. *Parade Magazine,* June 15, 4.

Shearer, L. 1977. Mentally ill Americans. *Parade Magazine,* Oct. 30, 12.

Sheps, M., and J. Ridley (eds.). 1965. *Public health and population change.* Pittsburgh:University of Pittsburgh Press.

Sherfey, J. 1955. Psychopathology and character structure in chronic alcoholism. In O. Diethelm (ed.), *Etiology of chronic alcoholism,* pp. 16–42. Springfield:Thomas.

Sherlock, S. 1955. *Diseases of the liver.* Oxford:Blackwell.

Shields, J., and E. Slater. 1967. Genetic aspects of schizophrenia. *Hospital Medicine,* **1,** 579.

Shulgin, A. 1971. Chemistry and sources. In S. Epstein (ed.), *Drugs of abuse,* pp. 3–26. Cambridge, Massachusetts:MIT Press.

Siegler, S. 1944. *Fertility in women.* Philadelphia:Lippincott.

Sills, D. 1973. Foreword. In J. Fawcett (ed.), *Psychological perspectives on population.* New York:Basic Books.

Silverman, C. 1968. *The epidemiology of depression.* Baltimore:Johns Hopkins Press.

Simmel, E. 1945. Significance of gynecology in psychoanalysis. *California and Western Medicine,* **63,** 169.

Slater, E., E. Hare, and J. Price. 1971. Marriage and fertility of psychiatric patients compared with national data. *Social Biology,* **Supplement 18,** S60.

Slaughter, C., and K. Krantz. 1963. Cirrhosis of liver complicating pregnancy. *American Journal of Obstetrics and Gynecology,* **86,** 1060.

Sloan, D., and L. Africano. 1976. Impotence. *Forum,* **5,** 13.

Smith, D., and J. Joffe. 1975. Increased neonatal mortality in offspring of male rats treated with methadone or morphine before mating. *Nature,* **253,** 202.

Smith, J., F. Lemere, and R. Dunn. 1972. Impotence in alcoholism. *Northwest Medicine Seattle,* **71,** 523.

Smith, K., D. Ulleland, and A. Streissguth. 1973. Pattern of malformation in offspring of chronic alcoholic mothers. *Lancet,* **1,** 1267.

Smithells, R. 1976. Environmental teratogens of man. *British Medical Bulletin,* **32,** 27.

Sobel, D. 1961. Infant mortality and malformations in children of schizophrenic women. *Psychiatric Quarterly,* **35,** 60.

Socarides, C. 1968. *The overt homosexual.* New York:Grune and Stratton.

Socarides, C. 1970. Homosexuality and medicine. *Journal of the American Medical Association,* **212,** 1199.

Soichet, S. 1959. Emotional factors in toxemia of pregnancy. *American Journal of Obstetrics and Gynecology,* **77,** 1065.

Spingarn, C. and M. Edelman. 1966. Parasitic diseases in relation to pregnancy. In J. Rovinsky and A. Guttmacher (eds.), *Medical, surgical, and gynecologic complications of pregnancy,* pp. 692–719. Baltimore:Williams and Wilkins.

Starkey, T., and R. Lee. 1969. Menstruation and fertility in anorexia nervosa. *American Journal of Obstetrics and Gynecology,* **105,** 374.

Statzer, D., and J. Wardell. 1972. Heroin addiction during pregnancy. *American Journal of Obstetrics and Gynecology,* **113,** 273.

Steinberger, E., R. Swerdloff, and R. Horton. 1977. The control of testicular function. In R. Greep and M. Koblinsky, (eds.), *Frontiers in reproduction and fertility control,* pp. 264–292. Cambridge, Massachusetts:MIT Press.

Stenchever, M., and M. Allen. 1972. The effect of delta-9-tetrahydrocannabinol on the chromosomes of human lymphocytes in vitro. *American Journal of Obstetrics and Gynecology,* **114,** 819.

Stenchever, M., T. Kunysz, and M. Allen. 1974. Chromosome breakage in users of marihuana. *American Journal of Obstetrics and Gynecology,* **118,** 106.

Sterling, T., and D. Kobayaski. 1975. The effect of smoking on sex: A critical review. *Journal of Sex Research,* **11,** 201.

Stern, R. 1966. The pregnant addict. *American Journal of Obstetrics and Gynecology,* **94,** 253.

Stevens, B. 1969. *Marriage and fertility of women suffering from schizophrenia or affective disorders.* London:Oxford University Press.

Stevens. B. 1970. Frequency of separation and divorce among women aged 16–49 suffering from schizophrenia and affective disorders. *Acta Psychiatrica Scandinavica,* **46,** 136.

Stewart, B. 1975. Drugs that cause and cure male infertility. *Drug Therapy,* **5,** 42.

Stoffer, S. 1968. A gynecologic study of drug addicts. *American Journal of Obstetrics and Gynecology,* **101,** 779.

Stone, A. 1954. Biological factors influencing human fertility. *Proceedings of the 1954 World Population Conference,* Rome, **1,** 737.

Straus, R. 1976. Alcoholism and problem drinking. In R. Merton and R. Nisbet (eds.), *Contemporary social problems,* pp. 181–218. New York:Harcourt Brace Jovanovich.

Straus, R., and S. Bacon. 1951. Alcoholism and social stability: A study of occupational integration in 2,023 male clinic patients. *Quarterly Journal of Studies on Alcohol,* **12,** 231.

Strecker, E., and F. Chambers. 1949. *Alcohol: One man's meat.* New York:Macmillan.

Stycos, J. 1963. Culture and differential fertility in Peru. *Population Studies,* **16,** 257.

Subak-Sharpe, G. 1974. Is your sex life going up in smoke? *Today's Health,* **52,** 50.

Suinn, R. 1970. *Fundamentals of behavior pathology.* New York:Wiley.

Sullivan, H. 1962. *Schizophrenia as a human process.* New York:Norton.

Sutherland, J., and I. Light. 1965. The effect of drugs upon the developing fetus. *Pediatric Clinics of North America,* **12,** 781.

Szulman, A. 1965. Chromosomal aberrations in spontaneous human abortions. *New England Journal of Medicine,* **272,** 811.

Tabbarah, R. 1971. Toward a theory of demographic development. *Economic Development and Cultural Change,* **67,** 25.

Takano, K., and J. Miller. 1972. ABO incompatibility as a cause of spontaneous abortion: Evidence from abortuses. *Journal of Medical Genetics,* **9,** 144.

Talkington, P. 1971. Impotence and frigidity. *West Virginia Medical Journal,* **67,** 25.

Taylor, C., J. Wyon, and J. Gordon. 1958. Ecologic determinants of population growth. *Milbank Memorial Fund Quarterly,* **36,** 107.

Taylor, E. 1969. *Essentials of gynecology.* Philadelphia:Lea and Febiger.

Taylor, H. 1962. Nausea and vomiting of pregnancy. In W. Kroger (ed.), *Psychosomatic obstetrics, gynecology, and endocrinology,* pp. 117–126. Springfield:Thomas.

Teitelbaum, M. 1975. The relevance of demographic transition theory for developing countries. *Science,* **188,** 420.

Tenbrinck, M., and S. Buchin. 1975. Fetal alcohol syndrome. *Journal of the American Medical Association,* **232,** 1144.

Thomas, H. 1965. The uterus. *Clinical Obstetrics and Gynecology,* **8,** 48.

Thomlinson, R. 1967. *Demographic problems.* Belmont, California:Dickenson.

Thomlinson, R. 1976. *Population dynamics.* New York:Random House.

Thompson, W., and P. Whelpton. 1933. *Population trends in the United States.* New York:McGraw-Hill.

Time. 1973. Crackup in mental care. Dec. 17, 74.

Time. 1975. The self starvers. July 28, 50. (a)

Time. 1975. Homosexuality: Gays on the march. Sept. 8, 32. (b)

Time. 1975. Pot and sex. Sept. 29, 54. (c)

Time. 1977. The chemistry of smoking. Feb. 21, 48. (a)

Time. 1977. Coke and angel dust. July 18, 49. (b)

Time. 1978. Sick again? Psychiatrists vote on gays. Feb. 20, 102. (a)

Time. 1978. Drinking as a way of life. May 22, 58. (b)

Titus, R. 1972. Lysergic acid diethylamide: Its effects on human chromosomes and the human organism in utero: A review of current findings. *International Journal of Addictions,* **7**, 701.

Tokuhata, G. 1968. Smoking in relation to infertility and fetal loss. *Archives of Environmental Health,* **17**, 353. (a)

Tokuhata, G. 1968. Smoker's risk of infertility and fetal loss greater. *Public Health Reports,* **83**, 225. (b)

Tourney, G., and L. Hatfield. 1973. Androgen metabolism in schizophrenics, homosexuals, and controls. *Biological Psychiatry,* **6**, 23.

Tourney, G., W. Nelson, and J. Gottlieb. 1953. Morphology of the testes in schizophrenia. *Archives of Neurology and Psychiatry,* **70**, 240.

Trimmer, E. 1972. Female homosexuality. In N. Morris (ed.), *Psychosomatic obstetrics and gynecology,* pp. 382–384. New York:Karger.

Trumbull, R. 1974. Eskimo mental ills tied to new life. *New York Times,* July 15, 8.

Tucker, B. 1975. Pregnancy and drugs. *Addictions,* **22**, 2.

Tupper, C., and R. Weil. 1968. The etiology of habitual abortion. In S. Behrman and H. Kistner (eds.), *Progress in infertility,* pp. 751–765. Boston:Little Brown.

Tupper, W. 1962. The psychosomatic aspects of spontaneous abortion. In W. Kroger (ed.), *Psychosomatic obstetrics, gynecology, and endocrinology,* pp. 144–152. Springfield:Thomas.

Tuthill, J. 1955. Impotence. *Lancet,* **1**, 124.

Tyler, E., J. Bonapart, and J. Grant. 1960. Occurrence of pregnancy following adoption. *Fertility and Sterility,* **11**, 581.

Uganda Atlas of Disease Distribution. 1968. Kampala:Makerere University College Press.

Ulleland, C. 1972. The offspring of alcoholic mothers. *Annals of the New York Academy of Sciences,* **197**, 167.

Underwood, P., L. Hester, T. Laffitte, and K. Gregg. 1965. The relationship of smoking to the outcome of pregnancy. *American Journal of Obstetrics and Gynecology,* **91**, 270.

Underwood, P., K. Kesler, J. O'Lane, and D. Callagan. 1967. Parental smoking empirically related to pregnancy outcome. *Obstetrics and Gynecology,* **29**, 1.

United Nations. 1973. *The determinants and consequences of population trends.* New York:United Nations.

United States Department of Health, Education and Welfare. 1973. *Alcohol and health.* New York:Scribner's.

United States National Institute of Mental Health. 1967. *Patients in state and county mental hospitals.* Washington, D.C.:U.S. Government Printing Office.

United States National Institute of Mental Health. n.d. *Alcohol and alcoholism,* Washington, D.C.:U.S. Government Printing Office.

United States Public Health Service. 1971. *The health consequences of smoking.* Washington, D.C.:U.S. Government Printing Office.

United States Public Health Service. 1972. *The health consequences of smoking,* Washington, D.C.:U.S. Government Printing Office.

United States Public Health Service. 1973. *The health consequences of smoking.* Washington, D.C.:U.S. Government Printing Office.

van de Walle, E., and H. Page. 1969. Some new estimates of fertility and mortality in Africa. *Population Index,* **35**, 3.

Van Thiel, D., H. Gavaler, and R. Lester. 1974. Ethanol inhibition of vitamin A metabolism in the testes: Possible mechanism for sterility in alcoholics. *Science,* **186**, 941. (a)

Van Thiel, D., J. Gavaler, R. Lester, D. Loriaux, and G. Braunstein. 1975. Plasma estrone, prolactin, neurophysin, and sex steroid-binding globulin in chronic alcoholic men. *Metabolism: Clinical and Experimental,* **24**, 1015.

Van Thiel, D., and R. Lester. 1974. Sex and alcohol. *New England Journal of Medicine,* **291**, 251.

Van Thiel, D., R. Lester, and R. Sherins. 1974. Hypogonadism in alcoholic liver disease: Evidence for a double effect. *Gastroenterology,* **67**, 1188. (b)

Veevers, J. 1972. Factors in the incidence of childlessness in Canada: An analysis of census data. *Social Biology,* **19**, 266.

Vero, T., and L. Szanyi. 1972. Role of individual resistance capability in pathogenesis of functional sterility and menstrual disturbances of psychosomatic origin. In N. Morris (ed.), *Psychosomatic medicine in obstetrics and gynecology,* pp. 429–432. New York:Karger.

Wahl, C. 1967. *Sexual problems.* New York:Free Press.

Wallach, R., E. Jerez, and G. Blinick. 1969. Pregnancy and menstrual function in narcotics addicts treated with methadone. *American Journal of Obstetrics and Gynecology,* **105**, 1226.

Wallgren, H., and H. Barry. 1970. *Actions of alcohol, vols. I and II.* New York:Elsevier.

Walton, R. 1972. Smoking and alcoholism: A brief report. *American Journal of Psychiatry,* **128**, 1455.

Ward, J. 1973. Towards a geography of alcoholism in Australia (abstract). *New Zealand Medical Journal,* **81**, 395.

Warner, R., and H. Rosett. 1975. The effects of drinking on offspring. *Journal of Studies on Alcohol,* **36**, 1395.

Webster, B. 1970. Venereal disease control in the United States of America. *British Journal of Venereal Diseases,* **46**, 406.

Weir, J. 1972. Drug addiction in pregnancy. The pregnant narcotic addict: A psychiatrist's impression. *Proceedings of the Royal Society of Medicine,* **65**, 869.

Weisbrod, B., R. Andreano, R. Baldwin, E. Epstein, and A. Kelley. 1973. *Disease and economic development—The impact of parasitic diseases in St. Lucia.* Madison:University of Wisconsin Press.

Wender, P. 1973. Genetics and schizophrenia. *Journal of the American Medical Association,* **223**, 1382.

West, D. 1968. *Homosexuality.* London:Duckworth.

Westoff, C., R. Potter, P. Sagi, and E. Mishler. 1961. *Family growth in metropolitan America.* Princeton:Princeton University Press.

Westoff, L., and C. Westoff. 1971. *From now to zero.* Boston:Little Brown.

Whelpton, M., and S. Sherlock. 1968. Pregnancy in patients with hepatic cirrhosis. *Lancet,* **2**, 995.

Whelpton, P., A. Campbell, and J. Patterson. 1966. *Fertility and family planning in the United States.* Princeton:Princeton University Press.

Whelpton, P., and C. Kiser. 1946–1958. *Social and psychological factors affecting fertility.* New York:Milbank Memorial Fund.

Whitehead, L. 1968. Altitude, fertility, and mortality in Andean countries. *Population Studies,* **22**, 335.

Whitelaw, M. 1960. Chlorpromazine in the infertile female. *International Journal of Fertility,* **5**, 175.

Wiedorn, W. 1954. Toxemia of pregnancy and schizophrenia. *Journal of Nervous & Mental Disease,* **120**, 1.

Wilde, M. 1973. The barren wives of Barama. *People,* **1**, 1, 26.

Wilkinson, P., A. Kornaczewski, J. Rankin, and J. Santamaria. 1971. Physical disease in alcoholism: Initial survey of 1000 patients. *Medical Journal of Australia,* **1**, 1217.

Williams, J. 1977. *Psychology of women: Behavior in a biosocial context.* New York:Norton.

Wilsnack, S. 1973. The needs of the female drinker; Dependency, power, or what? *Proceedings of the Second Annual Alcoholism Conference,* NIAAA, 65.

Winn, H. 1970. Contraception. *Clinical Obstetrics and Gynecology,* **13**, 701.

Witters, W., and P. Jones-Witters. 1975. *Drugs and sex.* New York:Macmillan.

Woerner, M., M. Pollack, and D. Klein. 1973. Pregnancy and birth complications in psychiatric patients. *Acta Psychiatrica Scandinavica,* **49**, 712.

Wolf, S. and B. Berle (eds.) 1976. The biology of the schizophrenic process. *Advances in Behavioral Biology* (special edition), **19**.

World Health Organization. 1969. Biological components of human reporoduction. *World Health Organization Technical Report Series,* **435**, 1.

World Health Organization. 1970. Spontaneous and induced abortion. *World Health Organization Technical Report Series,* **461**, 3.

World Health Organization. 1975. The epidemiology of infertility. *World Health Organization Technical Report Series,* **582**, 1.

World Health Organization. 1976. The epidemiology of infertility. *WHO Chronicle,* **30**, 229.

Wrong, D. 1977. *Population and society.* New York:Random House.

Yerushalmy, J. 1971. The relationship of parent's cigarette smoking to outcome of pregnancy. *American Journal of Epidemiology,* **93**, 443.

Yolles, S., and M. Kramer. 1969. Vital statistics. In L. Bellak and L. Loeb (eds.), *The schizophrenic syndrome,* pp. 66–113. New York:Grune and Stratton.

Zabriskie, J. 1963. Effect of cigarette smoking during pregnancy: Study of 2,000 cases. *Obstetrics and Gynecology,* **21**, 405.

Zellweger, H. 1974. Anticonvulsants during pregnancy: A danger to the developing fetus. *Clinical Pediatrics,* **13**, 338.

Zelson, C. 1973. Infant of the addicted mother. *New England Journal of Medicine,* **288**, 1393.

Zelson, C., E. Rubio, and E. Wasserman. 1971. Neonatal narcotic addiction: 10 year observation. *Pediatrics,* **48**, 178.

Zelson, C., J. Sook, and M. Casalino. 1973. Neonatal narcotic addiction: Comparative effects of maternal intake of heroin and methadone. *New England Journal of Medicine,* **289**, 1216.

Zinsou, R., C. Quennum, and E. Alihonou. 1966. Role of bilharziasis in female sterility. *Fertility and Sterility,* Fifth World Congress, 281.

Subject Index